Tuberculosis in the Americas, 1870–1945

This book focuses on the era during which the cause of tuberculosis had been identified, and public health officials were seeking to prevent it, but scientists had not yet found a cure. By examining tuberculosis comparatively in two Atlantic port cities, Buenos Aires and Philadelphia, it explores the medical, political and economic settings in which patients, physicians and urban officials lived and worked. Reber discusses the causes of tuberculosis, treatments and public health efforts to stop contagion, and how factors such as gender, age, class, nationality, beliefs and previous experiences shaped patient responses and often defined the type of treatment.

Vera Blinn Reber earned a PhD from the University of Wisconsin with specialization in Latin American and Comparative History. She taught World and Latin American History at Shippensburg University for 37 years. Her primary research interests are Argentine and Paraguayan nineteenth-century economic history and urban medical history.

Routledge Studies in the History of the Americas

1 **Memory of the Argentina Disappearances**
The Political History of Nunca Más
Emilio Crenzel

2 **Projections of Power in the Americas**
Edited by Niels Bjerre-Poulsen, Helene Balslev Clausen and Jan Gustafsson

3 **Mexico, 1848–1853**
Los Años Olvidados
Edited by Pedro Santoni and Will Fowler

4 **Tuberculosis in the Americas, 1870–1945**
Beneath the Anguish in Philadelphia and Buenos Aires
Vera Blinn Reber

For more information about this series, please visit: https://www.routledge.com/Routledge-Studies-in-the-History-of-the-Americas/book-series/RSHAM

Tuberculosis in the Americas, 1870–1945

Beneath the Anguish in Philadelphia and Buenos Aires

Vera Blinn Reber

Routledge
Taylor & Francis Group
NEW YORK AND LONDON

First published 2019
by Routledge
52 Vanderbilt Avenue, New York, NY 10017, USA

and by Routledge
2 Park Square, Milton Park, Abingdon, Oxon OX14 4RN

First issued in paperback 2020

Routledge is an imprint of the Taylor & Francis Group, an informa business

Library of Congress Cataloging-in-Publication Data
Names: Reber, Vera Blinn, 1941– author.
Title: Tuberculosis in the Americas, 1870–1945 : beneath the anguish in Philadelphia and Buenos Aires / by Vera Blinn Reber.
Description: New York : Routledge, 2019. | Series: Routledge studies in the history of the Americas ; 4 | Includes bibliographical references and index. |
Identifiers: LCCN 2018030661 (print) |
LCCN 2018040615 (ebook)
Subjects: LCSH: Tuberculosis—Pennsylvania—Philadelphia—History. | Tuberculosis—Argentina—Buenos Aires—History. | Public health—Pennsylvania—Philadelphia—History. | Public health—Argentina—Buenos Aires—History.
Classification: LCC RC309.P4 (ebook) | LCC RC309.P4 R43 2019 (print) | DDC 362.19699/500974811—dc23
LC record available at https://lccn.loc.gov/2018030661

ISBN 13: 978-0-367-58560-0 (pbk)
ISBN 13: 978-1-138-35950-5 (hbk)

Typeset in Sabon
by codeMantra

Tuberculosis in the Americas, 1870–1945

Beneath the Anguish in Philadelphia and Buenos Aires

Vera Blinn Reber

Routledge
Taylor & Francis Group
NEW YORK AND LONDON

First published 2019
by Routledge
52 Vanderbilt Avenue, New York, NY 10017, USA

and by Routledge
2 Park Square, Milton Park, Abingdon, Oxon OX14 4RN

First issued in paperback 2020

Routledge is an imprint of the Taylor & Francis Group, an informa business

Library of Congress Cataloging-in-Publication Data
Names: Reber, Vera Blinn, 1941– author.
Title: Tuberculosis in the Americas, 1870–1945 : beneath the anguish in Philadelphia and Buenos Aires / by Vera Blinn Reber.
Description: New York : Routledge, 2019. | Series: Routledge studies in the history of the Americas ; 4 | Includes bibliographical references and index. |
Identifiers: LCCN 2018030661 (print) |
LCCN 2018040615 (ebook)
Subjects: LCSH: Tuberculosis—Pennsylvania—Philadelphia—History. | Tuberculosis—Argentina—Buenos Aires—History. | Public health—Pennsylvania—Philadelphia—History. | Public health—Argentina—Buenos Aires—History.
Classification: LCC RC309.P4 (ebook) | LCC RC309.P4 R43 2019 (print) | DDC 362.19699/500974811—dc23
LC record available at https://lccn.loc.gov/2018030661

ISBN 13: 978-0-367-58560-0 (pbk)
ISBN 13: 978-1-138-35950-5 (hbk)

Typeset in Sabon
by codeMantra

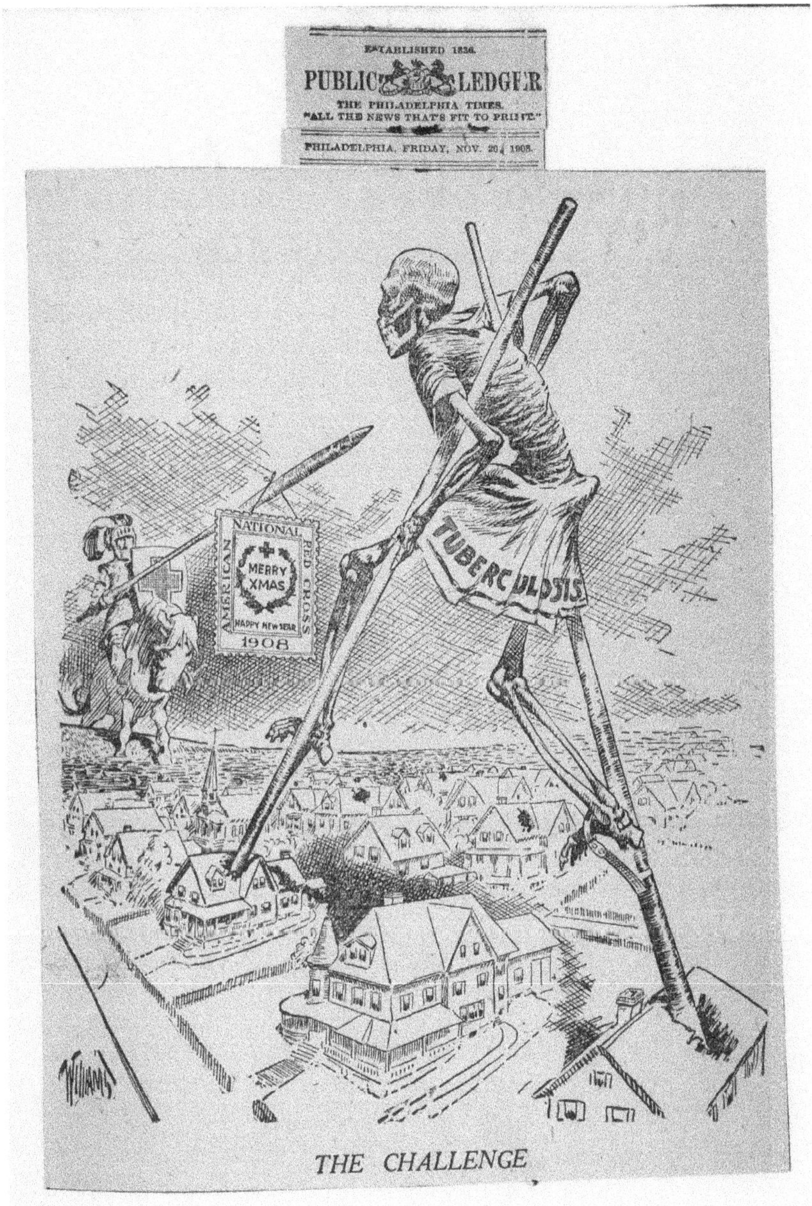

Frontispiece: "The Challenge," political cartoon, *Public Ledger* 20 Nov. 1908, from the John Seiser Mucklé papers [Coll. 0441], vol. II, Historical Society of Pennsylvania.

To Librarians and Library Staff

Contents

List of Figures

List of Tables

Acknowledgments

My students were the inspiration for *Beneath the Anguish in Philadelphia and Buenos Aires*. I regularly taught the Shippensburg University senior seminar on Comparative History and was often disappointed when choosing required books to discover few comparative works by historians. I often used monographs by anthropologists and political scientists. As I examined gaps in student knowledge, I realized how little they knew about the history of science and medicine; it was difficult to find historical monographs dealing with those subjects. In searching for a particular focus, I was struck by how little had been written on tuberculosis in Latin American history. Further, tuberculosis was a significant global disease in the nineteenth century, which required me to treat it within a broader context. Tuberculosis is also of current significance, as once again it is a major killer in underserved communities of the West and in the developing world.

A National Endowment for the Humanities Institute on the Contributions of the History of Medicine to Social Medicine, June 1995, under the direction of David J. Rothman at the College of Physicians and Surgeons of Columbia University provided me a broad background of theoretical readings in the history of medicine. During the summer, it became clear that I needed to turn to the work done by U.S. historians to develop the theoretical background for writing in the field of the social history of medicine. Since I had done much of my early historical work on Buenos Aires, I decided to return to historical research in a city I both knew and loved. I early chose the title, *Beneath the Anguish*, to indicate my interest in understanding patient perspectives. Research in Philadelphia represented a new challenge. My undergraduate students generally prefer U.S. history to that of other world areas. They worry about their ability to deal with scientific works. Many of my students had lived in Philadelphia and were familiar with the city. Philadelphia has long influenced the history of Pennsylvania. By choosing Philadelphia as my comparison city, I had a good match for examining tuberculosis and could interest my students in the social history of medicine.

Too often, the libraries and archives which make possible the research go unrecognized. So I want to thank the staff at the major centers for medical research in four cities: Buenos Aires, Philadelphia, Washington D.C. and London. In Buenos Aires, three institutions stand out. The Archivo General de la Nación Argentina provided the happy memories of my previous research in the city. The young staff at the Biblioteca Facultad de Medicina de Universidad de Buenos Aires readily brought me huge collections of books and newspapers and did much photocopying. But the most welcoming place was the Liga Argentina de Lucha contra la Tuberculosis where Dr. Jorge a. Phileu, who died in 2010, served as director. He introduced me to members of the Argentine Medical Association who did the first medical histories in Argentina and included me in their history seminars. He and his assistant at the Liga, Norma Arrizabalga, contributed to my understanding of tuberculosis in Argentina.

In Philadelphia, the Historical Library of the College of Physicians provided a welcoming atmosphere. The Philadelphia City Archives and Temple University's Special Collections provided the most significant historical source for Philadelphia, the Annual Messages of the Mayor of the City of Philadelphia. In Washington D.C., I thank the National Library of Medicine staff for preserving *Spunk,* the monthly magazine of the Mont Alto Sanatorium, from 1909 to 1963, sending me the microfilm, so that I could complete my research, and providing useful material on tuberculosis mortality. The Hispanic Reading Room is my favorite place to work at the Library of Congress. In London, my research home was the Wellcome Institute for the History of Medicine. Closer to home I thank the staff at the State Library of Pennsylvania in Harrisburg. My most significant support came from the staff and faculty at Ezra Lehman Memorial Library of Shippensburg University. I thank the interlibrary loan folks who searched diligently for requested material, the faculty who served at the "Ask Us Anything" desk and the staff who keep the library running. The history department secretary, Janice Reed, early in the process typed tables and continues to answer my Microsoft word questions.

During the twenty-two years of the research for *Beneath the Anguish,* many institutions supported me financially. I thank Shippensburg University for year-long sabbaticals, 1995–1996 and 2002–2003 which supported my research in Buenos Aires and Philadelphia. An SU Professional Development grant provided for travel to Madrid in July 1994, and another SU Professional Development grant in July of 2003 supported archival research in Philadelphia. A Wood Institute short-term fellowship supported research at the College of Physicians in Philadelphia in June 2003. A National Endowment for the Humanities Institute on the Contributions of the History of Medicine to Social Medicine in the summer of 1995 allowed for reading in comparative medical history.

I owe thanks to several individuals. In 2014–2015, Joe Schwartz did extensive copy-editing, focusing in particular on eliminating repetitions and in clarifying my argument. I am also appreciative of my editor at

Routledge, Max Novick, whose quick response to e-mails included the reassuring phrase, "nothing to worry about," and editorial assistant Jennifer Morrow, for her care with the details. The Routledge staff made the process to publication easy. There are two individuals I owe a special debt of gratitude. My friend, since graduate school at the University of Wisconsin, Mary C. Karasch, read several drafts of my manuscript and provided insight to reader comments; but most importantly she kept me from giving up in my efforts to find a publisher; thank you. My husband, John L. Offner, edited my writing, clarified my thinking, did additional chores to aid my research process and kept the house lights on during my many research trips. Finally, I want to thank my students at Shippensburg University from 1970 to 2008 in my Latin American and World History classes for keeping teaching and research challenging and exciting.

Introduction

Beneath the Anguish: Tuberculosis, 1870–1945

> (The Medicine) chokes me when I [Maria Kurtz] inhale it, and makes my head ache terrible and the phlegm does not flow from the nostrils, but from the throat... Since Friday my nose bleeds whenever I inhale the medicine.[1]

> Sra. N.C. de N. born in Buenos Aires... and married at 17 had a son. Three months after the birth of her son and with no appreciable cause developed a dry cough, was tired and had a fever... a few days later vomited blood.... Dr Rawson recommended she be taken directly to the Sierras de Córdoba... there was immediate improvement.[2]

Tuberculosis brings both pain and fear. Patients, including Maria Kurtz of Newark, New Jersey, and Sra. N.C. de N. of Buenos Aires, Argentina, frequently coughed, ran high fevers and imbibed foul-tasting medicines. They sought to prolong their lives by heeding their physicians and traveling to favorable climates. *Beneath the Anguish* examines the era in which the causes of tuberculosis were identified and the disease could generally be diagnosed but not cured. Patients suffered and hoped but ultimately realized that their lives would be shortened. Tuberculosis touched the lives of every community and every member within it.

"The Challenge" reflects that reality. A skeleton marked "Tuberculosis" and looking like death invades homes; it forces its stilts into the roofs of middle-class and wealthy homes. Tuberculosis attacked all peoples, not just the poor and immigrants. Riding to the protection is a knight in full armor on a white horse carrying a shield with an insignia of a Red Cross and wielding a lance; the lance carried a banner labeled "National American Red Cross Association, Merry Xmas 1908." The Red Cross Knight is prepared to fight against his opponent—tuberculosis. The first Red Cross national Christmas seal campaign was in 1908. The monies raised supported tuberculosis patients.[3]

Beneath the Anguish is a comparative history of tuberculosis from 1870 to 1945 that focuses on patient perspectives and public responses. Municipalities and states developed policies to prevent tuberculosis and assist the ill. Gender, age, class, nationality, beliefs and previous experiences shaped patient reactions to treatment and often defined the type and quality of treatment. Buenos Aires and Philadelphia provide the medical, political and economic settings in which patients, physicians and medical health professionals lived and worked. These two port cities, with diverse medical facilities, illustrate the growing international consensus between 1870 and 1920 as to the causes, prevention and treatment of tuberculosis. After the 1920s, Buenos Aires and Philadelphia exemplified growing international disagreements among physicians as to which specific medical therapies were most effective in preventing and curing tuberculosis. At the same time, urban public health programs demonstrated increasingly similar approaches to tuberculosis prevention.

From 1870 to 1945, scientists searched for a cure for tuberculosis, and health officials sought to prevent the public from contracting it. In those years, deaths from tuberculosis represented eight to fifteen percent of all deaths worldwide. Tuberculosis also debilitated and shortened the lives of millions more.[4] Furthermore, it weakened patients' immune systems and made them more susceptible to other diseases. In the 1870s, physicians had struggled to understand the cause of tuberculosis and sought primarily to ameliorate patients' symptoms. Initially, physicians and the general population defined, classified and named tuberculosis differently. By the early twentieth century, the western medical world generally agreed on the name, causes and effects of the disease. Physicians encouraged patients to follow a hygienic regimen of fresh air, nutritious food, rest and exercise. By the 1930s, physicians provided surgical treatment and experimental medications. It was only when streptomycin was discovered in 1943 that an effective cure was found for tuberculosis. By 1945, antibiotics effectively treated the disease.[5] But with the resurgence of tuberculosis in the 1990s, it has become clear that understanding the bacterial cause of tuberculosis does not in itself explain why some individuals but not others contract the disease. Because economic and social circumstances such as malnutrition, unsanitary living conditions and work environment also influence who is infected with the bacteria, tuberculosis is both a social and a biological disease.

Identification of the Tubercle Bacilli

By the 1940s, scientists had identified five varieties of tubercle bacilli of which only two cause disease in humans: one infects humans directly; the other infects cattle. Except for bovine tuberculosis, which is usually transmitted by unpasteurized milk, *Mycobacterium tuberculosis* reaches most humans through the air. Infected individuals produce airborne particles of bacilli through talking, coughing, sneezing, spitting and singing, which in a closed space may infect healthy individuals. In most cases, the bacillus reproduces slowly and may live in a person's lungs for years without the individual manifesting symptoms. Such an individual has latent tuberculosis and tests positive for the disease. Because the bacteria lie dormant such individuals are neither sick nor infectious but may subsequently become so.[6]

Recent research suggests that the ancestors of *M. tuberculosis* may have existed for three million years. The organism has been in existence long enough to evolve and spread at different rates. In 1979, an archaeologist, Michael Zimmerman, identified the oldest individual with tuberculosis, a six-year-old Egyptian child who lived in 1300 BCE. Since the 1940s, archaeologists have identified tuberculosis scars on the bones of ancient Americans. DNA analysis from a lesion on a lung of a thousand-year-old female mummy discovered in southern Peru in 1990 conclusively proved the existence of tuberculosis in the Americas before the arrival of the Spanish. Scientists who analyzed 483 skeletons from Chile and reviewed mummy dissection records suggested that tuberculosis was prevalent in one percent of the population between 200 BCE and CE 1500. Tuberculosis became a significant killer of indigenous populations only in the early seventeenth century when crowding, malnutrition and unsanitary conditions in the districts where Native Americans lived encouraged the spread of the disease.[7]

In the early 1990s, scientists concluded that *M. tuberculosis*, which causes the disease in humans, can be divided into six families of genetically related strains. Scientists used fragments of DNA of 875 strains from nationals of eighty countries to identify the main *M. tuberculosis* families still infecting humans. Three are ancient and found in Africa; three are modern and developed in Western Europe from African strains. (An additional seventh strain was found recently in the Horn of Africa.) In the nineteenth century, the European strains were carried to northern India, East Asia and the Americas. European strains replaced the original pre-Columbian strain, which now appears to be extinct. As the bacteria migrated with hosts, they have adapted and caused more severe illness. Treatment needs to adapt as well. The Beijing strain evolved from a European strain and is presently drug resistant: XDR-TB. Unfortunately, it is easily spread in a heavily populated interconnected world.[8]

Defining and Naming Tuberculosis

When most individuals consider tuberculosis, they think of pulmonary tuberculosis or tuberculosis of the lungs. This is the most common type of infection. However, the tubercle can also reproduce in other parts of the body including, bones, lymph glands, skin, kidneys and genitals. In the majority of cases, the body's immune system promotes healing and halts the infection, but leaves scar tissue. The nature of the bacilli capsule, which makes it impermeable to many antibacterial enzymes, explains why some humans may live with the tubercle with no observable effect. From 1870 to 1945, it is estimated that the bacilli infected up to ninety percent of the adult population in the western world, but on average only ten percent of those infected developed the disease.[9]

Although most people infected with *M. tuberculosis* never get sick or infect others, predicting who will become ill is complex. The resistance of individuals to infection depends on age, gender, the strength of the immune system and the particular strain. The elderly who get tuberculosis probably got it from reactivation of long-term latent tuberculosis. Infants, teenagers and pregnant women most likely received the bacteria through contact with infected individuals. Youths in their teen years and women at the beginning of menses and during pregnancies need additional protein in their diets, and when lacking it, are more vulnerable. Miliary tuberculosis may kill infants and young children in days. Environmental factors such as crowded living spaces, inadequate nutrition, and poor air quality also affect susceptibility. The growth of industrial societies expanded environmental factors that correlated with the spread of tuberculosis.[10]

The public, physicians and government officials sought to cope with a variety of epidemic diseases during the decades in which tuberculosis was most virulent. Between 1870 and 1912, both Buenos Aires and Philadelphia suffered epidemics of cholera, diphtheria, influenza, scarlet fever, smallpox, typhoid, typhus and yellow fever. In addition, Buenos Aires confronted epidemics of bubonic plague, dysentery and measles. In spite of the high death rates from tuberculosis, physicians viewed tuberculosis as a chronic disease (an ailment which was long-lasting, persistent and recurrent with periods of remission), not as an epidemic. Tuberculosis spread slowly and patients lived for a long time. Tuberculosis, similar to epidemic diseases, had a high mortality and afflicted cities; but its long incubation and confusing symptoms allowed authorities wrongly to equate it with pneumonia or the common cold.[11]

Politicians, not scientists, dated the beginnings and ends of epidemics and dictated how the citizenry should deal with the disease. Thus, communities were slow to acknowledge an epidemic and did so only when the death rate was so obvious that public authorities could no longer ignore it. Acknowledging an epidemic required the government to counter the public health threat. Managing an epidemic involved political considerations as to how to best protect the community without alienating it by extensive regulations. The result was that governments imposed quarantines and disinfections that primarily affected the poor. Eventually, the high mortality rates from tuberculosis encouraged public health officials to try to limit the spread of tuberculosis by controlling those infected, much as they did when epidemics such as cholera struck.[12]

Tuberculosis went by many English names including *phthisis* and *consumption*. A similar pattern of word usage existed in Spanish. In the 1850s, *tisis* and *consunción*, the Spanish words for *phthisis* or *consumption*, were commonly used. Then in 1882, Robert Koch (1883–1910), a

German physician proved the affliction to be bacterial and contagious. With Koch's discovery, the term *tuberculosis* emerged as the dominant English and Spanish name for the disease. This discovery of the cause of tuberculosis signaled scientific perspective on the disease. Renaming and explaining the disease, henceforth, affected how patients and public health professionals treated it. Within a global context, similar patterns of naming indicate a medical consensus on the classification of the disease and proposed treatments. The physicians and public health personnel in both Buenos Aires and Philadelphia adopted the name tuberculosis suggests that the disease was viewed similarly in the two cities.[13]

Images of Tuberculosis

The word "consumption" did not immediately disappear from popular usage, because the general public thought the term accurately described those infected. "Consumption" suggested a disease that dominated or devoured the individual. In the early nineteenth century, some in the western world considered it glamorous to look tubercular-flushed, thin, drained and melancholy. Alternating from gaiety to gloom, and from energetic activity to lethargy, the afflicted individual was often seen in life and literature as spiritually superior, creative and passionate. To many Europeans, those who died young of tuberculosis were romantic figures. Although tuberculosis infected individuals of all classes, the nineteenth-century European and American public often defined tuberculosis as the illness of intellectuals, writers, musicians and artists. Among the famous European and North American victims were Honoré de Balzac (1850), the Brontë Sisters (Emily 1847, Anne 1849, Charlotte 1855), Elizabeth Barrett Browning (1861), Anton Chekhov (1904), Frederick Chopin (1849), Fyodor Dostoyevsky (1881), Franz Kafka (1924), John Keats (1821), D. H. Lawrence (1930), Katharine Mansfield (1923), George Orwell (Eric Arthur Blair, 1950), Edgar Allan Poe (1849), Joseph Priestly (1804), Sir Walter Scott (1836), Robert Lewis Stevenson (1894) and Voltaire (François-Marie Arouet, 1778).[14]

Among the best-known individuals to die of tuberculosis in South America was Simón Bolivar, who was diagnosed with the disease prior to his death in December 1830. As early as 1818, he had a cough but even in 1829, his physician diagnosed a cholera attack. After his death, an autopsy of the lungs confirmed consumption.[15] Two of the most famous Río de la Plata tubercular invalids were intellectuals and writers. The Uruguayan playwright Florencio Sánchez spent most of his adult life in Buenos Aires and died in Milan, Italy, in 1910 while seeking a cure. The journalist and poet Evaristo Carriego died in Buenos Aires in October 1912; many were surprised at his death because he appeared to be healthy. The impressionist artist Fernando Fader, who lived in Córdoba and died in 1935, concealed his tuberculosis. As attitudes toward tuberculosis changed, and the elite viewed tuberculosis as the disease of the poor, artists and intellectuals hid their disease.[16]

Although nineteenth-century literature, plays and opera often romanticized tuberculosis, it also reflected changing attitudes. The opera *La Bohème*, by Giacomo Puccini, 1858–1924, first performed in Turin, Italy, portrays the seamstress Mimí who dies in poverty of tuberculosis. By the 1920s, writers and folk singers took a more nuanced attitude toward tuberculosis. Thomas Mann's, 1875–1955, novel, *The Magic Mountain*, is based on the experience of his wife, Katia, who spent several months in 1912 in a sanatorium for the wealthy in Davos, in the Swiss Alps. The Argentine author, Manuel Puig, 1932–1990, discusses fear of contagion and the fresh air treatment in his novel *Heartbreak Tango*. His main character, Juan Carlos Etchepare, spent his short life seeking cures for tuberculosis and lived sometime in Cosquin, Cordoba. He died at age twenty-nine.[17]

In the 1920s, tango lyrics told the stories of poor urban tubercular women and associated the disease with disappointment, disillusionment and estrangement. The country music which originated in the rural regions of the South in the 1920s sang of family, marriage, divorce, happiness, and finding and losing love. The lyrics of both tango and country music focused on the lives of the working class and thus, conveyed the difficulties of their lives. In the United States Jimmie Rogers, 1897–1933, recorded the autobiographical country song, "T.B. Blues"; "I've got the T.B. blues; I've been fightin' like a lion; Looks like I'm going to lose." In Argentina, Carlos Pesce wrote the lyrics to the tango "Muñeca de Percal"; "Early in the morning, you go to the workshop.... You're the girl who in a miserable attic suffers from incurable and cruel tuberculosis."[18]

Susan Sontag, a novelist and essayist, argued that tuberculosis, similar to cancer, came to represent the moral, social and political failures of society. She suggested that the tuberculosis metaphor provides two contradictory examples: that of an individual perceived as good, angelic and innocent because she died young and that of the diseased individual who was viewed as passionate and sexually decadent. The sick person was both the victim of the disease and responsible for her illness.[19] Sontag recognized that illness is not just a metaphor; it is real and involved pain. Sontag points to the complexities of analyzing tuberculosis. It can be both a metaphor and a complex tool for analyzing urban society, politics and policy. Individuals can both romanticize tuberculosis and feel its harmful effects.

Framing or Social Construction

Just as perspectives on tuberculosis changed from 1870 to 1945, so have intellectual approaches to the disease. Initially, most historians of medicine were medical professionals who focused on describing physician accomplishments. More recently, in order to understand and explain to the general public the various influences of disease, historians have used a variety of sources and approaches. The author utilized physician and patient accounts, governmental, medical, institutional and literary records, and a variety of historical methodologies to reconstruct the world of the tubercular ill. *Beneath the Anguish* also examines tuberculosis through the use of methodologies of framing, comparison and social history. For historians, the challenge is to understand the complexities of the disease, its social impact and the degree to which various groups experience and perceive it differently. Some medical historians have preferred to use the concepts of "social construction" or "framing" to describe a disease and emphasize its cultural dimensions. Scientists describe diseases and create definitions based on their research. However, the society and era in which scientists and historians live influence the questions they ask and how they describe and name diseases. Charles E. Rosenberg emphasizes that disease is "a complex intellectual construction, an amalgam of biological state and social definition." While illness impacts lives and real people experience maladies, the disease is also a social construction. Although the pathogen is real, patients and physicians tend to view the disease differently. The physician describes the symptoms of the disease and recommends treatments; the patient expresses frustrations over his or her limitations and infirmities and may accept or reject aspects of treatment.[20]

Phil Brown, a medical sociologist, suggests that "Social construction begins with social discovery—the ways in which people, organizations and institutions determine that there is a disease or condition. Other components of social construction follow: the experience of illness; decisions regarding treatment; social understandings of what constitutes outcome." Brown also suggests that the understanding of medical knowledge is separate from that of illness. The social construction of medical knowledge deals with the origins of professional beliefs and with medical diagnosis, while illness deals primarily with the experience of being sick. However, diagnosis is central to the understanding of illness, as it represents the medical professional's determination of the existence of the disease and is very much affected by social factors of class, race, sex, ethnicity and education. Public expressions and reactions to diagnosis are also socially constructed and influence treatment and patient responses. Diagnosis is a tool of social control, as it leads to labeling and changes a person's social roles and relationships.[21]

To be sick disrupts the normal aspects of life and threatens one's integrity. To be sick is to be abnormal. A man who was once the dominant person in the family and its financial support becomes dependent on his children. A mother accustomed to caring for sick family members must allow others to care for her when she becomes ill. But roles change not only within the family but within the broader social world. The employee's relationships to his co-workers and employer are altered. Co-workers may resent the ill person's inability to carry his own weight at the job. The employer is dissatisfied with the worker's performance. The patient is also subject to the requirements of his/her physician. These changing social relationships cause the patient anxiety and influence how the individual responds to the disease and those who try to heal it.[22]

The concept of "the social construct" of illness emerged within western society in the 1960s and represented efforts to see individuals as both biological and social. Too often it simply recognized that men and women define themselves culturally. Thus, Charles Rosenberg has preferred to use the model of "framing" as a way to explain and classify disease within a social/cultural setting. Class, race, gender, as well as political and economic institutions, influence group and individual assumptions about the treatment, prevalence and meaning of disease. Framing requires the historians of medicine to recognize that the individual's experience is time- and place-specific, that disease is defined in cultural terms and that disease itself helps shape culture. Health professionals and medical organizations respond to disease within a social setting. The state both defines the disease and reacts to it. What distinguishes the concept of "framing" from "social construct" is the recognition that disease is not just defined by society but molds and influences the character of the community. The name change from consumption to tuberculosis shaped both perceptions of the disease and how the community responded. According to Rosenberg, "Disease is both a fundamental substantive problem and an analytical tool, not only in the history of medicine but in the social sciences generally."[23] Tuberculosis is both the focus of the study and the means of examining society in Buenos Aires and Philadelphia.

Framing a disease is more than an individual action. Robert Aronowitz emphasizes that a "new consensus about illness is usually reached as a result of negotiations among the different parties with a stake in the outcome." Patients and their physicians continually navigate between two distinct views of ill health: "illness as a 'specific disease' and illness as 'individual disease.'" Individuals and social situations within a particular society and era define suffering, pain and disease. The physician's treatment reflects his/her knowledge of the disease and also recognizes that age, gender, race and ethnicity will influence a patient's response. Thus, diverse societies and various individuals in particular times have perceived different causes for tuberculosis and reacted accordingly. In the 1790s, the municipality of Buenos Aires thought that tuberculosis was contagious; city officials burned the belongings of the deceased and fumigated their homes. The United States medical schools in the 1860s taught students that consumption was non-contagious, inherited and usually incurable; this resulted in the spread of tuberculosis among family members.[24] Contemporary social historians of medicine provide the context for illness. Thus, Sheila M. Rothman, *Living in the Shadow of Death: Tuberculosis and the Social Experience of Illness in American History* (Baltimore, 1995), describes the world in which patients live. She also provides a model for the use of diverse sources, including general archives, family papers, diaries and memoirs, to discover patient voices. David Jones, *Rationalizing Epidemics: Meanings and Uses of American Indian Mortality since 1600* (Cambridge, 2004), uses four cases of Amerindians groups to describe and understand the responses to the suffering caused by the disease. Jones examined tuberculosis among the Dakota Sioux in the late nineteenth century and among the Navajo in the first half of the twentieth century. He emphasized the importance of noting the different perspectives of the ill from those who treated them. Government officials and physicians thought that the behavior and choices of the ill and their family contributed to increased mortality; they emphasized that limited economic opportunities exacerbated living conditions, including poor housing and inadequate food, and contributed to disease reception. In contrast, the Sioux and Navajo viewed taboos and spiritual transgressions as the cause of illness. Jones finds the voices of both the Amerindians (Sioux and Navajo) and Europeans (colonists, traders, physicians) and distinguishes among them. He emphasizes that the ill and the physicians viewed the disease differently.[25]

For Philadelphia, the voice of patients and their families can most easily be heard through *Spunk*, the magazine produced between 1909 and 1963 by the patients of Mont Alto sanatorium and through the extensive correspondence of Lawrence F. Flick. In comparison, the Porteño (resident of Buenos Aires) patients' voices were more muted. The Archivo General de la Nación Argentina holds papers on orphans and tubercular children, the Sanatorio Marítimo y Solarium in Mar del Plata, and the Hospital Vicente López y Planes in the Province of Buenos Aires. Patients' voices were located within the personal and policy information provided in physician treatment evaluations in the *Anales del Departamento Nacional de Higiene*, 1891–1914, *Anales del Círculo Médico Argentino*, 1877–1906 and the theses written by students to obtain the title of Doctor of Medicine at the National University of Buenos Aires between 1899 and 1936. In these, aspiring physicians described the diagnosis, prognosis and treatment of tubercular patients. The medical newspapers *Día Médico* and particularly *Semana Médica* (Argentina)—begun in 1894 and was still publishing in 1983—were useful in providing an understanding of social attitudes toward tuberculosis in Buenos Aires and the changing perspectives on tuberculosis.

Tuberculosis clearly affects patients and their families. Steady coughing makes it difficult to breathe; the chest hurts. Coughing up blood is frightening. Medications and drinking large amounts of milk often made patients sick to the stomach. Illness became anguish at many levels. Physically, the tubercular person found it increasingly difficult to bear the pain. Economically, the cost of treatment of an ill family member decreased savings and impoverished the family. Since tuberculosis frequently took those who were economically most productive, families regularly lost members who might have contributed to an improved standard of living. Socially, contagious individuals were viewed as outcasts. Psychologically, the ill were ashamed both because of the disease and because it was perceived that a weakness led to the disease. The issue of shame lingered on, so that even with modern antibiotics and cures some former patients did not want to discuss the disease or even admit to having had it.[26]

Tuberculosis Mortality Statistics

This monograph includes twelve tables which compare pulmonary tuberculosis deaths (mortality) in Philadelphia and Buenos Aires. There are no morbidity statistics; physicians had difficulty diagnosing tuberculosis and morbidity information is impossible to obtain for pre-1945 Buenos Aires and Philadelphia. There are conflicting data on the number of pulmonary tuberculosis deaths in many years. In the early years, physicians and public health officials viewed tuberculosis primarily as a lung disease and they failed to report other forms of tuberculosis. Tuberculosis may affect any organ or tissue including bones and joints, brain, eyes, abdomen, intestines, kidneys, larynx, lymph nodes and skin.[27] Eventually, public health officials divided tuberculosis into two major categories: pulmonary tuberculosis and other forms of tuberculosis. However, it is often unclear as to how compilers organized their data. For example, in 1920 on a table counting pulmonary tuberculosis deaths among Caucasians and African Americans in Philadelphia, the statisticians included acute miliary tuberculosis and tuberculosis of the larynx; other times these latter forms of tuberculosis represented separate categories.[28] Records also undercounted children who died of tuberculosis. During the first half of the twentieth century, physicians and public health officials evaluated children as thin, weak and unhealthy rather than tubercular; the deaths of those children were not attributed to tuberculosis. Although non-pulmonary forms of tuberculosis are undercounted in the nineteenth century, the number of mortalities increased in the twentieth century, most likely because of better diagnosis.

Statisticians did not even agree as to the total population of the city of Buenos Aires. Argentine censuses were taken in 1869, 1895, 1914 and 1947. The officials used growth rates to estimate the Buenos Aires populations between censuses. This resulted in the population estimates of Guillermo Rawson, Emilio R. Coni, Jacinto Veláquez, Juan Vaccaro and Nicolás Besio Moreno—all who were interested in the influence of disease on death rates and population growth—diverging by 0–25 percent. Variation in population size also resulted in different deaths rates. This monograph primarily utilized the statistics of Besio Moreno because he made the most careful study of both the city's growth rate and mortalities for 342 years (1594–1936). Jacinto Velazquez's statistics, calculated with a mathematical formula and published in the *Boletín mensual de estadística municipal,* were not as complete.[29] In comparison, the Philadelphia population and death statistics were more consistent; most historians utilized the *Annual Report of the Board of Health* published in the *Annual Message of the Mayor of the City of Philadelphia.* However, even Philadelphia statistics varied between formal censuses. Various sources disagreed on the numbers of tuberculosis deaths. There is as much as a twelve percent difference among death statistics for the same year.

Finally, the accuracy of tuberculosis figures for Buenos Aires and Philadelphia depended on correct medical diagnosis and complete government reporting. In many cases, tuberculosis deaths were undercounted. Deaths were not medically certified. Physicians not only regularly misdiagnosed, but often failed to report cases which were correctly identified as tuberculosis.[30] There was a stigma attached to tuberculosis, and families preferred that the causes of death be identified as pneumonia or some other illness. In spite of the questionable accuracy of tuberculosis mortality statistics, the available data provide new insight into four areas. Comparative statistics support the need for the revaluation of other types of mortality, for example, the accuracy of the number of pneumonia deaths. Tubercular deaths of adults and children provide insights into gender, class and ethnicity. A comparison of tuberculosis with epidemic diseases reinforces the evidence of tuberculosis as the major killer. The statistics confirm the rise and decline of tuberculosis as a dominant disease in Buenos Aires and Philadelphia between 1870 and 1945.

Comparison as Social History

Two cities—Buenos Aires and Philadelphia—are the focus of this comparative study. Between 1870 and 1945 both cities were large urban ports and manufacturing centers, had many immigrants and migrants from both Europe and rural areas within their respective countries. Buenos Aires was the capital of Argentina and the largest and economically most significant city of the nation, while Philadelphia was second only to New York City in its political and economic importance in the United States. Buenos Aires was the leading South American financial and commercial city with strong ties to Europe, and its economic growth contributed to the development of Argentina's hinterland. Philadelphia served a similar role in the United States. Philadelphia was larger than Buenos Aires during the nineteenth century, but by 1925 the population of Buenos Aires surpassed Philadelphia (see Table 2.1). The bureaucrats of both cities collected and recorded medical statistics that were utilized to manage their urban environments. The growth of a middle class in both cities changed the basis of economic and political power that affected public health policies and outcomes. Between 1870 and 1945, both cities changed from predominantly traditional port cities to modern ones with financial institutions that provided services to the public and transport systems that unified the central city and suburbs.

The era 1870–1945 was not only the period when tuberculosis was a major killer in both Buenos Aires and Philadelphia but was also the time when both cities developed new tuberculosis research institutions and undertook groundbreaking public health initiatives. Public health officials in both cities took action to improve the quality of food and housing of the poor, the ill and their families. By focusing on two significant international cities, it is possible to study patient experiences and to understand the rising global consensus on the nature and treatment of tuberculosis. The prevention efforts and treatment programs developed in Buenos Aires and Philadelphia illustrate how public health policies emerged in two very different cities. Philadelphia and Buenos Aires are important not because they prevented and treated tuberculosis more effectively than other cities but because they illustrate the challenges that cities in North and South America faced. They also provide two very specific environments in which physicians, health workers, and patients lived and worked.

Comparison provides an additional methodology to view the social environment of tuberculosis, its treatment, public policy and patient experiences. By evaluating the response to tuberculosis across time periods, regions and cultures, the comparative approach produces a more complete view of the disease's effects on individuals and society.[31] Historians regularly engage in comparison; in fact, they cannot avoid it, because general historical knowledge shapes the validity of questions asked and assumptions made. The issue is whether the comparison should be explicit. Ray Grew in "The Case for Comparing Histories" argues that comparison assists historians in four ways. Comparison helps define significant questions. It identifies important historical issues, provides a framework for research, and aids in the formation of conclusions.[32]

Social scientists, including political scientists, economists and cultural anthropologists, have utilized comparative methods, but historians have generally been slow to do so. Some professional historians argue that authors using the comparative method do not consider carefully enough the uniqueness of a society and see syntheses as superficial and oversimplified. In response, I would argue that a narrow focus on historical uniqueness undermines practical applications and useful conclusions.[33] Comparison keeps historians from overemphasizing the uniqueness of historical events and provides a broader context in which to examine specific case studies. Although comparison considers similarities and differences, my emphasis is on the commonalities of patient experiences within two societies.

In *Beneath the Anguish,* comparison framed the questions being asked and the research undertaken. Among the questions to be considered are the following: How did cities and the development of a global world shape public policies and programs? To what degree did gender, class, age and ethnicity influence the treatment of the tubercular and individual responses to it? How did treatment change with increased scientific understanding of tuberculosis and the emergence of new policies and institutions? What new institutions emerged to take care of the tubercular, and how do existing institutions change in response to the needs of tuberculosis patients? How does tuberculosis affect children? How and why did Buenos Aires and Philadelphia experience a decline in tuberculosis before antibiotics? Given medical successes, why do individuals continue to contract tuberculosis? Most importantly, how did physicians, public health officials and patients view and deal with tuberculosis?

Beneath the Anguish seeks to reconstruct the world of tubercular patients. It examines tuberculosis in social rather than biological terms. Disease and medical treatments will be viewed from the perspective of patient experiences, more than from that of physician observations. A study of disease as social history should be multidimensional. It should examine individual experiences of the disease in specific times and places, evaluate the various cultural influences on the disease and note the effects of the disease on society. It should also describe the role of the state and the importance of various institutions in dealing with the illness and recognize the global implications of the disease.[34]

Histories of Tuberculosis

There are no comparative histories of tuberculosis. However, there are both general literature and national histories of tuberculosis. Most important for my study are Barbara Bates, *Bargaining for Life: A Social History of Tuberculosis, 1876–1938* (Philadelphia, 1992) and Diego Armus, *The Ailing City: Health, Tuberculosis, and Culture in Buenos Aires, 1879–1950* (Durham, NC, 2011), a reorganized and revised revision of his Spanish monograph, *La ciudad impura: Salud, tuberculosis y cultura en Buenos Aires, 1870–1950* (Buenos Aires, 2007). Bates focuses on tuberculosis by examining the disease in Philadelphia through the experiences of Dr. Lawrence F. Flick, who had developed tuberculosis when a student, and his patients and their families. Unlike many tuberculosis sufferers, Flick regained his health. He went on to treat the tubercular and to become instrumental in founding both the Pennsylvania Society for the Prevention of Tuberculosis and the United States National Association for the Study and Prevention of Tuberculosis. But the challenges to families of dealing with tuberculosis and fighting the disease were similar to Flick's. Bates views patients and their families, physicians and tuberculosis institutions as bargaining with society for effective treatment for tuberculosis.

Diego Armus's study focuses on Buenos Aires, but—unlike most urban studies—disease and health issues are central to it. He convincingly argues that tuberculosis was central to understanding both the Porteño life and public health concerns, and he describes the uncertainties of those living with the disease in an urban environment. Three main arguments are central to his exploration of tuberculosis in Buenos Aires. First, tuberculosis was not just a biomedical issue but also offered a way of viewing all of the city's social and cultural issues. Second, he suggests that tuberculosis was a subculture that explained public health initiatives and political actions. Third, Armus reconstructs the tuberculosis experiences of both individuals and collective groups. He suggests that most Argentines voluntarily incorporated hygienic practices into their daily routine and sought to prevent the spread of tuberculosis.

My approach differs from that of both Diego Armus and Barbara Bateman in two ways. First, I place the tuberculosis patients and their families at the center of the narrative. Although I agree that physicians and families bargained for the tuberculosis patients, as Bates suggests, patients were more fatalistic than physicians. In the era 1870–1945, the tubercular and their families generally believed that they had little control over either their medical treatment or working conditions; but after 1945, the accomplishments of science and technology led the ill and their families to be less fatalistic and assume greater ability to control their world. Yet the Porteño working and middle classes continued to approach life more fatalistically than Philadelphians. This is reflected in the common usage of "Si Dios Quiere" (God willing). In contrast, North Americans increasingly believed that technology could triumph over human and natural disasters. I have not viewed the city as the central focus of my study as Diego Armus has done. He effectively used tuberculosis as an analytical tool to understand urban society. But in the process, Armus at times loses track of the ill and their families. It is doubtful that the sick and their families viewed their worlds only through the lens of tuberculosis. The working poor viewed illness as only one more challenge in their lives. Although the elite supported the hygienic efforts of the public health officials and sought to impose their views on the working class, the non-elite often found public health recommendations too costly. In order to provide a patient perspective with limited first-person accounts, I chose to emphasize the world of the tubercular patients and their families. In the case of both Bates and Armus, the reader is left wondering about the uniqueness of patient experiences as well as each city's tuberculosis institutions and policies. Most significantly, I place the ill and tuberculosis institutions and policies within a comparative and international perspective and connect them to a larger historical narrative.

This permits me to consider the universality of tuberculosis experiences and policies. I seek to combine the microhistorical and the global.[35]

Chapter Summaries

Chapter 1 explores how physicians, public health officials and patients viewed tuberculosis from the eighteenth to the twentieth century. From 1870 to 1945, an emphasis on the application of scientific approaches, the expansion of medical education, the formulation of national tuberculosis associations, the organization of international conferences, and the need to explain the disease to the public led to an international consensus on how to prevent and treat tuberculosis. This more global consensus, which shaped the views of Buenos Aires and Philadelphia patients and physicians, influenced specific treatments, transformed the role of hospitals and supported the development of preventoriums and sanatoriums. Over time, a growing number of physicians and public health personnel in Buenos Aires and Philadelphia became committed to preventing tuberculosis, treating those who contracted tuberculosis, and developing a cure.

Chapter 2 is the setting for understanding patient experiences within Buenos Aires and Philadelphia. The populations of both cities grew rapidly; the cities expanded geographically. The leadership provided by Francis Lawrence Flick (1856–1938) of Philadelphia and Emilio R. Coni (1854–1928) of Buenos Aires, spearheaded the development of new prevention and treatment efforts. Flick served as director of the Henry Phipps Institute for the study, treatment and prevention of tuberculosis in center-city Philadelphia. Emilio R. Coni organized the Buenos Aires municipal health services and supported the establishment of the Sanatorium and Hospital Municipal Doctor Tornú. Both men and their institutions illustrate the challenges of providing tuberculosis prevention and treatment for a growing urban population.

Chapter 3 relates tuberculosis prevention to gender, class, age and ethnicity in both Buenos Aires and Philadelphia. The diverse ethnicities and large numbers of immigrants in both Buenos Aires and Philadelphia added to the public health concerns of the upper classes and government officials. Unsanitary conditions and poorly ventilated living and laboring environments contributed to the spread of tuberculosis. Working conditions, rather than ethnicity, were a major determinant of who contracted tuberculosis. Workers recognized that work and home environments contributed to poor health and sought to improve conditions. Wealthy individuals could afford a choice of treatments, while the poor had to accept public health options. Women often rejected treatments that required travel and long absences from home. Many middle-aged individuals could not pay for time away from family and work.

Chapter 4 focuses on the treatment of patients. Diagnosis and care varied over time and according to gender, class and age. As was true globally, diet, medications, surgery and vaccination all became part of basic treatments in both Buenos Aires and Philadelphia. In the late nineteenth century, most families cared for ill relatives at home. With the growth of physician and institutional influence, hospitals and clinics became centers of patient care. Patients usually sought to maintain a normal life as long as possible. As Chapter 5 demonstrates, patients preferred home care, physician visits and public clinics, and sought to avoid institutions because of cost and their desire to remain with their families. Only when individuals became too sick to work and needed intensive care did they consider entering hospitals and sanatoriums.

Chapter 5 examines the organization and operation of public and private tuberculosis sanatoriums. Although many ill patients remained in their homes and attended nearby clinics and day camps, sanatoriums provided alternative options for residents of Buenos Aires and Philadelphia. During most of the twentieth century, sanatoriums offered both physicians and their patients hope for cures with a regimen of fresh air, diet and rest. Public health physicians and tuberculosis specialists emphasized that a cure was more likely if one spent time at public or private sanatoriums located in the city or countryside. However, the limited number of sanatorium beds meant that most of the poor and working class died at home or in hospitals.

Chapter 6 focuses on the children of Buenos Aires and Philadelphia. Public health officials thought that poor and malnourished children needed protection from tubercular adults. Both Buenos Aires and Philadelphia developed prevention programs in the public schools and open-air schools to improve the health of children who seemed susceptible to tuberculosis. Preventoriums built in the mountains or by the seashore were year-round institutions that sought to restore the bodies of unhealthy and pre-tubercular children. Medical treatments for children with tuberculosis were very similar to those for adults. Children faced the disruption of their education, the separation from parents and siblings, and the discipline of institutional treatment and requirements.

Chapter 7 evaluates tuberculosis in global and comparative terms. Tuberculosis policies of Great Britain, France, Germany, Spain, and continents of Africa and Asia are examined. Similarities and differences affected developments in Buenos Aires and Philadelphia. There was a growing consensus among physicians and public health officials on the causes and treatment of tuberculosis. Tuberculosis deaths declined erratically in Buenos Aires and Philadelphia in the early twentieth century before the introduction of effective drugs. Explanations for the decline in the number of tuberculosis cases include higher living standards that provided more balanced diets, improved living and working environments, the success of tubercular public education programs, the quarantine of the tubercular, and role of epidemics in the killing tubercular individuals.

Beneath the Anguish ends with the introduction of an effective cure for tuberculosis which emptied sanatoriums. Streptomycin, discovered in 1943, was initially produced in small amounts. Medical trials eventually determined that a combination of para-amino-salicylic acid (PAS) and streptomycin thwarted resistant strains of tubercle bacilli. In the late 1940s, chemotherapeutic agents and their adoption, globally as well as in Philadelphia and Buenos Aires, ended as a leading cause of death. The emergence of antibiotic-resistant strains of tuberculosis in the 1990s was connected to the AIDS epidemic that began in the 1980s.

Notes

1 Maria Kurtz to Lawrence F. Flick, Newark, N. J. 15 January 1905, Second Series, vol. 16, January–March 1905 (Lawrence F. Flick Papers, the American Catholic History Research Center and University Archives, The Catholic University of America, Washington, DC (hereafter cited as CUA). Lawrence F. Flick (1856–1938) was a Philadelphia tuberculosis specialist, founder of White Haven Sanatorium and organizer of the United States National Association for the Study and Prevention of Tuberculosis. Maria Kurtz was one of his many tuberculosis patients.

2 Fenelon Matorras, *Tisis tuberculosa y neumónica* (Buenos Aires: Imprenta a Vapor de la Nación, 1878), 87–88; translation by the author.

3 HSP, *Red Cross Letters*, 2, 22 June 1909 to John Seiser Mucklé; HSP, 1915, Red Cross Christmas Seals, 1915," Pennsylvania Society for the Prevention of Tuberculosis.

4 This statement is based on my analysis of a variety of reports, including world health statistics and a published material by Robert Koch.

5 Sheila M. Rothman, *Living in the Shadow of Death: Tuberculosis and the Social Experience of Illness in American History* (Baltimore: John Hopkins Press, 1995), 247–48.

6 William Johnston, "Tuberculosis" in *The Cambridge World History of Human Disease,* ed. Kenneth F. Kiple (New York: Cambridge University Press, 1993), 1059–62. This article should be the starting point for any understanding of tuberculosis. See also Courtney Humphries, "A Sleeping Giant," *Nature* 502 (10 October 2013): S14.

7 "Mummy autopsies reveal arthritis, cirrhosis, plaque – but little cancer," *Washington Post,* 29 January 2013, F5; Wilmar L. Salo et al., "Identification of Mycobacterium Tuberculosis DNA in a Pre-Columbian Peruvian Mummy," *Proceedings of the National Academy of Sciences* 91 (March 1994): 2091–94; Gail Dutton, "Pre-Columbian Tuberculosis," *Archaeology* 97, no. 4 (July/August 1994): 19; Gerald Conlogue, "More TB in Peruvian Mummies," *Archaeology* 55, no. 2 (March/April 2002): 14; Bernardo T. Arriaza et al., "Pre-Columbian Tuberculosis in Northern Chile: Molecular and Skeletal Evidence," *American Journal of Physical Anthropology* 98, no. 1 (September 1995): 37–45; Lois Wingerson, "Dark History of the White Death," *Archaeology* 97, no. 4 (September/October 2009): 43–47; Sally Lehrman, "The Diabolical Genius of an Ancient Scourge," *Scientific America* 309, no. 1 (July 2013): 82; Sebastien Gagneux, "Host-Pathogen

Co-evolution in Human Tuberculosis," *Philosophical Transactions of the Royal Society B: Biological Sciences* 367, no. 1590 (19 March 2012): 850–53.

8 Lehrman, "Diabolical Genius," 82–85 and Gagneux, "Host-Pathogen Co-evolution," 850–59.

9 Johnston, "Tuberculosis," 1060, 1065; for the percentage of infection, see Mark Harrison and Michael Worboys, "A Disease of Civilization: Tuberculosis in Britain, Africa and India, 1900–1939," in *Migrants, Minorities and Health: Historical and Contemporary Studies*, eds. Lara Marks and Michael Worboys (London: Routledge, 1997), 95.

10 Thomas Dormandy, *The White Death: A History of Tuberculosis* (Washington Square: New York University Press, 2000), 211, 223–24; Gumersindo Sayago, Juan B. Rocca and C. Ferrer Moratel, "Influencia del trabajo en el origen y en el desarrollo de la tuberculosis," *La Prensa Médica Argentina* 36, no. 39 (30 September 1949): 1972–1975; Courtney Humphries, "Sleeping Giant," *Nature* 502 (10 October 2013): S14–S15.

11 For the United States, see Richard Jensen, <rjensen@uic.edu> "Epidemics in American History," 18 February 1999, H-SCI-MED-TECH@H-NET.MSU.EDU (18 February 1999). For Buenos Aires, see Carlos Andrés Escudé, "Health in Buenos Aires in the Second Half of the Nineteenth Century," in *Social Welfare, 1850–1950: Australia, Argentina and Canada Compared*, ed. D.C.M. Platt (London: Macmillan Press, 1989), 60–69 and Victoria Mazzeo, *Mortalidad infantil en la ciudad de Buenos Aires 1856–1986* (Buenos Aires: Centro Editor de América Latina, 1993), 20–21.

12 Charles E. Rosenberg, "What Is an Epidemic?" in *Living with AIDS*, ed. Stephen R. Graubard (Cambridge: MIT Press, 1990), 1–7.

13 Other names utilized include wasting disease, weakness of the lungs and graveyard cough; individuals might refer to themselves as TBs or lungers. The enlargement of cervical lymph-nodes, also a form of tuberculosis, was known as The King's Evil or scrofula, while the spinal form of the infection was known as Pott's disease. See Helen Bynum, *Spitting Blood: The History of Tuberculosis* (London: Oxford University Press, 2012), 95–96; Katherine Ott, *Fevered Lives: Tuberculosis in American Culture since 1870* (Cambridge: Harvard University Press, 1996), 159–160; Rothman, *Living in the Shadow of Death*, 214. Robert A. Aronowitz, *Making Sense of Illness: Science, Society and Disease* (Cambridge: Cambridge University Press, 1998), 15, 173, 188, argues in great detail about the significance of naming diseases. For Spanish terms, see José Piñero, "Tisis tuberculosa" (MD diss., Universidad de Buenos Aires, Facultad de Ciencias Médicas, 1854), 1; *Diccionario Enciclopedia de Medicina y Cirugía Práctico escrito en Alemán bajo la Dirección del A. Guldenburg*, trans. Isidoro de Miguel y Viguri (Madrid: Sáenz de Jubera, Hermanos Editores, 1891), 33–34.

14 Linda Bryder, *Below the Magic Mountain: A Social History of Tuberculosis in Twentieth-Century Britain* (Oxford: Clarendon Press, 1988), 199; Leopoldo Cortejoso Villanueva, *Tuberculosis célebres: Grandes personalidades forjadas por la tuberculosis*, 2nd ed. (Barcelona: Editorial Mateu, 1958), has a long list of many less familiar tubercular deaths.

15 Oscar Beaujon, "La ultima enfermedad del Liberador," *Revista de la Sociedad de Bolivariana de Venezuela* 24, no. 82 (1965): 44–50.

16 For Sánchez, see Fernando García Esteban, *Vida de Florencio Sánchez* (Santiago, Chile: Ediciones Ercilla, 1939) and Ruth Richardson, *Florencio Sánchez and the Argentine Theater*, 1933 reprint (New York: Gordon Press, 1975); for Evaristo Carriego, see José Gabriel, *Evaristo Carriego* (Buenos Aires:

Agencia Sudamericana de Libros, 1921) and Jorge Luis Borges, *Evaristo Carriego* translated with introduction and notes by Norman Thomas Di Giovanni with the assistance of Susan Ashe (New York: E. P. Dutton, Inc., 1984); for Antonio Fernando Fader, see Loscano González Carbalho, *Fernando Fader* (Buenos Aires: Editorial Poseidon, 1943).

17 Thomas Mann, *The Magic Mountain*, trans. H. T. Lowe-Porter (New York: Vintage International, 1992); Manuel Puig, *Heartbreak Tango*, trans. Suzanne Jill Levine (New York: E. P Dutton & Co., Inc., 1975), 88–105.

18 Diego Armus, *The Ailing City: Health, Tuberculosis, and Culture in Buenos Aires, 1870–1950* (Durham: Duke University Press, 2011), 262–75; Diego Armus, "'Milonguitas' in Buenos Aires (1910–40): Tango, Social Ascent, and Tuberculosis," *História, Ciências, Saúde-Manguinhos* 9, no. 1 (2002): 187–207; Jimmie Rodgers, "TB Blues Lyrics," www.songlyrics.com/jimmie-rodgers/t-b-blues-lyrics/ (20 March 2018).

19 Susan Sontag, *Illness as Metaphor* (New York: Doubleday, 1990), 5–15, 25, 28–32, 38, 48–49.

20 Michel Foucault, *The Birth of the Clinic: An Archaeology of Medical Perception*, trans. A. M. Sheridan Smith (New York: Vintage Books, 1994), xix, 13 is often referred to in discussions of disease as a social construct. Charles E. Rosenberg, *The Cholera Years: The United States in 1832, 1849, and 1866* (Chicago: University of Chicago Press, 1962), 5 clearly defines in footnote 8 the social construction of disease.

21 Phil Brown, "Naming and Framing: The Social Construction of Diagnosis and Illness," *Journal of Health and Social Behavior*, 1995 (extra issue): 34–52. The quote is found on p. 38 and other ideas discussed on pp. 39–40, 45–46.

22 Harvard Brody, *Stories of Sickness* (New Haven: Yale University Press, 1987), 22–40.

23 Charles E. Rosenberg, "Introduction Framing Disease: Illness, Society and History," in *Framing Studies in Cultural History of Disease*, eds. Charles E. Rosenberg and Janet Golden (New Brunswick: Rutgers University Press, 1997), xxiii.

24 Aronowitz, *Making Sense of Illness*, 1, 8; R. M. Packard, "Tuberculosis and the Development of Industrial Health Policies on the Witwatersrand, 1902–1932," *Journal of Southern African Studies* 13, no. 2 (January 1987): 209, illustrates for South Africa how as the social and intellectual environment of the society changed along with its view of tuberculosis; David L. Ellison, *Healing Tuberculosis in the Woods: Medicine and Science at the End of the Nineteenth Century* (Westport: Greenwood Press, 1994), 8, 14, 32–33, 47; Horacio Rodríguez Castells, "Apuntes para la historia de la tuberculosis en la República Argentina," *Revista Argentina de Tuberculosis y Enfermedades Pulmonares* 31, no. 3 (1970): 123–26; Marta M. Zabatta and Patricia de Forteza, "El Protomedicato y la profilaxis de la tuberculosis en Buenos Aires Virreinal," *La Semana Médica* 152, no. 15 (19 May 1978): 479–83.

25 David S. Jones, *Rationalizing Epidemics: Means and Uses of American Indian Mortality Since 1600* (Cambridge: Harvard University Press), 17–18, 136–37, 158–62, 178–84.

26 Rothman, *Living in the Shadow of Death*, 8; Godias J. Drolet, "Tuberculosis Hospitalization," *Spunk* 18, no. 12 (March 1927): 18 suggested that the loss of life due to tuberculosis cost the United States a billion dollars annually; Marie K. Matteucci in an interview, 18 October 2004, Shippensburg, Pennsylvania, emphasizes the issue of shame felt by friends that have been cured.

27 Matthew R. Smallman-Raynor and Andrew D. Cliff, *War Epidemics: An Historical Geography of Infectious Diseases in Military Conflict and Civil Strife, 1850–2000* (New York: Oxford University Press, 2004), 58.

28 City of Philadelphia, *Annual Message of Mayor of Philadelphia* (Philadelphia, 1920), 582.

29 Nicolás Besio Moreno, *Buenos Aires: Puerto del Río de la Plata, Capital de la Argentina, estudio crítico de su población, 1536–1936* (Buenos Aires: Talleres Gráficos Tuduri, 1939), 405–9; 422–30.

30 Lawrence Francis Flick, "Differential Diagnosis between Tuberculosis of the Lungs and Diseases Which Resemble It," The Historical Medical Library of the College of Physicians of Philadelphia, Lawrence Francis Flick, collected reprints.

31 The following publications usefully discuss both the practical and theoretical issues of comparison: C. E. Black, *The Dynamics of Modernization: A Study in Comparative History* (New York: Harper & Row, 1966), 35–55, one of the earliest works to lay out a systematic approach for doing comparative history; Robert B. Bain, "Building an Essential World History Tool: Teaching Comparative History," in *Teaching World History: A Resource Book*, ed. Heidi Roupp (Armonk, NY: M.E. Sharpe, 1997), 29–34; Raymond Grew, "The Case for Comparing Histories," *American Historical Review* 85 (1980): 763–78; Peter Burke, "Models and Methods" in *History and Social Theory* (Ithaca: Cornell University Press, 1993), 22–43; Reinhard Bendix, "The Comparative Analysis of Historical Change," in *Social Theory and Economic Change*, eds. Tom Burns and S. B. Saul (London: Tavistock Publications, 1967), 67–86; Frederick Cooper, "Race, Ideology and the Perils of Comparative History," *American Historical Review* 101 (1996): 1122–1138. For a very interesting model of comparative history, see Roger Horowitz, Jeffrey M. Pilcher and Sydney Watts, "Meat for the Multitudes: Market Culture in Paris, New York City and Mexico City over the Long Nineteenth Century," *American Historical Review* 109 (2004): 1055–83.

32 Raymond Grew, "The Case for Comparing Histories," *American Historical Review* 85 (1980): 763–78.

33 Jared Diamond and James A. Robinson, eds., "Afterword: Using Comparative Methods in Studies of Human History," in *Natural Experiments of History* (Cambridge: Belknap Press, 2010), 272.

34 Rosenberg, *The Cholera Years,* provides an early example of the new medical social history. See his introduction in Rosenberg and Golden, *Framing Disease*, xvi–xxiii for an excellent discussion on medicine as social history.

35 Amy Stanley, "Maidservants' Tales: Narrating Domestic and Global History in Eurasia, 1600–1900," *American Historical Review* 121, no. 2 (April 2016): 439–40 discusses the challenges of combining a microhistorical and global approach.

1 Tuberculosis

Views and Perspectives

> If You Have Consumption
>
> 1 Be Hopeful and cheerful, for your disease can be cured if you have not neglected it too long.
> 2 Obey your physician's instructions. You may improve steadily for months, and then lose it all by carelessness.[1]

> A person who has had or is likely to have tuberculosis should choose an occupation demanding as little heavy physical labor, anxiety or wearing responsibility as possible, and affording the shortest hours, the most outdoor life or the best ventilation inside, with sufficient remuneration to provide sanitary quarters and plenty of good food.[2]

From 1870 to 1920, there were revolutionary changes in the western understanding of tuberculosis that resulted in a consensus among physicians and public health officials about the cause, prevention and treatment of tuberculosis. The quotations at the beginning of the chapter are from prize-winning pamphlets that were exhibited in 1908 at the Sixth International Congress on Tuberculosis. These pamphlets represented the efforts of state and local tuberculosis associations to inform the public on how to treat and prevent tuberculosis. They also reflected the consensus among health experts. Although patients considered the information presented in pamphlets, they often found the recommendations difficult to follow. New knowledge does not in itself assure accord and may lead to opposition. Furthermore, following the accepted advice on tuberculosis did not necessarily lead to a cure.

The growing consensus on the cause and treatment of tuberculosis emerged alongside new developments in the medical profession. Physicians and public health professionals organized and supported an increasing number of international conferences and the organization of national tuberculosis associations. American and Western European universities developed similar programs to train physicians. Hospitals became centers of physician training and treatment that provided an alternative option to home care. The growing similarity of medical education in America and Western Europe facilitated the exchange of ideas at international congresses because it assured that physicians spoke the same scientific language. Increased international communications, new organizations, and agreement as to how to train physicians facilitated the growing consensus on the prevention and treatment of tuberculosis.

Between 1870 and 1920, attitudes and policies toward tuberculosis converged in Argentina, the U.S., the Western European nations and nations influenced by the West. In this worldwide movement, Philadelphia and Buenos Aires were both important innovators, exemplifying the changing attitudes and policies. Nations, cities and nongovernmental institutions played key roles in transforming the new knowledge and medical practices in the effort to combat tuberculosis. Yet even with agreements among medical professionals, policies to prevent and treat tuberculosis often emerged slowly and haphazardly. The global public and tubercular patients only slowly accepted the germ theory of disease and that tuberculosis was contagious.

Historical Understandings of Tuberculosis

The history of the western understanding of tuberculosis begins with early Greek manuscripts. The ancient Greeks discussed the nature of the disease and whether it was hereditary or transmittable. They provided clinical descriptions of tuberculosis. Aristotle noted that phthisis (as the Greeks called the disease) was contagious, as did Galen who considered the most important diagnostic sign to be blood in the sputum. (Here, he agrees with early twentieth-century physicians.)[3] In the East, Chinese texts described symptoms of pulmonary tuberculosis as early as the western Jin period (265–316). By the twelfth century, Chinese Taoist medical texts viewed pulmonary tuberculosis as infectious in its final stage. The Japanese first described pulmonary tuberculosis in 984. Although eastern efforts to understand tuberculosis paralleled those of the West, the two regions did not influence one another's ideas before the modern age.[4]

By the seventeenth century, several European governments and cities viewed consumption as contagious and legislated to contain it; in 1669, the Consejo General de Sanidad of the Republic of Lucca (part of the Tuscany region of modern Italy) authorized autopsies and destroyed clothes worn by the deceased tubercular.[5] In the eighteenth and early nineteenth centuries, European attitudes toward phthisis varied. The French and British came to associate consumption with the literary and intellectual classes and often romanticized the disease in poems, novels and operas while viewing phthisis as hereditary. In contrast, Spaniards and Italians romanticized consumption less and continued to regard it as infectious. As a result, consumptive patients who traveled to warm climates often met hostility.[6]

In 1737, the municipal government of Valencia, Spain, ordered the expropriation of the possessions of those with phthisis. Fourteen years later, the Spanish government extended this directive to the entire country and required an inventory of all goods used by the tubercular, the burning of their clothes and the disinfection of their houses. For example, a Barcelona hotel in which Frederick Chopin had slept asked him to pay for his bed, because a police order required that it be burned. A Spanish patient's physician was responsible for enforcing these rules, and failure to carry out this responsibility might lead to the suspension of the physician's license. In Italian cities and the province of Tuscany, clothes of the tubercular were also burned. After the 1821 death of John Keats in Rome, Joseph Severn, who had cared for the poet, had to pay for the burning of the infected furniture in the Piazza di Spagna, and the cleaning and reconditioning of the death chamber.[7] The Spanish belief about the contagious nature of consumption and the edict of treatment through disinfection was applied to its American colonies. For example, in 1751 and 1752, the Spanish crown issued decrees governing the spread of contagious diseases. The municipality of Buenos Aires applied these decrees in the 1790s to tubercular cases, burning the belongings of the deceased and fumigating their houses. In 1794, the Brothers of Charity of Buenos Aires created a room for infectious patients in the Hospital de Mujeres. With the 1810 establishment of a revolutionary junta, Buenos Aires rejected Spanish colonial policy on tuberculosis.[8]

Throughout much of the nineteenth century, medical professionals in the Americas and Europe debated whether phthisis was hereditary or contagious. Before the acceptance of the germ theory of disease, practitioners and lay people viewed disease in personal terms, assuming that an illness was the result of an individual's religious, social, hereditary or economic circumstances. Until scientists developed the germ theory of disease and understood how the disease could be transmitted by water, air, food, and human and animal carriers, there was little understanding of infection or the spreading of diseases. In the nineteenth century, diseases were ascribed to "miasma": foul-smelling air or filthy water and decaying animal or vegetable matter were thought to cause diseases and lead to epidemics. When Edward Livingston Trudeau (1848–1915)—a tuberculosis physician and popularizer of the institution of the sanatorium in the U.S.—attended medical school in 1868, he learned that phthisis was non-contagious, inherited and usually incurable. Attitudes toward the treatment of tuberculosis changed gradually. By 1877, at the American Medical Association meeting in Chicago, the U.S. physicians generally agreed that consumption should be treated in the early stages and that patients benefitted by living in high altitudes.[9]

Modern attempts to bring tuberculosis under control began with Robert Koch's (1843–1910) 1882 proof of the bacterial nature of the disease. His work—along with that of Louis Pasteur and Joseph Lister—contributed to the modern definition of infection. Koch announced the identification of the tuberculosis bacillus on 24 March 1882 in his paper "On the Aetiology of Tubercular Disease," which was read to the Physiological Society in Berlin. The paper's publication was noted in an editorial in the medical journal *Lancet* on 22 April and in the *New York World* on 23 April 1882. The more politically conservative Philadelphians were slower than the residents of New York, Boston and Baltimore to accept the germ theory of disease and Koch's explanation of the cause of tuberculosis.[10] In spite of Koch's discovery, physicians, hygienists and practitioners continued to debate the degree of contagiousness of tuberculosis. Many Philadelphia and Buenos Aires physicians were unconvinced that Koch had found the cause; and only with the translation of his paper from German into English in 1884 did the U.S. medical establishment seriously consider his discovery. Leading medical colleges continued to propagate contradictory doctrines.[11]

During the 1870s, health professionals and the elite classes in the U.S., Argentina and Europe incorrectly associated tuberculosis with moral degradation—alcoholism and prostitution—thought to be caused by the new urban social order. For example, Gabriela de Laperriére de Coni, an Argentine social worker, was concerned with how the life and work of women and children influenced their health. She emphasized six contributors to pulmonary tuberculosis: alcoholism, unhealthy housing, deficient alimentation, excessive physical labor, poor hygiene, and moral and intellectual degradation.[12] In 1869, James Copland, a British physician, listed eighteen causes of consumption resulting from deviations from culturally accepted lifestyles. For example, he suggested that individuals were most inclined to consumption if exposed to cold air and damp clothes; if they had too many sexual partners, masturbated, or were celibate; women might contract consumption if they suffered physical abuses or rode astride horses rather than sidesaddle.[13]

The standard nineteenth-century European medical texts and dictionaries continued to emphasize that tuberculosis was a hereditary disease, whose onset was spurred by leading a sedentary, indoor life.[14] William Osler's original 1892 edition of *The Principles and Practices of Medicine* defined tuberculosis as "an infective disease, caused by the bacillus tuberculosis." The author further noted that "Tuberculosis unquestionably may be inherited, but in what way and how often are unsettled problems." This text, which went through multiple editions between 1892 and 1947, did not change its basic definition until the eighth edition in 1921. In 1895, however, the author muted his comments on the hereditability of tuberculosis, noting that "in extremely rare instance the disease is congenital."[15] As late as 1904, *Lippincott's Medical Dictionary* declared that pulmonary consumption was caused by heredity, family predisposition, sudden changes of weather, and "above all the presence of the tubercle bacillus."[16] Increasingly, conflicts over causes of tuberculosis were no longer along national lines but among specialists. Hygienists and sanitationists tended to view tuberculosis as communicable and spread by the poor and the working class; physicians and medical researchers continued to debate whether tuberculosis was inherited or contagious and the role of climate in causing, preventing and curing tuberculosis. These conflicts reflected contrasting political visions of how to use science to create a superior society.

Lawrence F. Flick (1856–1938),[17] who graduated from Jefferson Medical College of Philadelphia in 1879, focused his practice on tuberculosis patients. He never viewed tuberculosis as hereditary but did accept that an individual could be predisposed to it. Initially, he falsely saw the stomach as the usual mode of entrance of the bacilli and believed that there was little danger of contracting the disease through the lungs. As late as 1902, he observed no evidence that tuberculosis could be transmitted to human beings through milk and meat, suggesting that development of tuberculosis in children who drank milk from tubercular cows was purely coincidental. On the other hand, Flick correctly viewed climate as insignificant in preventing and curing tuberculosis, because the disease existed in all climates. Like many physicians of his day, Flick originally had an incomplete understanding of the causes of tuberculosis. Eventually, Flick's research, experience with patients and attendance at international conferences led him to become among the first Philadelphia physicians to accept that tuberculosis was an infectious disease caused by a microorganism.[18]

Flick had many heated discussions with his colleagues on the topic. To prove to other physicians that tuberculosis was contagious, he conducted a twenty-five-year study of tuberculosis in the fifth ward of the city of Philadelphia, a mostly poor immigrant community (twenty percent of whose residents were African-American). With mortality information provided by physicians and undertakers to the Board of Health, Flick located the phthisis cases on a map to show that cases appeared in the same houses and apartment buildings; less than ten percent of the cases were isolated. His evidence, presented to various professional groups, demonstrated not only that tuberculosis was contagious but also that houses in which the disease occurred remained a center of infection for an indefinite period. Flick's recommendations, correlating with international efforts, emphasized that the homes of tubercular individuals should be registered, so that health officials could track those who were ill.[19]

Argentine physicians, like their U.S. counterparts, debated the specific causes of tuberculosis and often agreed that it was difficult to prove the importance of any single factor. Some physicians argued that tuberculosis was hereditary, while others contended that the main culprits were factors such as climate, poor hygiene, an inadequate diet, crowded housing, poverty and lifestyle.[20] Debates over whether tuberculosis was hereditary, environmental or contagious had occurred worldwide for over 2,000 years. Between 1882 and 1902, the disputes among medical professionals over the causes of tuberculosis were particularly vociferous. Observations seemed to support that heredity and environment played a pivotal role because the disease did indeed run in families. People who lived at high altitudes and breathed clear cold air seemed rarely to contract tuberculosis. Attitudes slowly changed when evidence demonstrated that several cases occurred within a single family because the disease was contagious.

The different assumptions about the causes of consumption led to different treatments. Physicians who assumed a hereditary cause for tuberculosis concluded that there was little they could do to cure the ill. Sending a patient to a different environment was a treatment that physicians thought promising. Only anecdotal evidence suggested that a change of climate could cure tuberculosis. Because tuberculosis was thought to characterize the intellectual and artistic elites, North Americans and Europeans had romanticized the disease. But when consumption was viewed as contagious, the general public no longer romanticized it. Instead, the poor were viewed as the dominant carriers of tuberculosis.

As physicians, hygienists and practitioners accepted Robert Koch's proof of the bacterial nature of tuberculosis, an international consensus developed on the character and treatment of tuberculosis. By the 1890s, physicians hoped that tuberculosis could be cured, but efforts were limited by the difficulty of diagnosing the disease. Physicians initially hoped that sputum tests, based on new laboratory staining methods, would provide early diagnosis of tuberculosis. However, although the methods indicated the presence of *Mycobacterium tuberculosis*, it did not distinguish between those who had latent tuberculosis and those who had the disease. When patients began spitting blood or a doctor using a stethoscope detected cavities in the lungs, the disease was far advanced. The availability of the tuberculin skin test developed in 1907 and improved lung X-rays in the 1920s allowed physicians to diagnose the onset of pulmonary tuberculosis much earlier. Although physicians had a better understanding of tuberculosis by the 1920s, an effective cure remained elusive.[21]

At the beginning of the twentieth century, the general population remained uncertain as to the cause of tuberculosis. Ordinary people did not accept scientific interpretations of tuberculosis, because they did not understand the scientific arguments and because the medical profession offered no cures. The residents of Philadelphia and Buenos Aires initially reflected the general attitudes of their respective English and Spanish traditions. However, by the 1920s, educated elites were more inclined to accept a scientific perspective on the disease. As public health officials publicized the causes of tuberculosis and suggested cures, popular attitudes in Buenos Aires and Philadelphia began to reflect the view that tuberculosis was contagious rather than hereditary.

Associations for Tuberculosis Prevention and Treatment

Various national, state and municipal health associations helped create a commitment to founding of institutions combating tuberculosis and to preventing and treating it. In 1892, lay and medical citizens organized the oldest tuberculosis association in the U.S.—the Pennsylvania Society for the Prevention of Tuberculosis—at Lawrence Flick's office. The society sought to encourage the expansion of local tuberculosis prevention committees throughout the state. The Pennsylvania society emphasized cooperation with diverse organizations, including the Commonwealth Department of Health, community health agencies, baby welfare agencies, schools, county medical societies and local physicians.[22] The Pennsylvania Society warned about tuberculosis contagion. It issued circulars and public notices to discourage spitting in public places and sponsored lectures in churches, labor union halls, schools and clubs. Early prevention programs in Philadelphia were particularly focused on school children and African Americans. By 1935, the Pennsylvania Society had produced more than nine pamphlets, with titles such as "How to Avoid Contracting Tuberculosis" and "How Storekeepers and Manufactures Can Help to Prevent the Spread of Tuberculosis."[23]

Although other European countries had tubercular philanthropic programs, Pennsylvania was among the first societies to unite medical professionals and ordinary people in major public health campaigns. It raised funds to educate the public on tuberculosis prevention, to encourage the founding of a municipal hospital for patients suffering from advanced tuberculosis, to build sanatoriums for the impoverished in the initial stages of tuberculosis and to advocate enactment of laws that would help prevention of the disease. The programs also advocated improved ventilation in trolley cars, movie theaters and public buildings. Local communities began committees to support their own tuberculosis programs. For example, Shippensburg, a small community in South Central Pennsylvania, started a committee in 1917 to educate the public and initiate a visiting nurse program.[24]

Many national anti-tuberculosis associations were organized between 1890 and 1910. France established its association in 1891, followed by Germany in 1895, Belgium and Britain in 1898, Portugal and Italy in 1899, Canada in 1900, Denmark and Argentina in 1901, Sweden and the U.S. in 1904, Japan in 1908, and Norway and Russia in 1910. The U.S. leaders in the anti-tuberculosis campaign were stirred to action when they realized that European nations had developed effective national organizations. The 1904 creation of the National Association for the Study and Prevention of Tuberculosis enabled the U.S. to join with European nations in the international association which had been organized in 1902 with a central bureau in Berlin. The U.S. national association held its first annual meeting in 1905. The meeting focused on different sets of issues, including sociological factors, clinical and climatological practices, and pathological and bacteriological developments. From 1904 until 1945, the U.S. National Association for the Study and Prevention of Tuberculosis bound the various state and local tuberculosis associations together.[25]

The state and local associations then embarked on several major efforts: encouraging all states to organize associations, bringing these new associations and other diverse groups crusading against tuberculosis under national leadership, inaugurating tuberculosis exhibitions in large cities, and planning for the 1908 international congress to be held in Washington, D.C. By 1910, the national association had gotten organizations to register individuals with tuberculosis in nearly all large U.S. cities and in those states which had institutions for treating the disease. The national association also persuaded states to establish sanatoriums, hospitals and dispensaries to treat tuberculosis and encouraged the U.S. government to promote treatment for soldiers and sailors, to eliminate tuberculosis in cattle and to check immigrants for tuberculosis.[26]

The organizations supporting prevention efforts encouraged private individuals to take action. In 1907, a Wilmington, Delaware, woman, after she read about a program in Denmark, began the Christmas Seal campaign as a private endeavor to support indigent tubercular patients in her city. Eventually, the Christmas Seal campaign became a major fundraiser for the national association. Proceeds from seals purchased in Philadelphia were used for the tubercular work of the city, including financial support for hospitals, sanatoriums, visiting nurse programs and preventive education. In 1908, the Christmas Seal campaign supported many of Lawrence Flick's initiatives such as the Free Hospital for Poor Consumptives, White Haven Sanatorium and the Pennsylvania Society for the Prevention of Tuberculosis. In 1910, the National Tuberculosis Association and the Red Cross promoted the annual sale of Christmas seals, and in 1919, the national association assumed full sponsorship.[27]

By 1920, other nations recognized that the U.S. campaign against tuberculosis offered a model that could be replicated elsewhere. The national association effectively sought consensus on the diagnosis, prevention and treatment of tuberculosis with reports from standing committees at annual conferences and through coordinating with state associations. The national association also provided seminars for medical professionals and public health nurses on the nature and treatment of tuberculosis, surveyed sanatoriums and tuberculosis hospitals, promoted a tuberculosis crusade for children, provided motion pictures on tuberculosis, and published three journals. The local tuberculosis associations assured that necessary programs were maintained even when municipal health organizations were ineffective. Philadelphia passed an ordinance in 1915 requiring annual X-rays for food handlers, barbers and beauticians. The Philadelphia Tuberculosis Society took over the program and became among the first in the U.S. to take fluoroscopic images.[28]

The U.S. was not unusual in establishing organizations to support tuberculosis prevention policies. Emilio Coni and other physicians established the Argentine Anti-Tuberculosis League in Buenos Aires in 1901, three years before the U.S. established its national association. The Argentine by-laws emphasized a commitment to studying the various forms of tuberculosis, educating both professionals and the public and stressing prevention. Beginning in 1901, the league (supported by government financing) printed 200,000 leaflets of instructions for the tubercular and their families, emphasizing that tuberculosis was contagious but preventable if proper precautions were taken. Simple instructions, explaining for example how to use sputum cups or spittoons, were printed on matchboxes. Such materials were distributed in schools, churches, factories, workshops and public conferences. Efforts to educate the public were soon extended to Argentina's interior provinces. In the same year, the league began to publish a journal dealing with the struggle against tuberculosis. In 1902, the league established a dispensary for treating tubercular patients and sought legislative financing for a national sanatorium. The league was dedicated to the reform of unhealthy housing and drew the attention of municipal authorities to the relationship between unsanitary housing and tuberculosis. The league was also committed to improving working conditions and created popular kitchens to improve workers' nutrition. Although the Argentine Anti-Tuberculosis League had programs similar to those of the U.S. National Association, the Argentinean crusade against tuberculosis centered in Buenos Aires; provincial associations were limited or in some cases non-existent.[29]

The growing global uniformity of policies and attitudes among medical professionals led to the development of popular programs aimed at preventing tuberculosis. Various national associations against tuberculosis faced similar problems in educating the masses. In all countries, the general public was incapable of understanding complex discussions of tuberculosis and unwilling to spend much time reading medical discourses on tuberculosis. Agencies and countries produced leaflets for popular consumption that received medals and cash awards, and all delegates to international tuberculosis conference were exposed to this literature aimed at the broad public. Because no certain cure existed for tuberculosis, public health officials viewed prevention as the best means of reducing the incidence of tuberculosis. Commonwealth health organizations developed pamphlets on the causes and prevention of tuberculosis that provided information to local community groups, the tubercular and their families. Health educators had to be able to explain the causes, symptoms and treatment of tuberculosis in simple terms. "Tuberculosis is a communicable disease." "No spitting, no consumption." "Tuberculosis is curable."[30] Popular pamphlets were translated

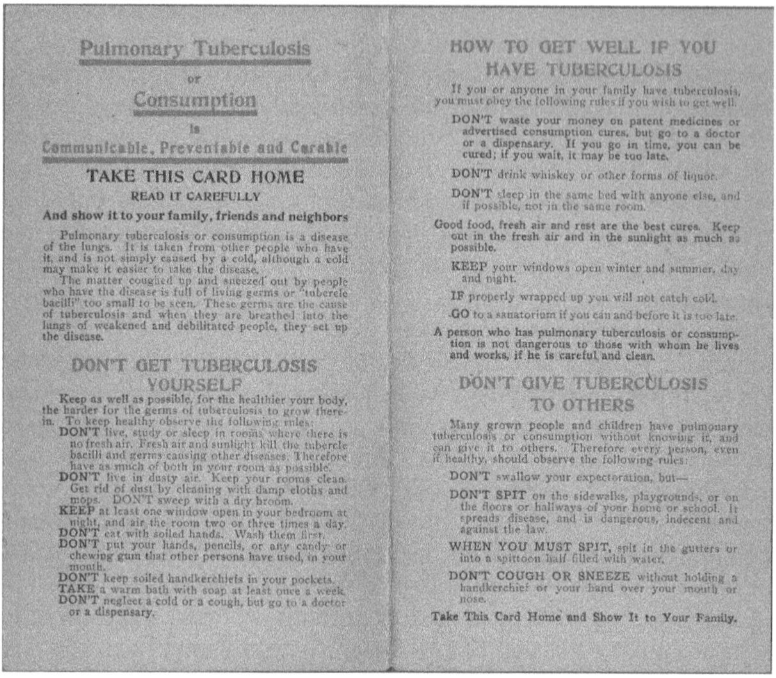

Pulmonary Tuberculosis

or

Consumption

is

Communicable, Preventable and Curable

TAKE THIS CARD HOME

READ IT CAREFULLY

And show it to your family, friends and neighbors

Pulmonary tuberculosis or consumption is a disease of the lungs. It is taken from other people who have it, and is not simply caused by a cold, although a cold may make it easier to take the disease.

The matter coughed up and sneezed out by people who have the disease is full of living germs or "tubercle bacilli" too small to be seen. These germs are the cause of tuberculosis and when they are breathed into the lungs of weakened and debilitated people, they set up the disease.

DON'T GET TUBERCULOSIS YOURSELF

Keep as well as possible, for the healthier your body, the harder for the germs of tuberculosis to grow therein. To keep healthy observe the following rules:

DON'T live, study or sleep in rooms where there is no fresh air. Fresh air and sunlight kill the tubercle bacilli and germs causing other diseases. Therefore have as much of both in your room as possible.

DON'T live in dusty air. Keep your rooms clean. Get rid of dust by cleaning with damp cloths and mops. DON'T sweep with a dry broom.

KEEP at least one window open in your bedroom at night, and air the room two or three times a day.

DON'T eat with soiled hands. Wash them first.

DON'T put your hands, pencils, or any candy or chewing gum that other persons have used, in your mouth.

DON'T keep soiled handkerchiefs in your pockets.

TAKE a warm bath with soap at least once a week.

DON'T neglect a cold or a cough, but go to a doctor or a dispensary.

HOW TO GET WELL IF YOU HAVE TUBERCULOSIS

If you or anyone in your family have tuberculosis, you must obey the following rules if you wish to get well.

DON'T waste your money on patent medicines or advertised consumption cures, but go to a doctor or a dispensary. If you go in time, you can be cured; if you wait, it may be too late.

DON'T drink whiskey or other forms of liquor.

DON'T sleep in the same bed with anyone else, and if possible, not in the same room.

Good food, fresh air and rest are the best cures. Keep out in the fresh air and in the sunlight as much as possible.

KEEP your windows open winter and summer, day and night.

IF properly wrapped up you will not catch cold.

GO to a sanatorium if you can and before it is too late.

A person who has pulmonary tuberculosis or consumption is not dangerous to those with whom he lives and works, if he is careful and clean.

DON'T GIVE TUBERCULOSIS TO OTHERS

Many grown people and children have pulmonary tuberculosis or consumption without knowing it, and can give it to others. Therefore every person, even if healthy, should observe the following rules:

DON'T swallow your expectoration, but—

DON'T SPIT on the sidewalks, playgrounds, or on the floors or hallways of your home or school. It spreads disease, and is dangerous, indecent and against the law.

WHEN YOU MUST SPIT, spit in the gutters or into a spittoon half filled with water.

DON'T COUGH OR SNEEZE without holding a handkerchief or your hand over your mouth or nose.

Take This Card Home and Show It to Your Family.

Figure 1.1 "Take this Card Home." Pennsylvania Society for the Prevention of Tuberculosis pamphlet, 1912, call number: UPA/Pam RA 644.T7 P46, Historical Society of Pennsylvania.

into many languages, thus contributing to the universality of basic ideas about tuberculosis. For example, a Philadelphia physician S. Adolphus Knopf published a popular booklet, *Tuberculosis as a Disease of the Masses and How to Combat It*, which went through seven editions between 1901 and 1913 and was translated into twenty-seven languages including Chinese.[31] Both private and public organizations sought to educate the public on how to deal with tuberculosis.

A good example of the educational material used in public health campaigns is the Pennsylvania Society for the Prevention of Tuberculosis's "Take this Card Home." The small pocket pamphlet "Pulmonary Tuberculosis or Consumption is Preventable and Curable" makes five major points. It informs the reader that tuberculosis was a germ passed through the air; it suggests a plan to prevent individuals from contracting tuberculosis; it explains how to get well if infected; and it emphasizes not giving the disease to others. The pamphlet urged recipients to take it home to show to family, friends and neighbors. The instructions were targeted at the working class. "Keep your windows open"; "don't sweep with a dry broom"; "take a warm bath with soap once a week"; "don't waste your money on patent medicine or advertised consumption cures"; "don't drink whisky or other forms of liquor"; and "don't spit." Some instructions such as "don't sleep in the same bed with anyone else, and if possible, not in the same room" would have been impossible for many families to follow. One instruction was partly false: "go to a doctor or a dispensary" (good advice since a physician can confirm if a person contracted tuberculosis and the infected individual can take action to prevent its spread); "if you go in time, you can be cured" (untrue); "if you wait, it may be too late." The worldwide development of associations to support patients and the local and national public health campaigns to prevent the spread of tuberculosis reflected a growing global consensus on the cause, prevention and treatment of tuberculosis.

International Conferences Contributions to Global Approaches

International conferences were important in standardizing global approaches toward tuberculosis and fostering worldwide agreement on how to prevent and treat tuberculosis. The rising international consensus on the nature and treatment of the disease began in 1851 in Paris at the first of fourteen International Sanitary Conferences held between 1851 and 1938. The conferences held in various European capitals in the nineteenth century (and a 1861 conference held in Washington, D.C.), focused primarily on cholera, although concerns went beyond quarantine issues to look at hygiene, sanitation and the causes of disease. Although throughout the nineteenth century conference delegates remained divided as to the causes and transmission of cholera, the International Sanitary Conferences laid the basis for international cooperation on disease prevention.[32]

In the 1890s, Germany took the lead in promoting international conferences on tuberculosis. Koch's discovery of the tuberculosis bacillus gave Germany the prestige to attract international experts on tuberculosis, many of whom had communicated with Koch or studied in Germany. The International Congress on Tuberculosis formally came into existence in Paris in 1898 with a second congress held in Berlin in 1899. In the early twentieth century, the international tuberculosis congresses convened in London in 1901, Berlin in 1903, Paris in 1905, Washington, D.C. in 1908 and Rome in 1911. In addition, international tuberculosis associations had annual conferences, in The Hague in 1906, Vienna in 1907, Stockholm in 1909 and Brussels in 1911.

These international conferences instructed medical practitioners, officials, politicians and the general populace on the origin, nature, prevention and general methods of the treatment for tuberculosis. The diverse conference representation, the scientific discussions, the presentation of statistical information on tuberculosis deaths and the various exhibitions laid the basis for a global consensus on the causes and treatment of tuberculosis. The British delegation to the 1899 International Congress in Berlin illustrates the conclusions reached concerning tuberculosis. In a report to their government, the British representatives emphasized that the bacillus discovered by Professor Koch caused consumption and all tubercular diseases; in most cases, the bacillus coughed up in phlegm was transmitted from sick to healthy people in dust that individuals inhaled into their lungs; milk and meat from tubercular cattle also caused tuberculosis; while the bacillus was present in all tubercular cases, whether an individual had active tuberculosis depended on his or her constitution. The continued disagreement among the conference participants over the cause of tuberculosis is recognized in the final conference report. The delegates acknowledged that tuberculosis was rarely transmitted by inheritance, while concluding that a specific child could have less resistance than another. Attendees further recommended that a child's health should be strengthened through wholesome food and a well-ventilated house.[33]

The fifth International Congress of Tuberculosis in Paris in 1905, with some 3,000 delegates from all parts of the world, reached a consensus on the treatment of tuberculosis. Joseph Walsh, President of the Pennsylvania Society for the Prevention of Tuberculosis and Medical Director of White Haven Sanatorium from 1916 to 1935, stated that no new methods for the treatment of tuberculosis were proposed but that "it was generally agreed that sufficient rest, sufficient fresh air and sufficient good nourishment were the only elements in the treatment at present known to science." He also reported that "The official seal... of the congress was put on various efforts toward the cure and prevention of tuberculosis, namely sanatoria for adults and children, hospitals for advanced cases, and supporting dispensaries, park convalescent camps (day camps) and societies for education of the public."[34]

The largest contingent of physicians and health worker presenters at these international conferences came from the host country. Over seventy percent of the five hundred presentations at the 1905 Paris conference were made by the French delegates. Under the leadership of Lawrence F. Flick, the U.S. became a participant in the International Congress in Paris in 1905. The U.S. delegates, with the second largest number of participants, made less than three percent of the presentations. Both official delegates representing their countries and volunteers came from most of the European countries, including Sweden, Denmark, Great Britain and Rumania. Persia, Turkey, Algeria, Tunisia, Egypt and China also sent representatives as did Argentina, Brazil, Cuba, Mexico and Uruguay.[35] In 1908, at the Sixth International Conference in Washington, D.C., U.S. delegates delivered almost fifty percent of the presentations, while the French delivered only seventeen percent.[36] Although not all countries sent delegates to all meetings, about the same numbers of countries were represented at both the 1905 and 1908 international conferences.

The conferences were held in many different countries, and each of the host countries expanded its understanding of how best to prevent and treat tuberculosis. As for the countries that did not host the conferences, they too benefited. For example, Guatemala sent two representatives to the 1905 conference, who reported to the Minister of Foreign Affairs. The government then published a report providing data from the sessions that the delegates had attended, which included information on the causes of tuberculosis, new diagnostic methods, dispensaries and sanatoriums, social and health programs, and tuberculosis in animals.[37] All the conferences featured a similar range of presentations. Thus, those attending international conferences could participate in sessions dealing with the latest research on the pathology and bacteriology of tuberculosis; clinical studies and tuberculosis therapy in sanatoriums, hospitals and dispensaries; surgery and orthopedics; prevention and treatment of tuberculosis in children; the economic, social and industrial aspects of tuberculosis; state and municipal action to combat tuberculosis; and tuberculosis in animals. Although presenters read papers in French, German or English, summaries were provided in the languages not used.[38]

There were also exhibits on the prevention and identification of tuberculosis, including examples of anti-tuberculosis leaflets; statistics on mortality, summarized in graphs, tables and maps; scientific information on anatomy, bacteriology, surgery, and formalin-preserved samples of body parts, particularly the lungs; descriptions and photographs of tuberculosis dispensaries, hospitals and sanatoriums; and corporate presentations of medical equipment for sale. Fourteen countries, fifteen U.S. states, and seven U.S. government departments exhibited at the 1908 Washington conference. Pennsylvania had an extensive exhibition with eighty-five displays. These included charts on the number of deaths for the year 1907; maps indicating tuberculosis by county and with locations of dispensaries; state funding plans for tuberculosis; models of tents, cabins, open-air pavilions, dispensaries, and sanatoriums; examples of a physician's dispensary coat, a disinfector's suit, disinfecting apparatus and sputum cups; laboratory samples, equipment and photographs of infected body parts; and sample tuberculosis applications for treatment, reports on numbers of treatments and photographs of tuberculosis institutions.[39]

The international conferences encouraged common statistical measures, particularly related to tuberculosis deaths. For example, beginning in 1891, the Buenos Aires city government began publishing the *Anuario estadístico de ciudad de Buenos Aires*. Not all statistics were accurate or comparable. Numbers differed, depending on whether only pulmonary tuberculosis was counted (or all varieties of tuberculosis), or whether children under fifteen were counted. Finally, the value of the statistics rested on the accuracy of diagnosis and the completeness of the reporting of numbers of tuberculosis cases. Nevertheless, these statistics—not withstand their deficiencies—allowed for comparisons across countries and contributed to an understanding of the worldwide impact of tuberculosis. The national exhibitions, as well as presentations describing national prevention programs, made use of such statistical evidence. Information about declining tuberculosis mortality in one country served as an incentive for others to adopt similar prevention programs.[40]

Lawrence F. Flick was the prime organizer who brought the 1908 international congress to Washington, D.C. He hoped that having an international conference in the U.S. would encourage politicians and the public to provide more support for the campaign against tuberculosis. Flick was particularly impressed by the strength of the campaign against tuberculosis in the smaller countries whose prevention programs were superior to the U.S. programs. He stated that Buenos Aires's "crusade against tuberculosis (was) the most advanced in the Western Hemisphere and perhaps of the World" and that even if the U.S. had "been represented at its best, it could not have competed with Buenos Aires." Flick hoped that the examples of smaller countries similar to Argentina might encourage the U.S. to develop better prevention efforts.[41]

Planning an international congress was a major enterprise.[42] The congress drew more than 4,000 attendees and lasted three weeks—one week for scientific work and two for city visits. Local, state and national groups had to unite to call attention to issues related to tuberculosis. The organization of the 1908 Washington conference began with Flick's vision. He secured the endorsement of President Theodore Roosevelt, who offered Washington, D.C. as the location for the 1908 conference. With the help of state associations, Flick sought to raise $100,000 in gifts of $5,000 from each of twenty men to provide a fund for the scientific and philanthropic part of the congress. The interest from these funds paid for prizes for exhibitions, while the funds themselves supported a secretary general, staff, translators, rental of exhibition space, transport of foreign exhibitions, and honoraria for speakers. Translators had to be hired, so that presentations could be printed in English, German and French. All participants expected to receive the six volumes of conference transactions. States were asked to bear the cost of hosting international visitors who might visit tuberculosis institutions as well tour the U.S. Many states and cities had difficulty finding donors who would help pay the conference costs.[43] There also needed to be coordination of the international exhibits which traveled from the conference to other large cities, including New York and Philadelphia. Diplomacy was required in credentialing groups. For example, John Fulton, the General Secretary for the Congress, received a letter from Emilio Coni (1855–1928), the Buenos Aires Director of Public Assistance, who proposed that the Liga

Argentina Contra Tuberculosis become Argentina's organizing committee. Flick agreed to this proposal but emphasized that since the league would be the official representative of the Argentine Republic, members of public health societies, medical services and all groups interested in tuberculosis should be included.[44]

These international congresses led to a standardized understanding of tuberculosis for several reasons. The hosting of an international tuberculosis conference forced organizers to reach an agreement on what was an effective tuberculosis program. The host country could advertise to a wider audience in its own country and to foreign delegates its successes in combating tuberculosis and in solving health problems. Better national programs were developed, because of growing awareness of the types of prevention programs in different countries and their varying degrees of effectiveness. Moreover, the interactions among leading experts on tuberculosis enabled the world's health specialists to share information on scientific discoveries and ideas to reform. This shared information led to a consensus on the nature of tuberculosis and its prevention. The visual exhibitions, excursions to tuberculosis institutions and informal conversations resulted in common understandings.[45] The result was that when delegates returned to their home countries, they sought to initiate the most effective prevention programs and treatments.

Consensus on Medical Education

The western world's growing consensus on the educational requirements necessary for the training of physicians led to doctors having similar understandings of various diseases. In particular, a consensus arose on how to prevent and treat tuberculosis. England, where physicians were members of the elites, distinct from those in the trade guilds such as surgeons and apothecaries, served as the model for U.S. doctors. By establishing medical schools in the U.S., physicians hoped to develop a professional corps. In 1765, the University of Pennsylvania, then known as the College of Philadelphia, opened the first medical college in the U.S. The only eligible applicants were men. As of 1850, women could also train to become doctors with the founding of the Female Medical College of Pennsylvania. Whereas France had only three medical schools in 1850, the U.S. offered medical training in forty-two institutions.[46]

Beginning in the 1870s, physicians recognized the need to increase the number of doctors who received rigorous academic training. Women initially benefited by reforms in medical education. During the 1880s, the percentage of women physicians doubled. There were 7,000 women physicians in the U.S. at the turn of the century, whereas England had 258 and France had only ninety-five. In 1893, Johns Hopkins University opened a four-year medical school to which both men and women were admitted. (Wealthy women endowed Johns Hopkins in return for the admission of women to university programs.) All entering students were required to have a college degree. By 1910, medical professionals agreed that perspective physicians should have a bachelor degree and that medical training required scientific study, laboratory experience and practical hands-on training. If possible, physicians followed their formal training with a tour of the important European medical and research centers in Heidelberg, Vienna, Berlin and Paris to familiarize themselves with European practices. New requirements lengthening the medical education decreased the number of medical schools and increased class-gender-racial homogeneity and knowledge of the graduating physicians.[47]

The new trends in medical practice and education were not confined to Europe and the U.S.[48] The medical education in Argentina was heavily European. In 1822, the National Legislature in Buenos Aires authorized the creation of the Academia Nacional de Medicina. In that year, the Universidad de Buenos Aires offered its first program in medicine and two years later graduated its first student. In 1852—when the Facultad de Medicina graduated twelve students—courses covered anatomy, pathology, gynecology, pediatrics, obstetrics and public health. An 1877 national law mandated the establishment of a second medical school in Córdoba.[49]

Between 1870 and 1920, the Buenos Aires medical school added courses on contagious diseases.[50] The Facultad de Medicina introduced Emilio Coni, Enrique Tornú, Samuel Gache and José Penna, who would be instrumental in the development of Argentine health policies, to contemporary European social and medical theories and gave them experience with tubercular patients in the medical clinic. Like their counterparts in the U.S., Argentine medical school graduates traveled to Europe and particularly France. After 1900, some students interested in tuberculosis might go to Robert Koch's laboratory in Berlin, whereas others preferred the Institut Pasteur in Paris.[51] The first woman graduate from the Facultad de Medicine, Cecilia Grierson, 1859–1934, traveled to Europe in 1889 to become familiar with the most recent medical treatments.[52]

Within Latin American, Argentina's approach to medicine was not unique. After Mexico gained independence, physicians sought non-Spanish European models and soon absorbed French traditions and new cures through European medical publications. After the 1880s, Mexican physicians increasingly traveled abroad to visit the Institut Pasteur, study at European medical schools, attend medical conferences and tour municipal sanitary operations in Paris, Berlin and Rome. By the end of the nineteenth century, Mexican physicians presented their accomplishments at international conferences, hosted hygiene congresses in Mexico City and developed site-specific strategies and campaigns to deal with the disease.[53] Similarly, in the second half of the nineteenth century, Brazilians began to set up rural sanitation clinics, supported urban campaigns against specific diseases and extended the role of the state in public health. Although Latin American medical professionals benefited from international contacts and influences, they also contributed to new approaches to the disease. National medical and political leaders' efforts led to the expansion of scientific medicine and new public health approaches in Latin America.[54]

Because the nineteenth-century medicine was often ineffective, ordinary people were initially skeptical of its claims. As a result, medical practice paid too little, so doctors were unwilling to invest in a lengthy professional education. Bitter feuds among physicians as to methods of cure further weakened their standing with the public. Many families were accordingly reluctant to make use of medical professionals. In Philadelphia, patients sometimes complained about doctors, noting that the cost of an examination for tuberculosis might exceed a patient's weekly salary. In the absence of automobiles and phones, obtaining a physician's services required time and effort. Although nurses were available, families often chose not to hire them, because of the cost or class prejudice against the lower-class women who usually filled those positions. The professionalization of nursing began with the establishment of nursing schools in the 1870s.[55]

In spite of cultural factors that led to some national differences in medical education in the U.S., Europe and Latin American countries, developments followed similar patterns.[56] The establishment of medical colleges supported professionalization. Medical education was reformed with an emphasis on scientific study, laboratory experience and practical hands-on training. New requirements lengthened medical education and improved the ability of physicians to care for their patients. Similarities in medical education contributed to a growing consensus on how to treat tuberculosis.

Changing Roles of Hospitals

From 1870 to 1920, U.S. and Argentine hospitals changed their focus from emphasizing long-term charity care for the chronically ill to using new technologies and medications to cure specific illnesses. In Philadelphia, the use of X-ray and laboratory reports required patients to go to hospitals. As a result, physicians assumed more control over their patients. Medical efficiency and scientific advances legitimized both physicians and hospitals. The increased concentration of populations, growing wealth and new medical equipment encouraged the movement of patients from care in the home to care in hospitals. The dependence on hospital care occurred most rapidly in cities. As hospital care gained greater acceptance and the ill could choose between private and public facilities, the middle classes were more inclined to go to hospitals. With greater pressure for admission, hospitals began to focus on providing care for surgical patients and the acutely ill. Recuperating patients were discharged more promptly. Furthermore, the evolution of the hospital and the role of the physician occurred, while the cause of tuberculosis was being defined and new treatments and approaches to it were being developed.[57]

In the nineteenth-century, in Argentina and the U.S., the norm was to care for the sick in the home. Women were the major care givers. Patients went to a hospital only to die, or if they had no supporting family to care for them. In 1873, there were only 120 U.S. hospitals; their main function was to provide for the poor. Lower-class families reluctantly sent their sick members to hospitals. By contrast, families of middle-class patients cared for them at home. Often, hospitals did not have space for tubercular patients. In 1899, St. Agnes Hospital of Philadelphia refused entrance for one of Flick's patients, while noting that "if all the Catholic Hospitals did as much for consumptives as St. Agnes, there would not be a problem." In 1904, in Philadelphia, the total number of private and public beds for tuberculosis patients was under 400. (In the same year, 3,117 patients died of pulmonary tuberculosis.) Although the lack of beds for tuberculosis patients continued into the 1950s, Philadelphia hospitals were radically reformed by the 1920s. They evolved from a focus on the care of the chronically ill to facilities that provided acute intervention with new technology.[58]

The same factors that contributed to the evolution of hospital functions in the U.S. contributed to the transformation of Buenos Aires hospitals. Typical Buenos Aires hospitals, such as the Hospital de Hombres and the Hospital de Mujeres, managed by Catholic orders, were taken over by the government in 1822. These hospitals were not medically advanced, but they did provide the basis for state operation of hospitals. In the first few decades of the nineteenth century, Argentina's hospitals deteriorated because of war, social anarchy, and the political and economic difficulties of the independence era. The hospitals lacked sufficient professional personnel to care for the ill and were primarily custodial institutions for housing the poor, the indigent and the chronically ill. Until the middle of the nineteenth century, few infectious patients, including those with tuberculosis, entered the hospitals. In the 1840s, Argentina's French, English and Irish communities established local hospitals, and in 1868, the government established the 240-bed Lazareto San Roque for contagious diseases. Because initially tubercular patients were not considered contagious, they were admitted to general hospital wards.[59] The hospitals were managed by diverse constituencies: the city, the national government, charity institutions and foreign communities. Eighty-one percent of the hospitals were totally or almost completely state-funded. In addition to hospitals, in the late nineteenth century, Buenos Aires had twenty small private clinics.[60]

During the 1870s and 1880s, the poor went to the public hospitals expecting little medical help; many died under unhealthy and crowded conditions with little medical treatment. From 1870 to 1878, between 45.9 and 82.1 percent of tuberculosis patients in the Hospital General de Mujeres died.[61] In 1875 and 1879, the majority of the hospital tubercular cases were cooks, ironers, seamstresses, servants and launders. Most were unmarried, Argentine-born and ranged between ages sixteen and thirty.[62] An exposé of city hospitals in 1877 noted the following deficiencies: beds lacked sheets and pillow cases, the latrines were full, the food was poor, doctors did not have the needed instruments for operations and patients did not receive appropriate medicines. As late as 1881, the general municipal hospitals were so crowded that some patients slept in the corridors, and even the most ill were often refused admittance due to the lack of space. Hospital personnel did not follow hygienic practices, lacked laboratory facilities, rarely performed autopsies, failed to disinfect the rooms, bedding, and clothing, and did not separate the contagious from other patients. As a result, infectious diseases such as tuberculosis spread rapidly. Inadequate state and municipal funding assured substandard hospital care and a lack of available beds for the ill.[63] To obtain admittance with free care to the hospitals, patients had to receive a certificate of poverty signed by a municipal doctor and a member of the hygiene commission. Patients ineligible for free care needed to pay minimum hospital expenses. A very few people fraudulently received free care by providing a false address in a poor neighborhood. But in general, because of the poor reputation of the public hospitals, only patients of limited means chose to enter.[64]

The quality of hospitals in Buenos Aires improved over time, as new hospitals replaced old ones and modern public health practices were implemented; the Hospital San Roque replaced the Hospital de Hombres in 1882, and five years later the Hospital Rivadavia supplanted the underfunded and obsolete Hospital General de Mujeres.[65] Beginning in 1892, Asistencia Pública, a Porteño municipal agency which administered the city's public assistance programs and regulated its health practices, made provisions to concentrate infectious patients at the Hospital Francisco Javier Muñiz, the city's contagious disease facility. In 1891, Muñiz assisted thirty-one tubercular patients. By 1908, the number had increased to 1088; sixteen to eighteen percent of the infectious patients whom the hospital received were tubercular.[66] As of 1895, fifty-three percent of tubercular patients died in their own homes. In many cases, families preferred to provide home care. At the same time, there were a limited number of beds for tubercular patients in hospitals. The Hospital Rivadavia similarly to Philadelphia General Hospital turned away many tubercular patients because there was no bed space.[67]

Within Argentina, medical professionals were increasingly influenced by ideas from abroad, particularly from France. Central to their interest was the professionalization of hospital staff. With more middle-class patients entering hospitals and the increasing influence of trained physicians, the organization of hospitals changed. Physicians were initially paid for their hospital work only when working with contagious or mental patients. When doctors received pay for all hospital work and hospitals provided services unavailable in the home, physicians increasingly recommended hospital care for their patients. With the expansion of hospitals came a need for additional trained staff to care for the ill. The Buenos Aires municipal government accordingly established a nursing school in 1885 to provide needed medical personnel. It was no longer enough to construct hospitals and asylums for the poor and ill; it was also necessary for the government to provide social services to improve the poor's hygienic conditions, their health and their morality.[68]

In both the U.S. and Argentina, the transformation of hospitals reflected changes in the view of disease. Laboratory analysis contributed to identifying and treating of the disease. With new technologies, diseases were microbiologically examined rather than clinically observed. Patients themselves could choose from various institutions. Increased patient choice, a more professional medical staff and the ability of hospitals to offer services that homes could not provide led more of the ill to enter hospitals. The hospitals with improved diagnostic facilities increased the physicians' influence over their patients. The changes in the role of hospitals and the professionalization of the medical staff were occurring while researchers were proposing new cures for tuberculosis. Similarities in the quality of medical education and changes in the type of hospital treatment in Buenos Aires and Philadelphia provided a basis for the international consensus on the prevention and treatment of tuberculosis.

Family and Patient Perspective

Despite the significant professional changes in physician training and hospital development and the growing popular support for medical science, many patients remained hesitant to accept new medical practices. Tuberculosis sanatoriums began operating at the end of the nineteenth century but became an optimum choice in Argentina and the U.S. only in the 1920s. The result was that hospitals in both Buenos Aires and Philadelphia were initially the only alternatives to home care. Wives and mothers bore the brunt of caring for tubercular husbands and children in both the U.S. and Argentina, but still often opposed sending a family member to a hospital. Families also resisted sending relatives to sanatoriums, because of distance and the extended separation.[69] With the increased gravity of illness, the strain on family members increased. Thus, the parents of Sarah Calliagham, an eighteen-year-old Philadelphia resident suffering from terminal pulmonary tuberculosis, requested that she be transferred to a hospital. She was a member of a large family; both parents worked, and there was no one but a younger sister at home to care for her. In another instance, the wife of a tubercular man living in a poor Philadelphia neighborhood in a house that "[was] not a place for a respectable person" desired that he be admitted to the hospital.[70] Thirty-one-year-old Pedro Clemente, an Argentine farm laborer, chose to go to the hospital in January 1873 rather than have his family care for him, because he had lost strength, had a cough, and ran a temperature at night. Diagnosed with advanced tuberculosis, he died several months later.[71]

Even with the challenges of caring for tubercular patients, many families preferred to care for the ill in their homes. John Anconca, an ex-marine who worked in the Philadelphia office of the Continental Cotton Oil Company, was in 1907 in the last stages of tuberculosis. His wife took care of him, even though he was able to leave his bed for only short times each day. If Anconca went to the hospital, his wife and daughter could both work to make ends meet. In spite of being twelfth on the charity list of the Phipps Institute, which would have paid for his care, he rejected his physician's recommendation that he go to a Philadelphia hospital. Anconca stated that he "would rather die where he is."[72] Also in 1907, a Spanish immigrant, a railroad gatekeeper in Buenos Aires, was cared for by his wife. Given the reputation of the hospital, his wife preferred to care for him at home, even though she was responsible for cooking, washing, ironing and caring for five children.[73]

Once at the hospital, families and patients often complained about the food and treatment. Mrs. McManus noted that she subsisted on the food brought by her husband and kept meat under her bed to show the doctor when he made the rounds. While the physician agreed that it was poor, he remarked that the meat "was the identical quality we had on our own table" and that unpalatable food could be exchanged. On hearing her complaints, the Mother Superior at St. Agnes, a Catholic institution, ordered her dismissed. Her husband decided to take a house in the country, so that he could provide both her and the children with milk, nourishing stews and chicken. As in the hospital, Mrs. McManus continued to experience night sweats, chills, coughs, trouble with her bowels and pain in her abdomen. Nevertheless, she appeared happier.[74] At times, patients took advantage of the hospitals to continue their previous lifestyles. Henry Devere of Philadelphia was discharged from a hospital for drunkenness as well as disobeying hospital rules. He had gone for walks every night and had returned intoxicated and with liquor for other patients.[75]

As some of these examples indicate, tubercular patients did not always adapt easily to the new institutions that cared for them or followed their physicians' instructions. Non-skilled workers could not easily change their occupations. Individuals in the working class expected their jobs to involve heavy physical labor, long hours and poor pay. If they were fortunate, they might work outdoors. Low salaries further limited the possibility of living in a well-ventilated home or eating nutritious food. If the major family earner became ill, he, of course, was anxious and concerned about both his family and himself. A family with an ill member was even less likely than most to be able to afford to follow the doctor's advice or meet the additional expenses of a hospital stay. The public awareness of the contagious nature of tuberculosis led to additional anxieties and concerns.

Although physician knowledge and hospital care improved by the early twentieth century, tubercular patients still had to deal with painful medical procedures, loss of autonomy, enforced inactivity, isolation from family and society's discriminatory practices. Tubercular patients might be shunned by neighbors and evicted from their homes. All who knew the Argentine poet and journalist, Evaristo Carriego, realized the cause of his death at age twenty-nine in 1912. Yet his parents tried to conceal the fact that he had died of tuberculosis.[76] Those who survived the disease to return to their home communities often preferred that no one learn of their diseases, because tuberculosis was contagious, associated with the poor and stigmatized. As we have seen, tuberculosis had been transformed from being considered a romantic illness in the nineteenth century to being thought a shameful infirmity in the twentieth century.

Consensus on Tuberculosis Treatment

A common western heritage unified Europe and the Americas and laid the basis for similar approaches to medicine. The development of reformed medical institutions and new treatments were encouraged by major nineteenth-century transformations. In the Americas and Europe, the expansion of industrialization contributed to a rapid change in social structure, which strengthened the working and middle classes. These new groups had a growing respect for science and demanded new institutions for their care. Government and private institutions in the Americas responded with efforts to organize and provide for health care. Important scientific discoveries caught the popular imagination and awakened people to the possibilities of medical science.

Families became aware of the contagiousness of tuberculosis and of the means for preventing it. Nevertheless, patients and their families were slow to accept the new scientific understanding of tuberculosis. But at the same time, patients benefited from the efforts of state and national tuberculosis associations to prevent tuberculosis and to provide free treatment for the poor. The improved training of physicians and reformed hospitals encouraged patients to opt increasingly for professional care. The growing agreement on how to prevent and treat tuberculosis in Buenos Aires and Philadelphia gave physicians and hospitals the needed prestige to get patients to follow preventive methods and to accept professional care.

Between 1890 and 1920, a consensus emerged among both the public and medical professionals as to the nature and treatment of tuberculosis. The organizations of national associations and international conferences held between 1880 and 1911 were central to promoting uniform attitudes and policies among medical professionals and national public health officials. The physicians who organized the national tuberculosis associations and who attended the international conferences were increasingly being trained at new medical schools and obtained practical experience in reformed hospitals. The acceptance of European models of medical education in the Americas contributed to similar curriculums. Furthermore, when physicians met at national or international conferences, they spoke the same scientific language. The national and state tuberculosis associations' efforts effectively contributed to increasing medical services for poor tuberculosis patients and to shaping attitudes toward the disease. At the same time, the implementation of scientific medicine and the development of modern public health programs that occurred in Philadelphia and Buenos Aires beginning in the second half of the nineteenth century were the work of national medical and political leaders and not the result of European efforts. Local initiatives were encouraged by the international conferences, tuberculosis associations and hospitals, which created opportunities to discuss the nature and treatment of tuberculosis. The consensus as to the causes, prevention and treatment of tuberculosis in both Buenos Aires and Philadelphia occurred in spite of the cities' differences.

Notes

1 O. D. Wescott, "Consumption Is the Most Common Form of Tuberculosis and Is a Germ Disease," in International Congress on Tuberculosis, *Transactions of the Sixth International Congress on Tuberculosis*, Washington, September 28 to October 5, 1908 *with an Account and Catalogue of the Tuberculosis Exhibition* (Philadelphia: W.F. Fell Company, 1908), 5: 277. Although the tubercle bacilli multiply slowly, they may remain alive in the body for years; except for the bovine variety, individuals contract tuberculosis almost entirely by aerial transmission; tubercle bacilli are spread by respiratory actions of talking, coughing, sneezing or spitting. For a general discussion of tuberculosis, see F. M. Burnet and David O. White, *Natural History of Infectious Disease* (Cambridge: Cambridge University Press, 1972), 213–15 and William Johnston, "Tuberculosis," in *Cambridge World History of Human Disease,* ed. Kenneth F. Kiple (New York: Cambridge University Press, 1993), 1059–67.

2 H. S. Goodall, "Tuberculosis: A Leaflet for Teachers," in International Congress on Tuberculosis 1908, *Transactions* 5: 291.

3 Owsei Temkin, "An Historical Analysis of the Concepts of Infection," in *The Double Face of Janus and Other Essays in the History of Medicine* (Baltimore, London: Johns Hopkins University Press, 1977), 460; Horacio Rodríguez Castells, "Apuntes para la historia de la tuberculosis en la República Argentina," *Revista Argentina de Tuberculosis y Enfermedades*

Pulmonares 31, no. 3 (1970): 121; Thomas Dormandy, *The White Death: A History of Tuberculosis* (Washington Square: New York University Press, 2000), 2–3.

4 William Johnston, "A Genealogy of Tubercular Diseases in Japan," *Social History of Medicine* 7, no. 2 (1994): 248–49.

5 Antonio Albert Guerrino, "Las primeras legislaciones antituberculosas," *Orientación Médica* 15, no. 713 (15 July 1966): 230.

6 J. N. Hays, *The Burden of Disease: Epidemics and Human Response in Western History* (New Brunswick, NJ: Rutgers University Press, 1998), 156–58; Linda and Michael Hutcheon, *Opera: Desire, Disease, Death* (Lincoln: University of Nebraska Press, 1996), 218–19; F. B. Smith, *The Retreat of Tuberculosis*, 1850–1900 (New York: Crom Helm), 77.

7 Guerrino, "Las primeras legislaciones antituberculosas," 230; Enrique P. Aznarez, "La Polémica contagionista de la tuberculosis en el siglo XIX y su repercusión in Córdoba, 'La memoria en contestación del Dr. Francisco Martinéz Doblas (1831),'" *Anales de Tisiología y Climatología* 3 (1944); Dormandy, *White Death*, 52–54; John Evangelist Walsh, *Darkling I Listen: The Last Days and Death of John Keats* (New York: St. Martin's Press, 1999), 129, 131.

8 Castells, "Apuntes para la historia," 123–26; Marta M. Zabatta and Patricia de Forteza, "El Protomedicato y la profilaxis de la tuberculosis en Buenos Aires Virreinal," *La Semana Médica* 152, no. 15 (19 May 1978): 479–83. For a more detailed discussion of attitudes toward contagion in Buenos Aires, see Vera Blinn Reber, "Misery, Pain and Death: Tuberculosis in Nineteenth Century Buenos Aires," *The Americas* 56, no. 4 (April 2000): 499, 502–4.

9 For examples of disagreements, see Erin H. Ackerknecht, "Anticontagionism between 1821 and 1867," *Bulletin of the History of Medicine* 22 (1948): 565–68 and Roger Cooter, "Anticontagionism and History's Medical Record," in *The Problem of Medical Knowledge: Examining the Social Construction of Medicine*, eds. Peter Wright and Andrew Trecher (Edinburgh: Edinburgh University Press, 1982), 90–91; David L. Ellison, *Healing Tuberculosis in the Woods: Medicine and Science at the End of the Nineteenth Century* (Westport: Greenwood Press, 1994), 8, 14, 32–33, 47.

10 Michael Worboys, *Spreading Germs: Disease Theories and Medical Practice in Britain, 1865–1900* (Cambridge: Cambridge University Press, 2000), 205–9; D. M. Fox, "Social Policy and City Politics: Tuberculosis Reporting in New York, 1880–1900," *Bulletin of the History of Medicine* 49, no. 2 (summer 1975): 176 and Frank Ryan, *The Forgotten Plague: How the Battle Against Tuberculosis Was Won and Lost* (Boston: Little Brown and Company), 9–15.

11 Ellison, *Healing Tuberculosis in the Woods*, 30; J. Woodrow Savacool, "Philadelphia and the White Plague," *Transactions and Studies of the College of Physicians* ser. 5, 8, no. 3 (1986): 153–54, 179.

12 Georgina D. Feldberg, *Disease and Class: Tuberculosis and the Shaping of Modern North American Society* (New Brunswick: Rutgers University Press, 1955), 29–35, 45–46; Héctor Recalde, *Vida popular y salud en Buenos Aires, 1900–1930* (Buenos Aires: Centro Editor de América Latina, 1994), 46.

13 Dormandy, 42–43; Feldberg, *Disease and Class*, 29–35, 44–46; Smith, 25–55; J. Copland, *Forms, Complications, Causes and Treatment of Bronchitis* (London: Longmans, Green and Co., 1866), 57–66. Elizabeth Lomax, "Heredity or Acquired Diseases? Early Nineteenth Century Debates on the

Causes of Infantile Scrofula and Tuberculosis," *Journal of the History of Medicine and Allied Sciences* 32, no. 4 (July 1997): 356–74 notes the various causes of tuberculosis.

14 Pedro Luis Napoleón Chernoviz, *Diccionario de medicina popular y ciencias accesorias* (Paris: em Casa de autor, 1879), 1021. Susan Sontag, *Illness as Metaphor and AIDS and Its Metaphors* (New York: Farrar, Straus and Giroux, 1989), 54.

15 William Osler, "Tuberculosis," in *Principles and Practice of Medicine*, 2nd ed. (New York: D. Appleton and Company 1895), 184, 188, 206.

16 R. W. Green, *Lippincott's Medical Dictionary: A Complete Vocabulary of the Terms Used in Medicine and the Allied Sciences* (Philadelphia: J.B. Lippincott Company, 1897), 786.

17 The Strittmatter Award provides a concise bibliography of the accomplishments of Dr. Lawrence F. Flick. See The Historical Medical Library of the College of Physicians of Philadelphia (hereafter CPP), Lawrence Francis Flick, Collected Reprints (hereafter FCR), 'The Strittmatter Award, 1933 to Dr. Lawrence Flick', privately printed for The Philadelphia County Medical Society, March 1933.

18 CPP, FCR, Francis Lawrence Flick, "Hygiene of Phthisis," *Transactions of the Philadelphia County Medical Society*, 11 January 1886; Charles Winslow Dulles, "Consumption Not Contagious," read 2 June 1897, *Transactions of the College of Physicians*, Third series, 19 (1897): 178–90; CPP, FCR, Lawrence F. Flick, "The Mode of Entrance of the Bacillus Tuberculosis into the System," *Times and Register*, 19 October 1889 (Philadelphia: Medical Press Company, Limited 1889): 9; CPP, FCR Lawrence Francis Flick, "Are Meat and Milk a Source of Seed Supply for Human Tuberculosis," *Journal of Tuberculosis*, October 1902, 5.

19 CPP, FCR, Lawrence Francis Flick, "Contagion of Phthisis (Tubercular Pneumonitis)," *Transactions of the Medical Society of the State of Pennsylvania* (June 1888): 12–17; CPP, FCR, Lawrence Francis Flick, "A Review of the Cases of Tuberculosis which terminated in Death in the Fifth Ward of the City of Philadelphia during the Year 1888," read before the Philadelphia County Medical Society, 22 May 1889. For a detailed discussion of Flick's efforts to prove tuberculosis contagious and to convince the Philadelphia Board of Health to adopt mandatory notification, see Samuel Kelton Roberts, Jr., *Infectious Fear: Politics, Disease and the Health Effects of Segregation* (Chapel Hill: University of North Carolina, 2009), 89–92.

20 The following Argentine sources published between 1843 and 1890 illustrate the debate: Eugenio Pérez, "Opúsculo sobre la tisis pulmonar" (MD diss., Facultad de Medicina, Universidad de Buenos Aires, 1843), 27–28; Ismael Carrillo, "La tisis y el clima de nuestras provincias," *Revista Médico-Quirúrgica* 14, nos. 13–14 (8 October 1877): 314–18; J. P. Riera, "Influencia de las costumbres en las enfermedades" (MD diss., Facultad de Medicina, Universidad de Buenos Aires, 1878), 21; Pedro J. Frías, "Estudio de algunas cuestiones sobre la herencia de la tisis" (MD diss., Facultad de Medicina, Universidad de Buenos Aires, 1879); G. N. Chaves, "Consideraciones generales sobre la herencia, el contagio, la profilaxis y el tratamiento de la tuberculosis pulmonar," *La Semana Médica* 6, no. 35 (31 August 1899): 314.

21 Donald G. McNeil, Jr., "New Tuberculosis Test May Soon Be Possible," *New York Times*, 2 January 2018, D6; Feldberg, 47.

22 CP, Lawrence Francis Flick Papers (hereafter LFP), Tuberculosis Letters, Miscellaneous, 170. Pennsylvania Society for the Prevention of Tuberculosis,

Yearbook 1918, 7; Pennsylvania Society for the Prevention of Tuberculosis, *Annual Report 1896* (Philadelphia, 1897), 2 and *Annual Report of the Pennsylvania Society for the Prevention of Tuberculosis for the Year Ending April 1, 1908* (Philadelphia, 1908), 4–6; CP, FCR, "The Crusade against Tuberculosis in Pennsylvania," Annual Address of the President of the Free Hospital for Poor Consumptive delivered on 9 March 1908," 3.

23 CPP, FCR, Pennsylvania Society for the Prevention of Tuberculosis, Pennsylvania Conference of Tuberculosis Workers, *Annual Report 1914* (Philadelphia, 1914).

24 CPP, FCR, Pennsylvania Society for the Prevention of Tuberculosis, "Program of Work for the Coming Year," *Annual Report 1915* (Philadelphia, 1915), 16–17; CPP, FCR, Pennsylvania Society for the Prevention of Tuberculosis, "Preventive Work by Local Anti-Tuberculosis Societies in Pennsylvania," *Annual Report 1917* (Philadelphia, 1917).

25 Linda Bryder, *Below the Magic Mountain: A Social History of Tuberculosis in Twentieth-Century Britain* (Oxford: Clarendon Press, 1988), 15–16; "First Annual Meeting of the National Association for the Study and Prevention of Tuberculosis," *Transactions of the National Association for the Study and Prevention of Tuberculosis*, 1, 1905 (New York: Irving Press, 1906), 9; Herman M. Biggs: "Address of the President," *Transactions of the National Association for the Study and Prevention of Tuberculosis* 3 (Philadelphia, 1907), 17–18.

26 CPP, JWP, *Letters and Programmes, National Association for the Study and Prevention of Tuberculosis*, vol. 3 (1904–1912), deals with the efforts of the association to organize state associations and develop consensus on the most effective prevention programs in the U.S. Lawrence F. Flick, "Present Status of the Tuberculosis Campaign and the Essentials for Thorough and Prompt Success," *New York Medical Journal* 91 (1910): 261–64; Edward L. Trudeau, "Address of the President," National Association for the Study and Prevention of Tuberculosis, *Transactions of the National Association for the Study and Prevention of Tuberculosis*, 1 (New York, 1905), 13–19. Lawrence F. Flick, "Address of the Vice-President: The Duties, Responsibilities and Opportunities of the National Association for the Study and Prevention of Tuberculosis," *Transactions of the National Association for the Study and Prevention of Tuberculosis* 2 (1906): 15–20; Livingston Farrand, "Report of the Executive Secretary, *Transactions of the National Association for the Study and Prevention of Tuberculosis* 5 (1909): 17–20.

27 Historical Society of Pennsylvania, hereafter HSP, *Red Cross Letters*, 2, 22 June 1909 to John Seiser Mucklé; "Red Cross Christmas Seals, 1915," Pennsylvania Society for the Prevention of Tuberculosis, The Historical Society of Pennsylvania, 1915; Savacool, 177.

28 Charles Hatfield, "Report of the Executive Office for the Year Ending May 1, 1920," Transactions of the National Association for the Study and Prevention of Tuberculosis, Sixteenth Annual Meeting, St. Louis, Mo., April 22, 23, and 24 1920 (New York, 1920), 31–41. Although comments from U.S. members may be self-serving, their comparative evidence from international conferences suggests that U.S. prevention programs were well respected; Savacool, 173.

29 "Resumen de los trabajos realizados en el primer año de su existencia," *La Lucha Antituberaculosa* 2 (May 1901–1902): 29–30; S. Gache, "La lucha antituberculosa en la República Argentina," *La Lucha Antituberculosa* 4, nos. 1,2,3 (June/July/August 1904): 3–19; Emilio R. Coni, "La lucha antituberculosa en la República Argentina," *La Lucha Antituberculosa* 5, nos.

4–8 (1905): 147–50; Emilio R. Coni, "Campaña contra la tuberculosis en la República Argentina," *La Semana Médica* 16, no. 40 (7 October 1909): 1399–1400, 1406.

30 See International Congress on Tuberculosis, *Transactions of the Sixth International Congress on Tuberculosis, Washington, September 28 to October 5, 1908* (Philadelphia: William F. Fell, 1908), 5: 271–305, for examples of the prize-winning essays and leaflets.

31 S. Adolphus Knopf, *Tuberculosis as a Disease of the Masses and How to Combat It* (New York: M. Firestack, 1901); Dormandy, *White Death*, 174.

32 Paul Weindling, ed., "International Sanitary Conference," *International Health Organizations and Movements, 1918–1939* (New York: Cambridge University Press, 1995), 7; CPP, Joseph Walsh Papers (hereafter JWP), vol. 4 (1906–1912), *International Conference on Tuberculosis and International Congress on Hygiene*, "Provisional Program of IXth International Tuberculosis Conference, Brussels, 5th to 8th, October, 1910"; CPP, FCR, L. F. Flick, "Report on the International Congress on Tuberculosis: Made to the National Association for the Study of Tuberculosis on May 7, 1907"; Harvard University Library Open Collections Program, "International Sanitary Conferences," http://ocp.hul.harvard.edu/contagion/sanitaryconferences.html, March 2011.

33 Herbert Maxwell and P. H. Pye-Smith, "Report of the Delegates of Her Majesty's Government on the International Congress on Tuberculosis held at Berlin from 24th to 27th May 1899," Great Britain, Parliament, House of Commons, *Command Papers* (London: Majesty's Stationery Office, 1899), 4–8.

34 CPP, JWP, vol. 10, *European Trips, 1896, 1900, 1905, 1907, 1910*, "Tuberculosis Work in Europe," Paper read before the Luzerne County Medical Society, 20 June 1906, 1.

35 Congrès International de la Tuberculose, *Rapports présentés au congrès, Paris 2–7 octobre, 1905* (Paris, 1906), three volumes, served as the basis of the analysis of the representatives at the 1905 conference.

36 International Congress on Tuberculosis, *Transactions* 1908, six volumes.

37 Julián Rosal and Manuel Arroyo, Informe sobre el Congreso Internacional de la Tuberculosis, verificado en Paris del 2 al 7 de Octubre de 1905, presentado al Señor Ministro de Relaciones Exteriores (Guatemala, 1906).

38 See International Congress on Tuberculosis, *Transactions*, 5: 9–15 and Congrés International de la Tuberculose, *Rapports*, 1: 15–17 for the focus of the congresses.

39 Congrès International de la Tuberculose, *Rapports*, vol. 3; International Congress on Tuberculosis, *General Catalogue of the European and American Exhibits* (Philadelphia: William F. Fell Company, 1908), 5–25; "Descriptive Catalogue, the Exhibit of the State Department of Health of Pennsylvania at the International Congress on Tuberculosis, Washington, D.C., September 21 to October 12, 1908," in *Third Annual Report of the Commissioner of Health of the Commonwealth of Pennsylvania*, 1908 (Harrisburg: C.E. Aughinbaugh, 1909), 486–517.

40 Buenos Aires, *Anuario estadístico de la ciudad de Buenos Aires* (Buenos Aires: Compañía Sud-Americana de Billetes de Banco, 1885), 95; Buenos Aires, *Statistical Year-Book of the City of Buenos Aires*. (Buenos Aires: Compañía Sud-Americana de Billetes de Banco, 1910), 119–123; See particularly, Emilio R. Coni, "The Campaign against Tuberculosis in Argentina," *Transactions 1908,* 4: 49–61. Coni used statistics on disinfections, hospital admissions and mortality to point to a successful prevention program while

at the same time suggesting a need for improvement in working-class housing and sanitation.

41 Lawrence Francis Flick, "Crusade against Tuberculosis," *John Hopkins Hospital Bulletin* 18 (1907): 304–9, quote 306.

42 CPP, FCR, "Report on the International Congress on Tuberculosis: made to the National Association for the Study and Prevention of Tuberculosis on May 7, 1907," 2–3, 6–8; CPP, LFP, vol. 54 (November–December 1908) has a great deal of correspondence dealing with the organization of the conference. For details on the organization of the congress, see CPP, JWP, vol. 5, 1908, Letters and Minutes of the Secretary of the International Congress of Tuberculosis.

43 There are large numbers of letters dealing with fund raising in CPP, LFP, vol. 36, 37; see, for example, vol. 36 (January–February 1906), 19 January 1906, George Gordon to Flick; vol. 37 (March–May 1906), 5 March 1906, C.O Probst to Flick; vol. 52 (September 1908), September 1, 1908, John Fulton to Flick.

44 CPP, LFP, vol. 45 (November–December 1907), 9 November 1907, John S. Fulton to Flick.

45 Edgar M. Green wrote Flick concerning the 1908 conference: "Is there any special hotel which is to be used as the headquarters of the tuberculosis conference in Washington? I should prefer staying in one of the hotels where many of the men will be because in that way there would be more opportunity of meeting them." See CPP, LFP, vol. 51 (August 1908), 4 August 1908.

46 The most significant work providing an overview of the history of medicine in the U.S. is Paul Starr, *The Social Transformation of American Medicine* (New York: Basic Books, 1982), 40–44, 93–97.

47 Starr, *Social Transformation*, 114–17, 123–25. Ott, *Fevered Lives*, 60, 137.

48 The westernization and internationalization of medical education is noted also in China and Japan. The translation of English and American medical texts beginning in 1868 and the introduction of European-trained Japanese physicians at the Tokyo University Medical School prepared Japan to modernize its medical education. Protestant missionaries and the education of Chinese students in Japan conveyed western understandings of the causes of disease to the Chinese. By 1905, Chinese interest in science could be seen in the large number of Chinese publications dealing with western medicine. Although the culture of China and Japan continued to influence the scientific and diagnostic techniques that physicians utilized in their respective countries, Chinese and Japanese nationals participated when their governments sent representatives to international congresses. See Johnston, "Genealogy of Tubercular Diseases," 260–63; William Johnston, *The Modern Epidemic: A History of Tuberculosis in Japan* (Cambridge: Harvard University Press, 1995), 70–72, 194–95; Bridie J. Andrews, "Tuberculosis and the Assimilation of Germ Theory in China, 1895–1937, *Journal of the History of Medicine and Allied Sciences* 52, no. 1 (January 1997): 114, 132, 136–40, 149.

49 For discussions of medical education in Argentina, see Eliseo Cantón, *Historia de la medicina en el Río de la Plata desde su descubrimiento hasta nuestras días, 1512 á 1925* (Madrid: Imp. G. Hernández y Galo Sáez, 1928), 3, 93, 224; Juan Túmburus, *Síntesis história de la medicina argentina* (Buenos Aires: El Ateneo, 1926), 71–83; Samuel Gache, "Rese a histórica de la medicina Argentina: 1891–1904," in *Guía Médica de la República Argentina*, ed. Congreso Internacional de Medicina e Higiene (Buenos Aires, 1910), 3–38. The number of graduates between 1824 and 1891 is given in

Diogène Decoud, *Les sciences médicales dans la République Argentine* (Buenos Aires, 1933), 21–22.

50 Raúl Vaccarezza, *Vida de médicos ilustres* (Buenos Aires: Editoral Troquel, 1980), 126–27; Decoud, *Les sciences médicales*, 69–77.

51 E. Wilde, Archivo de Protomedicato, Facultad de Medicina de Buenos Aires (hereafter cited as AFM) 6997; D. Decoud, AFM 2743; J. M. Penna, AFM 5386; "Enrique Tornú," *Archivos Argentinos de Tisiología y Neumonología* 53, nos. 1–4 (1987): 5–8.

52 Gregorio Araóz Alfaro, "Bodas de plata," *La Prensa Médica Argentina* 1, no. 1 (10 June 1914): 13; Carolina Barry, "Cecilia Grierson: Argentina's First Female Doctor," *Irish Migration Studies in Latin America* 6, no. 3 (November 2008): 213–18.

53 Paul Ross, "Mexico's Superior Health Council and the American Public Health Association: The Transnational Archive of Porfirian Public Health, 1887–1910," *Hispanic American Historical Review* 89, no. 4 (November 2009): 574, 577–78, 599.

54 Nancy Leys Stepan, "The National and the International in Public Health: Carlos Chagas and the Rockefeller Foundation in Brazil, 1917–1920," *Hispanic American Historical Review* 91, no. 3 (August 2011): 474–76.

55 Starr, 56, 60, 136–37, 155; Emily K. Abel, *Hearts of Wisdom: American Women Caring for Kin, 1850–1940* (Cambridge, MA: Harvard University Press, 2000), 40–44.

56 T. N. Bonner, *Becoming a Physician: Medical Education in Britain, France, Germany and the United States*, 1750–1945 (New York, 1995), 3–10, 347.

57 Charles E. Rosenberg, "Inward Vision & Outward Glance: The Shaping of the American Hospital, 1880–1914," *Bulletin of the History of Medicine* 53 (1979): 346–91; Joel D. Howell, "Machines and Medicine: Technology Transforms the American Hospital," in *The American General Hospital: Communities and Social Context*, eds. Diana Elizabeth Long and Janet Goldens (Ithaca, NY: Cornell University Press, 1989), 109–34; David Rosner, *A Once Charitable Enterprise: Hospitals and Health Care in Brooklyn and New York, 1885–1915* (Cambridge: Cambridge University Press, 1982), 13–35.

58 See Abel, *Hearts of Wisdom*, for an excellent study of care giving; see 40–43 and 37–67, which gives an overview of the nineteenth century; for quote, CPP, LFP, Tuberculosis Letters, vol. 9 (1899); CPP, LFP, vol. 36 (January–February 1906), Philadelphia 13 January 1906, Mary Williams to Lawrence Flick; Savacool, 168; see Table 2.2 for deaths in 1904.

59 Ricardo González Leandri, "Sujeción y carencia cambio y continuismo en los hospitales de Buenos Aires (1870–1900)," *Asclepio* 42, no. 1 (1990): 299; Rodríguez Castells, "Apuntes para la historia," 126; José Penna and Horacio Madero, *La Administración sanitaria y asistencia pública en la ciudad de Buenos Aires* (Buenos Aires: Guillermo Kraft, 1910), 2, 70–83; Cynthia Jeffres Little, "The Society of Beneficence in Buenos Aires, 1823–1900" (PhD diss., Temple University, 1980), 183.

60 Carlos Andrés Escudé, "Health in Buenos Aires in the Second Half of the Nineteenth Century," in *Social Welfare, 1850–1950: Australia, Argentina and Canada Compared*, ed. D. C. M. Platt (London: Macmillan Press, 1989), 63; Emilio R. Coni, *Higiene Social: Asistencia y previsión social. Buenos Aires caritativo y previsor* (Buenos Aires: Imprenta de Emilio Spinella, Ed., 1918), 7.

61 Juan B. Arini, *Estudio estadístico del Hospital General de Mujeres* (Buenos Aires: Imprenta de M. Biedma, 1879), 16–17, 39, 41.

62 Reber, "Misery," 510.

63 "La Municipalidad y la higiene pública," *El Porteño* (Buenos Aires), 16 February 1877: 1; Ernest Allen Crider, "Modernization and Human Welfare: The Asistencia Pública and Buenos Aires, 1882–1910" (PhD diss., Ohio State University, 1975), 31.

64 Crider, "Modernization and Human Welfare," 182–183.

65 Penna and Madero, *La administración sanitaria* 2: 129; Rodriguez Castells, "Apuntes para la historia," 126–27.

66 Coni, "La campaña contra la tuberculos," (14 October 1909): 1438; Emilio R. Coni, "La lucha antituberculosa en la República Argentina," *La Lucha Antituberculosa* 5: 156–57.

67 Alberto B. Martínez, *Censo general de población, edificación, comercio e industrias de la ciudad de Buenos Aires, levantado en los días 11 y 18 de septiembre de 1904* (Buenos Aires: Cia. Sudamericana de Billetes del Banco, 1906), 323; Beneficencia 1897–1900 (Buenos Aires: Imprenta Litografía y Encuadernación G. Kraft, 1900), 18. For problems in the Hospital Rivadavia, Little, 208. "Mortalidad por enfermedades infecciosas en la ciudad de Buenos Aires durante los años 1895 y 1996." *Anales del Departamento Nacional de Higiene* 2, no. 25 (1 July 1896): 403–10; 425–28; 6, no. 27 (16 July 1896): 494–97; 6, no. 30 (8 August 1896): 522–24; 6, no. 34 (8 September 1896): 610–12, 721–22; 6, no. 42 (8 November 1896): 800–801, 862–66; 7, nos. 1, 2 (1 and 8 January 1897): 21–23; 7, nos. 5, 6 (1 and 8 February 1897): 86–89.

68 Ricardo González Leandri, *Curar, persuadir, gobernar: La construcción histórica de la profesión médica en Buenos Aires, 1852–1886* (Madrid: Consejo Superior de Investigaciones Científicas Centro de Estudios Históricos, 199), 295–95, 303–6.

69 For U.S., Sheila M. Rothman, Living in the Shadow of Death: Tuberculosis and the Social Experience of Illness in American History (Baltimore: John Hopkins Press, 1995), 198; for Argentina, José Mazzini, "Profilaxis de la tuberculosis en las sierras de Córdoba," Segunda Conferencia Nacional de Profilaxis Antituberculosa, Rosario 6–8 de Septiembre 1919, Actas y Trabajos, vol. 3 (Rosario de Santa Fé: Taileres de la Biblioteca Argentina, 1920), 155–56.

70 CP, LFP, Tuberculosis Letters, vol. 7 (1897, pt. 4), 4 June 1897, W. P. Grough to Sister Superior; CP, LFP, Tuberculosis Letters, vol. 8: 421, 24 December 1898, R. Hamagan to Flick.

71 Alejandro Albarracín, *Consideraciónes sobre la tisis pulmonar*, MD diss., Facultad de Medicina, Universidad de Buenos Aires, 1875 (Buenos Aires: Imprenta de Luis L. Pintos, 1875), 89–90.

72 CP, LFP, vol. 41 (February–March 1907) Philadelphia 16 February 1907 Henry P. Smith to Bromley Wharton.

73 Gabriela de L. de Coni, "El Barrio de las ramas," *Alianza de Higiene Social* 7 (1907–1908): 80.

74 CP, LFP, Tuberculosis Letters, Vol. 14 (1901, pt. 3); October 22. St. Agnes to Flick; CP, LFP, Tuberculosis Letters, vol. 14 (1901, pt. 3), 26 October 1901 P. MacManus to Flick.

75 CP, LFP, Tuberculosis Letters, vol. 10 (1900, pt. 3), October 1900 Charles W. Naulty to Flick; CP, LFP, vol. 10 (1900, pt. 1), 26 April 1900. Charles W. Naulty to Flick,

76 Jorge Luis Borges, *Evaristo Carriego,* translation with introduction and notes by Norman Thomas DiGiovanni with the assistance of Susan Ashe (New York: E.P. Dutton, Inc., 1984), 60–61.

2 Two Cities and Their Medical Establishments

Buenos Aires and Philadelphia, 1870–1945

> Buenos Aires deserves its name, for its air is clear as well as keen, there being no large manufacturing works to pollute it with coal smoke. The streets are well kept; everything is fresh and bright. The most striking buildings besides those of the new Legislative Chambers with their tall and handsome dome are the Opera-house, the interior of which equals any in Europe, and the Jockey Club, whose scale and elaborate appointments surpass even the club-houses of New York.[1]

> Wonderful changes have taken place in the physical appearance of Philadelphia in the last generation, but in spite of the widened streets, the great boulevards, and the constant growth in population, wealth, and importance, the true lover of the old town can still discover the traces of that elusive charm which gave the place distinction in the days of our fathers.[2]

As can be seen in the quotes above, between 1923 and 1925, observers of Buenos Aires[3] and Philadelphia[4] described the two cities in glowing terms. Both were seen as prosperous modern cities with new buildings and expanding populations. Both were old colonial river port cities with manufacturing sectors. Buenos Aires was the capital of Argentina and the largest and economically most significant city of the nation, while Philadelphia was second only to New York City in its political and economic importance. Buenos Aires was the leading South American financial and commercial city with strong ties to Europe and its economic growth contributed to the development of its hinterland. Philadelphia served a similar role in the U.S. Philadelphia was larger than Buenos Aires during the nineteenth century, but by 1925, the population of Buenos Aires surpassed Philadelphia. (See Table 2.1.) Internal and foreign migrations contributed to the population growth of both cities.

Between 1870 and 1945, both cities changed from predominantly traditional port cities to modern ones with financial institutions that provided services to the public and transport systems that unified the central city and suburbs. The prosperity of both supported educational and cultural institutions. The growth of a middle class in both cities changed the basis of economic and political power that affected public health policies and outcomes. Both urban metropolises faced similar sanitary and health issues. Because of the large number of deaths due to tuberculosis, public health experts in Buenos Aires and Philadelphia supported building hospitals and creating new institutions to serve tuberculosis patients. Improvements in the standard of living in both cities contributed to the decreasing number of deaths from tuberculosis. Although the problems that the populations of both cities faced were surprisingly similar, their different colonial and cultural traditions help explain the differences in residents' responses to living and working in Buenos Aries and Philadelphia. At the same time, the differences between the two cities underline the significance of the growing international consensus on the cause and treatment of tuberculosis.

The Setting: Buenos Aires

Travelers to Buenos Aires had diverse views about the city. Constructed on the gridiron plan as a port city of the Rio de la Plata, visitors between 1890 and 1910 were less favorably impressed than later ones. In a short visit to the city, Frank Vincent described the streets and sidewalks as "narrow, badly paved and dirty" and criticized the condition of the public buildings, monuments and large plazas. By 1910, however, some people held that Buenos Aires was one of the most beautiful cities of the world, the Paris of the Americas; it won praise for its size, luxurious homes, diverse architectural designs, numerous well-supplied shops, broad boulevards, many plazas and parks, and social and cultural activities.[5]

When travelers moved beyond the center of the city, they often found urban ugliness. James Bryce, whose quote begins the chapter, also noted: "If the best parts of Buenos Aires are as tasteful as those of Paris, there is plenty of ugliness in the worst suburbs. On its land side, the city dies out into a waste of scattered shanties...dirty and squalid with corrugated iron roofs....These are inhabited by the newest and poorest of the immigrants from southern Italy and southern Spain."[6] Even though some foreign visitors observed slum housing, their understanding of the city's problems was superficial. They often missed the depth of the economic challenges and the complexities of the social issues faced by Porteños. Tourists were not in Buenos Aires during epidemics, and they also failed to note the impact of tuberculosis. Visitors did not fully comprehend the significance of the tenements, the ethnic diversity of the city's population and the shifts of population within the city. Sightseers to Buenos Aires were unfamiliar with the rapid population growth, the difficulty of finding affordable housing, the poor working conditions in homes and factories, and reform efforts to improve the quality of living.

As a result of the yellow fever epidemic of 1870–1871, many wealthy citizens seeking better urban services moved to the north from the southern district. The colonial-style homes that the wealthy vacated were often torn down or converted into tenements. By the 1880s, Buenos Aires began to lose its Spanish colonial character. Single-storied, flat-roofed houses made of crude bricks were replaced with larger two-story buildings. In 1886, there were a few houses of four floors; in 1898, twenty-two percent of newly constructed houses had more than one floor. Although early tenement houses were often built cheaply of wood and zinc, in the twentieth century, brick became the main construction material. The moderate climate cut the cost of house construction, but building materials and land were expensive. Central Buenos Aires, however, retained some wealthy residences as well as tenements. It has remained the commercial, governmental and cultural center of Argentina.[7]

Between 1870 and 1945, foreign immigration and internal migration transformed Buenos Aires into a major metropolis. Table 2.1 indicates for the nineteenth century and the first twenty-five years of the twentieth century that Buenos Aires was a smaller city than Philadelphia; during the first part of the twentieth century, Buenos Aires grew more rapidly than Philadelphia. By 1905, the population of Buenos Aires was over a million and twenty years later Buenos Aires with a population of 1,914,400 surpassed Philadelphia in size. After 1914, internal migration began to outpace foreign immigration but became massive in the 1930s. Internal migration assured the continued growth and economic influence of the city of Buenos Aires in both Argentina and the world.[8] By 1947, the population of Buenos Aires (2,981,043) was one and a half times that of Philadelphia (1,991,368).[9]

The city was initially unprepared to house or provide services for a large influx of European immigrants. Rapid population growth resulted in substandard housing and the limited availability of piped water, sewage disposal, gas, electricity and medical assistance. New arrivals who took unskilled jobs found the cost of living in Buenos Aires to be very high. By 1887, twenty-five percent of the city's population lived in conventillos (tenement houses), deteriorated colonial-style buildings with poor ventilation and without running water, toilets and electricity. These one-to-two-story tenement buildings contained many rooms built around a courtyard. Entrepreneurs also built cheap new housing of wood and tin in the parishes of Balvanera, Pilar and Barracas in central Buenos Aires. Newly arriving immigrants crowded into buildings subdivided for use among various families. It was not unusual for a family with three to six children or four men to occupy one room measuring three by four meters. Conventillos housed more men than women, because many single men came to Buenos Aires searching for employment. The tenements were crowded and unsanitary; wells were polluted because of their location near latrines. Communal kitchens rarely existed, so families did their cooking on charcoal braziers which led to smoke-filled rooms. These conditions spread illnesses such as diphtheria, typhoid, typhus and tuberculosis. Moreover, half of the conventillo population was under the age of fifteen. Although a given building might house predominantly one ethnic group, a specific parish included residents of diverse nationalities.[10]

Poor housing and living conditions encouraged the rapid spread of tuberculosis among the lower class. In 1909, the percentage of all deaths from tuberculosis among the various Buenos Aires parishes varied between 1.9 percent in Balvanera Norte, which was socially diversified, to nine percent in Palermo, a middle-class neighborhood; La Boca, the poor densely populated port area, had a lower mortality rate than Catedral Norte, a wealthy neighborhood. However, the working-class districts of Balvanera Sud, Pilar, San Cristóbal and Santa Lucía had the highest tuberculosis mortality. Note, though, that the percentage of those dying of tuberculosis as reported by the various parishes is far lower than the autopsy results. The conflicting statistics point to misdiagnosis and underreporting of tuberculosis. Furthermore, the parishes' social and ethnic diversity suggests the difficulty of documenting that a particular ethnic group or class was more susceptible to tuberculosis than others. Finally, some local circumstances mitigated the number of tuberculosis cases. La Boca, an Italian community, is an interesting case; not only were the houses more flimsy (so that rooms received more air and light), but also the residents had more access to proteins that increased resistance to *Mycobacterium tuberculosis;* on the other hand, residents were too poor to afford medical treatment and tuberculosis cases were certainly underreported.

From 1906 to 1911, the number of deaths due to tuberculosis surpassed deaths from epidemic diseases in all Buenos Aires parishes; no matter what the neighborhood, people were more likely to die of tuberculosis than of any other disease.[11]

Table 2.2 shows that in Buenos Aires, the total deaths from diphtheria, measles, scarlet fever, smallpox, typhoid and whooping cough surpassed tuberculosis deaths in all but eight years from 1869 through 1895. This was a time when the rapid spread of contagious disease in an urban environment killed large numbers of people. Diphtheria was endemic from 1887 to 1893, typhoid was widespread in 1869 and 1888–1891, measles was epidemic in 1893 and scarlet fever was virulent from 1895 to 1901. But it was smallpox that often killed the most individuals; from 1869 to 1906, there were nine major outbreaks. Although epidemic deaths declined in Buenos Aires in the twentieth century, individuals continued to die from diphtheria, measles, scarlet fever, typhoid and whooping cough.

Although Buenos Aires housing often did not meet municipal hygiene standards, there were gradual improvements. By 1900, most tenement houses had concrete patios and offered some form of bathing facilities. Nevertheless, twenty to seventy people often shared a single latrine. In spite of the failure of housing to meet higher standards, the housing shortage made it impossible to decrease overcrowding. A construction boom provided more housing for laborers, but the high cost of construction—which rose forty percent from 1891 to 1897—and continued demand for housing in the center of the city kept rents high. The result was an increase in the number of squatter settlements on the outskirts of the city. While rent in outlying urban settlements was cheaper than in center-city conventillos, lack of water and sewage made for worse living conditions. In 1904, only half of the city's population had piped water and one-third had access to sewers. The municipal government recognized that providing piped water and extending the sewer system was needed to improve the quality of life. By 1914, the Buenos Aires government provided seventy-three percent of the population with running water, but two-thirds still remained without a sewer system. Those neighborhoods more distant from the center of the city were most likely to lack water and sewage services.[12]

Urban reformers emphasized that improved housing would help to prevent tuberculosis; they believed that the densely populated tenements contributed to the rapid spread of contagious diseases and high mortality. Thus, municipal authorities and private charities attempted to solve the housing problem. As early as 1887, the Buenos Aires municipal government proposed building houses for workers and permitted charity organizations to construct low-cost housing. In the same year, the Department of Public Works began building 116 row houses of four rooms with kitchens, baths and running water, which by 1889 were completed and rented to workers. In 1912, the Señoras de San Vicente de Paul, a private Catholic organization, opened ninety-six new two-bedroom homes for the city's neediest families. Railroad companies also build some housing for workers. The city government supplemented such efforts, realizing as it did that the private sector and charity could not provide all the housing that was needed. Catholic reformers considered it a moral mandate to build affordable housing, and the country's legislators thought it politically advantageous to support housing reform. By 1919—even as the urban population continued to increase—less than ten percent of the population lived in conventillos. Families increasingly were able to own their own homes or to afford to rent better housing. Perhaps, as a result, the number of deaths from tuberculosis declined.[13]

Three developments encouraged workers to move to the city's outskirts to acquire cheaper housing: subsidized train and bus transport, less expensive land and new financial institutions that made it possible for workers to borrow money to buy urban lots and building materials. Railroad links to the interior lowered the cost of building materials. By 1910, the city was not only the terminus of an extensive railroad system but also had 400 miles of streetcar track carrying over 300 million passengers per year. In 1911, the Anglo-Argentine Tramway began constructing a subway. Thus, early in the twentieth-century the majority of urban working-class people resided in small plain two-and-three room houses on the periphery of Buenos Aires. The outward movement of the working class intensified during the next three decades. The working class was encouraged to find housing on the outskirts of Buenos Aires, while the bourgeoisie preferred to remain in the center of the city near entertainment locations, educational institutions and their white collar jobs. Beginning in the early twentieth century, the Buenos Aires government began improving transportation, sanitation and public services such as gas, water and electricity to make the historic center more attractive for its residents.[14]

Buenos Aires also benefited from a substantial number of world-class hospitals. In 1895, Buenos Aires had close to twenty hospitals to serve a population of 649,680. Most of the facilities were relatively new. At least fifteen hospitals took tubercular patients and provided both experimental treatment and terminal care. The national government hospitals included Rawson, Rivadavia and San Roque. The municipality operated the Hospicio Las Mercedes, which was nationalized in 1903. The Hospital Clínicas was associated with the School of Medicine. The British, Spanish, French, Italian and German communities supported hospitals; in 1910, these immigrant-run hospitals treated 20.4 percent of all hospitalized patients in the city. The government also had a military hospital, the Hospital Militar, a children's hospital, Hospital de Niños, an insane asylum for women, Hospital Mujeres Dementes, and a hospital for contagious diseases, Casa de Aislamiento. Four hospitals treated only an occasional tubercular patient: Hospital Norte, Pirovano, Oftalmológico and the Asilo de Las Mercedes. In the early twentieth century, the government took control of several hospitals that had once been operated by the Sociedad de Beneficencia de la Capital. These included Casa de Huérfanos de la Merced y Sucursal, Hospital Nacional de Alienadas, Hospital Rivadavia, Asilo de Huérfanos, Casa de Expósitos y Sucursal, Hospital de Niños, Hospital y Consultorio Oftalmológico, Asilo de Mercedes and Hospital y Asilo Marítimo. By 1945, thirty-two hospitals operated to serve a population of 2,595,861. The list included the addition of approximately ten municipal hospitals and several specialized hospitals.[15]

International trade and foreign investment contributed to the rapid economic growth of Buenos Aires. But in spite of the city's dependence on the export of meat and wheat, during most of the nineteenth century, the port remained inadequate; large ships had to anchor as much as sixteen miles from the quay. Construction of a deep-water port began only in the mid-1890s. By 1910, 15,000 ships came to Buenos Aires per year, and nine million tons of cargo were unloaded at dockside, three times the tonnage of 1895. No longer did immigrants need to wade ashore or take small boats to reach the land.[16]

Between 1910 and 1914, the number of industrial establishments in the city grew from 8,119 to 10,275. Small-scale family workshops, often located in the living quarters of the tenements, each employed a handful of people to produce clothing, furniture, and metal works and to process food. These small businesses could be found throughout the city. Larger enterprises—usually located in the southern and far western districts of the city—expanded, as the number of family workshops declined. Between 1920 and 1929, the manufacturing sector grew at a rate of 4.3 percent per year. The number of industrial establishments, primarily producers of textiles and processed foods, almost doubled. Large companies manufactured shoes, woolen textiles, tobacco products, metal tools and agricultural implements. From the mid-1930s to the mid-1940s, industrial production in textiles and metals continued to expand rapidly, while the oil by-products industries, electrical appliance production companies and road construction also employed a large labor force. In the 1930s, the government adopted a policy discouraging imports that greatly benefited the Argentine industry.[17]

At the beginning of the century, the small size of industrial firms—characterized by limited capital investment and primitive technology—often resulted in poor working conditions. However, an increasing number of larger firms paid higher salaries, which supported workers' upward mobility. Although reformers argued for legislation to protect workers' health and to limit the number of hours worked, both the national and city governments were slow to approve enforceable legislation to protect workers. Thus, the majority of buildings used for industrial work did not meet sanitation standards. For example, workers in bakeries, cotton mills, printing establishments and coal mines inhaled dust that caused lung infections. Public health officials viewed poor air quality as a major contributor to pulmonary tuberculosis. Reformers recommended the periodic whitewashing of walls, the provision of adequate light and ventilation, the addition of more latrines and wash basins and the supplying of adequate drinking water.[18]

The government recognized that the facilities employing women and children were often worse than those employing men. As a result, legislation was enacted to protect women and children in factories and shops by limiting their working hours and prohibiting them from working in dangerous industries. By 1910, the municipality fined the companies breaking the law, yet only a small percentage of work sites were inspected. Government officials could require health and safety standards for large factories, but improvements were too costly for home workshops.[19]

Although immigrants arriving in Buenos Aires found many opportunities, it was an expensive city. The cost of living often increased three to four percent per year. The problem for many was that salaries—although two to three times higher than in Spain, Italy and France—did not keep up with expenses and were particularly low for unskilled workers. From 1910 to 1917, the average cost of basic articles increased by twenty percent, while salaries increased by only ten percent. The cost of living was influenced by various factors: for example, rent increased substantially between 1910 and 1914 (but then declined); the cost of bread and meat rose over twenty-six percent in 1915, and the cost of clothes increased ninety-eight percent between 1910 and 1917. Low income, rising costs and limited savings made it difficult for workers to deal with substantial health problems. The proportion of Buenos Aires' deaths stemming from tuberculosis increased from 10.25 percent in 1910 to 15.49 percent in 1918 before beginning to decline. When a parent contracted tuberculosis, families were often forced to turn to social services; a sick child, who could not contribute to the family income, further reduced the standard of living.[20]

Increased economic growth during the 1920s improved the life for Porteños, but worker purchasing power remained below that of the U.S. workforce. Working-class families frequently required their children to work in domestic sweatshops or as street vendors to help support the family. Migrants from the provinces increasingly moved to the city and its suburbs. The middle class expanded in numbers and prosperity, finding employment in commerce, government and service industries. The upper class continued to enjoy a high standard of living, spending lavishly on trips to Paris, Rome, London and Madrid.

Between the world wars, Buenos Aires modernized, as broad new avenues, parks and plazas were constructed. By 1940, its population reached 2,488,069. Central Buenos Aires contained wealthy residences and remained the commercial, governmental and cultural center of Argentina. The number of industrial firms in the capital nearly doubled from the mid-1930s to the mid-1940s, rising from 13,440 to 25,156. The number of commercial establishments also escalated from 27,761 to 92,877 in forty years. As the seat of the national government, cultural center of the nation and a major dispenser of medical services and educational opportunities, Buenos Aires supported the growth of the middle class and after the 1920s, the increased standard of living of the working class. The years 1935 to 1948 were prosperous for the Porteños, as the city benefited from European importation of Argentinean products during the war and reconstruction in the postwar years.[21] The growing prosperity of the city correlated with a decline in tuberculosis, supporting the contention that an improved standard of living explains declining tuberculosis mortality. Tuberculosis as a percent of total deaths dropped from 11.45 in 1920 to 9.48 in 1938.

The Setting: Philadelphia

Like Buenos Aires, Philadelphia was a planned city with streets initially laid out in a gridiron with parks, plazas and open spaces reserved for public use. For a short time, at the end of the eighteenth century, Philadelphia served as the capital of the U.S. In 1800, Philadelphia was the largest city in the U.S. During the nineteenth century and the first half of the twentieth century, Philadelphia was second only to New York City in size and importance.[22] Table 2.1 indicates that throughout the nineteenth century Philadelphia was larger than Buenos Aires; in 1870, Philadelphia's population was more than three and a half times that of Buenos Aires. By 1888, Philadelphia had a population of over a million.

The climate of Philadelphia is temperate, with hot humid summers similar to those of Buenos Aires. Because Philadelphia is above the equator and Buenos Aires is below it, the cities experience the seasons at a different time of the year. Philadelphia has colder winters, which require more substantial construction for housing, and families must spend more on warm clothing. Before the Civil War, although there was some concentration of immigrant groups in the city, Philadelphia did not have African-American ghettos. After the Civil War, the temperate climate and economic opportunities made Philadelphia attractive to both internal migrants and foreign immigrants. By the end of the 1860s, the original grid street plan changed, as the commercial district expanded and workers traveled to their jobs via streetcars. Center-city housing conditions grew worse as population density increased. As was true of Buenos Aires, neighborhoods included residents of diverse classes.[23]

Philadelphia was a river port and a transportation center. The Delaware River flows along the eastern side of the city and provides Philadelphia with a link to the Atlantic Ocean. During the eighteenth century, Philadelphia was the major international port of the colonies. By the end of the nineteenth century, there were five miles of continuous wharves along the Delaware and four along the Schuylkill River. By the turn of the twentieth century, Philadelphia's port served as a gateway for iron, steel, coal and oil. Because land was unavailable near the city center, early industrial growth in Philadelphia developed along the rivers near the port area.[24]

Immigrants from abroad and migrants from elsewhere in the U.S. settled first in the city center in three-story houses on narrow alleys. There was little light and air in these houses, which also lacked sewage and piped water. The overcrowded housing served as both home and workspace. Between the 1870s and 1920s, Philadelphia expanded north, south and west, incorporating outer suburbs as part of the city. Families found housing in row houses or back-alley shanties. Three or more families, each doing their own cooking but sharing inadequate toilets, occupied partitioned tenement buildings. As in Buenos Aires, slum residents faced problems such as the absence of paved streets, inadequate sewer and toilet facilities, overcrowding and unsanitary conditions. Although there was increased piped water, outhouses remained a fixture.[25] Congested housing and the lack of sanitation contributed to the spread of chronic diseases such as tuberculosis and epidemics of cholera, scarlet fever, typhoid and smallpox. As indicated in Table 2.2, Philadelphians died in large number from diphtheria in 1883 and 1891–1900, scarlet fever in 1875, smallpox in 1871–1872 and 1881; typhoid remained a constant threat to lives until 1918 when its influence decreased.

Between 1887 and 1902, builders constructed nearly one hundred thousand two- and three-story, brick row houses. The city government prohibited construction of high-rise tenements and wooden buildings. After 1870, there were to be not more than six unrelated individuals per single dwelling. Building and loan associations (the first building and loan association in the U.S. was founded in Philadelphia in 1831) encouraged individual home ownership in the suburbs. While Philadelphia reformers expressed interest in building worker housing to decrease the impact of contagious diseases, they were less successful than their Buenos Aires counterparts, because Philadelphia's government saw housing construction as the purview of the private sector. Wages did not increase much in the early part of the century, but combined family wages gradually allowed many families to purchase homes in the suburbs.[26]

By 1890, twenty-five percent of the population of mostly—clerks, teachers and skilled workers—owned their own home. There were more such homeowners in Philadelphia than in any other U.S. city. By 1905, people increasingly bought homes in the suburbs. At the same time, many unmarried men and women lived in the urban center in inexpensive rented rooms. Until World War I, workers tended to locate in high-density areas near their jobs. A particular ethnic group might dominate a block, but seldom constituted even half the population of a particular neighborhood. Many African Americans lived in Philadelphia, but in 1938 they represented only 14.04 percent of the city's population.[27]

Beginning in 1858, Philadelphia introduced horse-drawn streetcars; and in the 1890s, it added electric trolleys. Supplementing the urban trams were the steam railroad commuter lines. With this extensive transport system, center-city commerce prospered. Expansion of the rail and trolley system encouraged workers to buy property in the suburbs since they could easily get to the center of the city for shopping and work. In the twentieth century, access to downtown Philadelphia continued to improve. In 1907, the first subway opened, and bus routes were expanded. The city created large diagonal boulevards in 1908 to open space in the congested city center, so as to improve the flow of traffic and to beautify the city. World War I and political disagreements within the city council delayed further city improvements until the 1920s when additional boulevards were constructed; many new buildings were also completed in the 1930s.[28]

Although the population was shifting more rapidly toward the suburbs by the 1920s, the inner city dominated Philadelphia social life until after World War II. Even with improved transportation, new immigrants and unskilled workers preferred to live in areas of the city that had cheap older housing, close to their friends and their jobs. By 1930, Philadelphia's historical city was primarily home to the poor and low-skilled families. With the decline of transportation costs, the working and middle classes could afford to build homes further out along commuter train lines. Employment grew in greater Philadelphia to service a diversified economy. For Philadelphians, living in the suburbs represented upward mobility; suburban life was always more attractive to them than to the Porteños. The center of Buenos Aires attracted all classes because cultural activities and business never deteriorated as they did in Philadelphia in the 1930s.[29]

Because Philadelphia was the capital of the U.S. for only a short time and was not the capital of Pennsylvania, government employment had less of an impact on Philadelphia's economy than on Buenos Aires's. From 1870 to 1914, Philadelphia enlarged its transportation and commercial base by adding both large and small industrials. Located near iron and coal mines, Philadelphians profitably manufactured iron and steel products, including locomotives and ships. As in Buenos Aires, textiles were a major Philadelphia industry; it was more important than coal, iron or railroads in employing capital and workers. During the 1880s, forty percent of laborers worked in clothing and textile firms, and by 1904, Philadelphia produced more textiles (including woolens, clothing and carpets) than any other U.S. city.[30] In 1915, textile and clothing manufacturers employed one-third of all Philadelphia wage earners. Food products, such as sugar refining, meat processing and baking ranked second in number in the provision of jobs, and was followed by printing, publishing and metal fabrication. Just as in Buenos Aires, the whole family often worked ten to twelve hours a day to make ends meet, and women and children earned much less than men.[31]

Philadelphia supported distinguished educational institutions, world-renowned cultural institutions and large green spaces. The University of Pennsylvania (Penn) traces its origin to 1740 and to Benjamin Franklin's concept of nonsectarian education. Penn is thought by some to be the fourth oldest institution of higher education in the U.S. and the country's first university. Although established somewhat later than the University of Córdoba, Argentina (1613), Penn was established earlier than the University of Buenos Aires (1821). The Philadelphia Museum of Art was founded in 1877 and the Free Library in 1891. Coinciding with international movements in the 1890s to create large urban spaces to make cities more healthy and attractive, Philadelphia's city planners proposed a mile-long parkway that took thirty years to complete. In 1928, the Philadelphia Museum of Art opened to the public in a new building at the end of the parkway.[32]

As the city was expanding, so did its medical institutions. The oldest hospital in the city and the U.S. was Philadelphia General, which began as an almshouse in 1732 and was closed in 1977. In the nineteenth century, philanthropists founded most of the Philadelphia medical institutions which provided for the city's ill, including Jefferson Hospital in 1825, the University of Pennsylvania Hospital in 1851 and the Children's Hospital of Philadelphia in 1855. Four Catholic hospitals (St. Joseph founded 1849, St. Mary's founded 1860, St. Agnes found 1888 and Misericordia founded 1918) served many immigrant patients. The German Hospital and Presbyterian Hospital served a diverse community. Three Jewish hospitals (Mt. Sinai founded 1899, Lebanon Hospital founded 1907 and Northern Liberties founded 1920) initially focused on Jewish patients but soon responded to the needs of other Philadelphia residents as well. The House of Mercy, Chestnut Hill and the Rush Hospital for Consumption and Allied Disease opened to serve tuberculosis patients between 1877 and 1895. African Americans founded the Frederick Douglass Memorial Hospital and Training School to meet the needs of their community in 1895 and Mercy Hospital in 1907. The Phipps Institute, the Kensington Dispensary and Eagleville Home opened in the early 1900s, specifically to serve the tubercular.[33]

The 1920s through the 1940s—years that included the Great Depression and World War II—challenged Philadelphia's prosperity. During the 1920s, more than half of the city's residents owned their own homes, but large mortgages led to one-fifth of the homeowners losing their homes between 1928 and 1932. In 1933, forty percent of the city's population was unemployed. The New Deal programs of Franklin D. Roosevelt aided the unemployed with jobs and programs to assist homeowners facing eviction. Prosperity returned when World War II brought increased manufacturing jobs for both women and minorities and promoted full employment. But the peace in 1945 led to cutbacks in government contracts and the loss of war industry jobs. Eventually, the growth of educational institutions provided new vocational opportunities.[34]

Buenos Aires and Philadelphia Confront Tuberculosis

Between 1870 and 1938, families in Buenos Aires and Philadelphia faced increased possibilities that loved-ones would die of tuberculosis. Table 2.1 provides comparative data for tuberculosis deaths for Buenos Aires and Philadelphia and confirms the reality of family concerns. The data on pulmonary tuberculosis deaths as a percent of total deaths for Philadelphia and Buenos Aires takes into consideration the difference in city size to provide a comparison of pulmonary tuberculosis deaths for the two cities. From 1873 to 1902, tuberculosis deaths in Buenos Aires were lower than those in Philadelphia with two exceptions (1876 and 1898) by a ratio of 0.32–5.62. From 1898 through 1914, Buenos Aires' mortality rates are comparable with those of Philadelphia. However, Philadelphia tuberculosis began to decline in 1904 when it accounted for twelve percent of total deaths.

Table 2.1 Comparative Demographics, Buenos Aires and Philadelphia, 1870–1938

Year	Phila Total Pop	BA Total Pop	BA % of Pop of Phila	Phila Total Deaths	BA Total Deaths	Phila No Pul TB Deaths	BA No Pul TB Deaths	Phila Other TB Deaths	BA Other TB D	Phila	BA	PhilaNo Total TB D	BA No Total TB D	Phila Pul	BA Pul
										% of Pul D of Total TBD				% of Total Deaths	
1870	674,022	186,650	27.69	15,317	6,010	2,308	274	8	0	99.65	100	2,316	274	15.07	4.56
1871	700,000	175,912	25.13	15,485	21,466	2,237	495	10	0	99.55	100	2,247	495	14.45	2.31
1872	725,000	181,500	25.03	8,987	5,682	2,330	597	25	0	98.94	100	2,355	597	25.93	10.51
1873	750,000	191,500	25.53	15,224	5,891	2,291	755	0	0	100	100	2,291	755	15.05	12.82
1874	775,000	202,200	26.09	15,238	7,190	2,304	685	18	25	99.22	96.48	2,322	710	15.12	9.53
1875	800,000	213,700	26.71	17,805	6,751	2,359	858	45	22	98.13	97.5	2,404	880	13.25	12.71
1876	825,594	226,100	27.39	18,892	5,277	2,676	783	21	30	99.22	96.31	2,697	813	14.16	14.84
1877	850,856	239,500	28.15	16,004	5,538	2,349	716	20	27	99.16	96.37	2,369	743	14.68	12.93
1878	878,118	254,000	28.93	15,743	5,536	2,491	756	19	30	99.24	96.18	2,510	786	15.82	13.66
1879	901,380	269,700	29.92	15,473	6,794	2,481	776	17	28	99.32	96.52	2,498	804	16.03	11.42
1880	847,170	286,700	33.84	17,711	7,073	2,692	774	18	22	99.34	97.24	2,710	796	15.20	10.94
1881	868,000	305,100	35.15	19,515	6,316	2,768	782	18	23	99.35	97.14	2,786	805	14.18	12.38
1882	886,539	325,000	36.66	20,259	7,[illegible]96	2,809	808	14	19	99.5	97.7	2,823	827	13.87	11.23
1883	907,041	346,500	38.20	20,076	8,501	2,798	932	14	21	99.5	97.8	2,812	953	13.94	10.96
1884	927,995	369,700	39.84	19,999	8,142	2,801	1,053	33	36	98.84	96.69	2,834	1,089	14.01	12.93
1885	849,432	394,700	46.47	21,392	9,295	2,821	1,017	22	25	99.23	97.6	2,843	1,042	13.19	10.94
1887	993,801	450,500	45.33	21,719	12,938	2,800	1,041	37	25	98.7	97.65	2,837	1,066	12.89	8.05
1888	1,016,758	481,000	47.31	20,372	12,367	2,695	1,069	49	29	98.21	97.36	2,744	1,098	13.23	8.64
1889	1,040,245	514,200	49.43	20,536	14,736	2,532	1,245	49	104	98.1	92.29	2,581	1,349	12.33	8.45
1890	1,046,964	526,900	50.33	21,732	16,417	2,764	1,168	30	87	98.93	93.07	2,794	1,255	12.72	7.11
1891	1,069,264	516,880	48.34	23,367	14,332	2,624	1,024	53	118	98.02	89.67	2,677	1,142	11.23	7.14
1892	1,092,168	550,080	50.37	24,305	14,692	2,709	1,078	23	103	99.16	91.28	2,732	1,181	11.15	7.34
1893	1,115,562	583,280	52.29	23,655	14,290	2,671	1,103	35	167	98.71	86.85	2,706	1,270	11.29	7.72
1894	1,139,457	616,480	54.10	22,680	13,702	2,513	1,283	47	136	98.16	90.42	2,560	1,419	11.08	9.36
1895	1,163,864	649,680	55.82	23,796	14,947	2,449	1,166	64	156	97.45	88.2	2,513	1,322	10.29	7.80
1896	1,888,797	682,880	36.15	23,982	13,545	2,514	1,268	55	100	97.86	92.69	2,569	1,368	10.48	9.29
1899	1,266,832	782,480	61.77	23,796	13,567	2,818	1,450		225		86.57		1,675	11.84	10.69
1900	1,293,697	815,680	63.05	25,078	16,504	2,717	1,672	12	226	99.56	88.09	2,729	1,898	10.83	10.13
1901	1,321,408	840,880	63.64	24,137	15,807	2,946	1,675	44	218	98.53	88.48	2,990	1,893	12.21	10.60
1903	1,373,414	924,480	67.31	25,510	13,996	3,053	1,689	72	226	97.7	88.2	3,125	1,915	11.97	12.07

(Continued)

Year	Phila Total Pop	BA Total Pop	BA % of Pop of Phila	Phila Total Deaths	BA Total Deaths	Phila No Pul TB Deaths	BA No Pul TB Deaths	Phila Other TB Deaths	BA Other TB D	Phila	BA	PhilaNo Total TB D	BA No Total TB D	Phila Pul	BA Pul
										% of Pul D of Total TBD				% of Total Deaths	
1904	1,399,268	967,280	69.13	25,976	14,313	3,117	1,771	384	274	89.03	86.6	3,501	2,045	12.00	12.37
1905	1,425,122	1,013,680	71.13	24,807	15,916	2,838	1,914	377	231	88.27	89.23	3,215	2,145	11.44	12.03
1906	1,450,976	1,063,880	73.32	27,768	17,916	3,161	2,011	105	270	96.79	88.16	3,266	2,281	11.38	11.22
1907	1,476,830	1,118,080	75.71	27,750	18,616	3,157	2,115	449	279	87.55	88.35	3,606	2,394	11.38	11.36
1909	1,528,540	1,239,280	81.08	25,029	18,959	2,863	1,964	26	306	99.1	86.52	2,889	2,270	11.44	10.36
1910	1,554,902	1,306,680	84.04	27,045	20,968	2,873	2,150	393	335	87.97	86.52	3,266	2,485	10.62	10.25
1911	1,583,190	1,378,880	87.10	26,276	22,869	2,960	2,304	142	367	95.42	86.26	3,102	2,671	11.27	10.07
1912	1,611,478	1,456,080	90.36	25,660	22,982	2,654	2,253	395	378	87.3	85.63	3,040	2,631	10.34	9.80
1913	1,639,766	1,538,480	93.82	25,612	23,009	2,692	2,435	459	422	85.43	85.23	3,151	2,857	10.51	10.58
1914	1,668,054	1,553,805	93.15	26,918	23,486	2,684	2,849	356	425	88.29	87.02	3,040	3,274	9.97	12.13
1915	1,696,342	1,563,082	92.14	26,287	23,904	2,754	2,857	423	452	86.69	86.34	3,177	3,309	10.48	11.95
1916	1,724,498	1,575,643	91.37	27,621	23,289	3,013	3,122	425	472	92.23	86.87	3,267	3,594	10.91	13.41
1917	1,753,058	1,589,926	90.69	29,681	22,337	3,019	3,254	262	554	92.01	85.45	3,281	3,808	10.17	14.57
1918	1,781,346	1,604,693	90.08	42,643	23,805	3,350	3,688		503		88		4,191	7.86	15.49
1920	1,829,983	1,629,016	89.02	26,516	24,123	2,219	2,761		655		80.83		3,416	8.37	11.45
1921	1,842,391	1,664,780	90.36	23,704	23,860	1,912	2,790	253	746	88.31	78.9	2,165	3,536	8.07	11.69
1922	1,854,799	1,704,400	91.89	25,103	23,691	1,893	2,849	269	694	87.56	80.41	2,162	3,543	7.54	12.03
1923	1,867,207	1,774,400	95.03	26,654	24,353	1,867	2,888	195	715	92.79	80.16	2,012	3,603	7.00	11.86
1924	1,879,615	1,844,400	98.13	24,980	25,186	1,777	3,253		462		87.56		3,715	7.11	12.92
1925	1,892,023	1,914,400	107.18	26,061	25,421	1,781	3,374		485		87.43		3,859	6.83	13.27
1927	1,916,839	2,054,400	110.06	24,801	26,531	1,508	3,075		536	86.72	85.16	1,739	3,611	6.08	11.59
1928	1,930,247	2,124,400	110.06	26,930	26,313	1,607	3,117	235	569	92.14	84.56	1,744	3,686	5.97	11.85
1929	2,011,655	2,194,400	109.08	25,346	28,702	1,361	3,391	220	496	81.45	87.24	1,671	3,887	5.37	11.81
1930	1,954,063	2,254,400	115.37	24,541	27,095	1,396	3,037	194	568	87.8	84.24	1,590	3,605	5.69	11.21
1932	1,978,879	2,319,400	117.21	23,777	26,177	1,234	3,244	163	575	88.33	84.94	1,397	3,819	5.19	12.39
1933	1,991,287	2,347,400	117.88	23,916	25,768	1,238	3,080		541	89.84	85.06	1,378	3,621	5.18	11.95
1934	2,003,695	2,373,400	118.45	24,984	26,173	1,258	2,766	146	509	89.28	84.46	1,409	3,275	5.04	10.57
1936	2,028,511	2,419,400	119.27	25,015	26,106	1,194	2,603	155	474	88.18	84.6	1,354	3,077	4.77	9.97
1937	2,040,919	2,418,835	118.52	25,239	27,377	1,190	2,535	125	439	90.49	85.24	1,315	2,974	4.71	9.26
1938	2,053,327	2,444,126	119.03	24,309	28,308	1,104	2,684	133	455	89.25	85.5	1,237	3,139	4.54	9.48

Sources: Beso Moreno, Buenos Aires: 96–97, 173–175, 430–1; Buenos Aires, Revista de Estadística (January–March 1945): 4; Philadelphia, Annual Message of the Mayor, various years, particularly 1912, 3: 109; 1920: 482; 1938: 450.
Abbreviations: BA = Buenos Aires; Phila = Philadelphia; Pop = Population; D = Deaths; Pul = Pulmonary TB.

Beginning in 1915, tuberculosis as a percent of total deaths declined more rapidly in Philadelphia than Buenos Aires and decreased from 10.48 percent in 1915 to 4.54 percent in 1938. Buenos Aires tuberculosis deaths were more erratic; pulmonary tuberculosis deaths declined substantially from 10.94 in 1885 to 7.80 in 1895 before beginning a steady increase and varied between 9.29 percent in 1896 and 13.27 in 1925 in an era when the city's population more than doubled. (The large number of deaths from 1916 to 1918 are outliers due to World War II and the 1918 influenza epidemic.) Only from 1926 do pulmonary tuberculosis deaths again begin a slow decline in Buenos Aires from 11.76 to 9.26 percent of all deaths in 1938. From 1870 to 1938, the number of tuberculosis deaths continued to rise in both cities, but they are quite small in comparison to pulmonary tuberculosis.

From 1870 to 1938, non-pulmonary tuberculosis deaths vary between 0 and 14.5 percent of all tuberculosis deaths in Philadelphia and between 0 and 19.8 percent of all tuberculosis deaths in Buenos Aires. Non-pulmonary tuberculosis deaths, however, were 3.3 times more common in Buenos Aires than Philadelphia. For example, in the nineteenth century, non-pulmonary tuberculosis deaths were never higher than 2.6 percent of all tuberculosis deaths in Philadelphia, but in Buenos Aires non-pulmonary tuberculosis deaths increased to 13.4 percent of all tuberculosis deaths in 1899. Most likely, because of better diagnosis, the number of reported non-pulmonary deaths increased in the twentieth century. From 1900 to 1938 in Buenos Aires, tuberculosis mortality, as a percent of all tuberculosis deaths, varied between eleven percent in 1900 and twenty-one percent in 1921. In the same period, non-pulmonary tuberculosis deaths averaged 14.48 percent of tuberculosis mortality deaths in Buenos Aires. In Philadelphia between 1900 and 1938, tuberculosis mortality, as a percent of all tuberculosis deaths, varied between 0.44 percent in 1900 and 14.6 percent in 1913, while non-pulmonary tuberculosis deaths averaged 8.98 percent of tuberculosis mortality deaths in Philadelphia.[35]

Because of population growth in both cities, the annual number of deaths from pulmonary tuberculosis continued to increase in Philadelphia until 1920 and in Buenos Aires until 1926. From 1904 onward the population of Buenos Aires increased far more rapidly than Philadelphia's. This rapid growth overwhelmed public health efforts in Buenos Aires, making it increasingly difficult to improve living conditions within the city. Unsanitary conditions promoted the spread of tuberculosis. At the same time, tuberculosis victims in Buenos Aires lived in both elite and poor districts. The data suggests a correlation between a rise in the standard of living and a decline in the number of tuberculosis deaths. For example, the rise of homeownership in Philadelphia was a reflection of increased living standards.

Table 2.2 Comparison of Number of Deaths due to Epidemic Diseases and Tuberculosis in Buenos Aires and Philadelphia, 1869–1938

Year	*Diphtheria & Cough*		*Measles*		*Scarlet Fev*		*Smallpox*		*Typhoid*		*Whooping Cough*		*Total Epid Deaths*		*Pulmonary Deaths*		*All Types TB*		*TB Deaths as % of Epid D*	
	BA	*Phila*	*BA*	*Phila*	*BA*	*Phila*	*BA*	*Phila*	*BA*	*Phila*	*BA*	*Phila*	*BA*	*Phila*	*BA*	*Phila*	*BA*	*Phila*	*BA (%)*	*Phila (%)*
1869	176	182	5	85	2	799	183	6	600	373	20	74	986	1,519	370	1,975	370	1,991	38	131
1870	83	172	1	48	11	956	195	9	165	409	36	105	491	1,699	274	2,308	274	2,316	56	136
1871	79	145	12	43	12	262	1,656	1,879	159	313	12	81	1,930	2,723	495	22,37	495	2,247	26	83
1872	126	143	5	143	18	174	836	2,585	176	369	29	163	1,190	3,577	597	2,330	597	2,355	50	66
1873	131	110	71	30	0	319	76	39	161	364	24	97	463	959	755	2,291	755	2,291	163	239
1874	202	179	125	117	0	461	525	15	205	491	24	74	1,081	1,337	685	2,304	710	2,322	66	174
1875	212	652	8	12	21	1,032	1,041	54	140	419	63	125	1,485	2,294	858	2,359	880	2,405	59	105
1876	206	706	11	53	24	328	22	407	134	761	13	88	410	2,343	783	2,676	813	2,697	198	115
1877	136	458	39	69	6	379	12	155	106	542	56	81	355	1,684	716	2,349	743	2,369	209	141
1878	240	464	19	12	13	554	7	0	114	404	11	109	404	1,543	756	2,491	786	2,510	195	163
1879	369	321	62	8	50	336	429	6	147	344	30	103	1087	1,118	776	2,481	804	2,498	74	223
1880	335	323	3	108	15	291	832	424	163	498	32	101	1,380	1,745	774	2,692	796	2,710	58	155
1881	241	457	43	17	14	486	7	1,336	216	645	22	113	543	3,054	782	2,768	805	2,786	148	91
1882	221	933	93	91	12	310	362	314	212	650	42	63	942	2,361	808	2,809	827	2,823	88	120
1883	193	1,006	5	58	12	561	1,510	173	180	579	17	86	1,917	2,463	932	2,798	953	2,812	50	114
1884	253	680	194	3	25	540	142	35	193	662	30	5	837	1,925	1,053	2,801	1,089	2,834	130	147
1885	336	609	17	131	67	375	736	6	209	610	51	132	1,416	1,863	1,017	2,821	1,042	2,843	74	153
1887	995	816	141	131	62	159	1,299	0	280	621	35	130	2,812	1,857	1,041	2,800	1,066	2,837	38	153
1888	1385	623	99	24	17	235	657	80	388	785	67	140	2,613	1,887	1,069	2,695	1,098	2,744	42	145
1889	905	727	261	92	17	298	185	0	509	736	85	146	1,962	1,999	1,245	2,532	1,349	2,581	69	129
1890	1037	943	80	106	26	189	2,198	0	628	666	57	205	4,026	2,109	1,168	2,764	1,255	2,794	31	132
1891	623	1,362	54	25	11	341	275	5	408	683	93	141	1,464	2,557	1,024	2,624	1,142	2,677	78	105
1892	609	1,707	188	85	12	485	30	0	214	440	29	140	1,082	2,857	1,078	2,709	1,181	2,732	109	96
1893	658	1,159	812	88	59	267	14	5	214	456	64	212	1,821	2,187	1,103	2,671	1,270	2,706	70	124
1894	445	1,394	104	132	149	153	15	13	217	370	65	190	995	2,252	1,283	2,513	1,419	2,560	143	114
1895	381	1,340	204	84	598	79	277	45	208	469	42	151	1,710	2,168	1,166	2,449	1,322	2,513	77	116

1896	230	1,155	61	191	303	61	176	0	207	402	100	158	1,077	1,967	1,268	2,514	1,368	2,569	127	131
1900	245	1,042	193	382	359	163	110	0	193	449	53	124	1,153	2,160	1,672	2,717	1,898	2,729	165	126
1901	237	643	80	26	409	220	1,227	156	173	444	56	261	2,182	1,750	1,675	2,946	1,893	2,990	87	171
1903	113	608	88	141	53	189	207	278	157	957	28	291	646	2,464	1,689	3,053	1,915	3,125	296	127
1904	86	541	54	220	52	201	522	229	113	744	53	73	880	2,008	1,771	3,117	2,045	3,501	232	174
1905	74	452	83	53	25	57	484	0	142	684	47	136	855	1,382	1,914	2,838	2,145	3,215	251	233
1906	100	546	84	344	60	56	970	0	266	1063	57	387	1,537	2,396	2,011	3,161	2,281	3,266	148	136
1907	120	509	118	65	89	100	76	0	219	890	78	194	700	1,758	2,115	3,157	2,394	3,606	342	205
1909	126	512	78	229	39	133	169	0	220	331	33	135	665	1,340	1,964	2,863	2,270	2,889	341	216
1910	207	492	69	148	49	152	543	5	195	272	62	327	1,125	1,396	2,150	2,873	2,485	3,266	221	234
1911	274	498	79	305	69	195	169	1	347	230	92	116	1,030	1,345	2,304	2,960	2,671	3,102	259	231
1912	79	388	76	50	8	123	5	1	654	205	95	100	917	867	2,253	2,654	2,631	3,040	287	351
1913	339	359	201	199	30	172	18	0	427	257	80	106	1,095	1,093	2,435	2,692	2,857	3,151	261	288
1914	254	329	118	77	32	129	1	0	488	124	119	266	1,012	925	2,849	2,684	3,274	3,040	324	329
1915	402	317	353	184	36	26	1	0	171	109	105	47	1,068	683	2,857	2,754	3,309	3,177	310	465
1916	230	390	39	102	7	40	0	0	235	128	97	129	608	789	3,122	,3013	3,594	3,267	591	414
1917	215	441	126	87	29	31	0	0	144	108	58	168	572	835	3,254	3,019	3,808	3,267	666	391
1918	195	384	38	119	65	43	0	0	202	85	74	337	574	968	3,688	3,350	4,191	3,281	730	339
1920	220	413	116	166	60	115	0	0	170	60	53	95	619	849	2,761	2,219	3,416		552	0
1921	157	318	20	1	58	104	2	0	153	42	27	141	417	606	2,790	1,912	3,536	2,165	848	357
1922	157	281	111	0	23	86	9	0	156	53	150	39	606	459	2,849	1,893	3,543	2,162	585	471
1923	172	270	55	2	31	34	1	0	142	29	41	103	442	438	2,888	1,867	3,603	2,012	815	459
1927	238	220	131	3	145	34	0	0	123	29	67	31	704	317	3,075	1,508	3,611	1,739	513	549
1928	225	230	160	150	174	22	0	0	93	17	82	132	734	551	3,117	1,607	3,686	1,744	502	317
1929	353	69	90	9	413	26	0	0	57	14	20	81	933	199	3,391	1,361	3,887	1,671	417	840
1930	171	48	128	16	94	34	0	0	61	18	112	24	566	140	3,037	1,396	3,605	1,590	637	1136
1932	119	16	83	1	14	48	0	0	60	26	39	57	315	148	3,244	1,234	3,819	1,397	1212	944
1933	170	13	29	12	17	33	0	0	50	12	44	9	310	79	3,080	1,238	3,621	1,378	1168	1744
1934	166	22	107	17	13	28	0	0	37	17	107	59	430	143	2,766	1,258	3,275	1,409	762	985
1936	137	10	56	15	6	7	0	0	31	18	17	30	247	80	2,603	1,194	3,077	1,354	1246	1693
1937	170	7	33	5	28	17	0	0	39	29	91	29	361	87	2,535	1,190	2,974	1,315	824	1511
1938	171	10	25	22	28	10	0	0	56	16	27	29	307	87	2,684	1,104	3,139	1,237	1022	1422

Sources: Besio Moreno, Buenos Aires, 173–5; Buenos Aires, Revista de estadistica municipal de la ciudad (January–March 1945); Buenos Aires, Year-Book 1910–1911, 112–8 Philadelphia, Annual Message of the Mayor of Philadelphia, various years, particularly 1900, 1912, 1928, 1936.
Abbreviations: Fev = Fever; Epid = Epidemics; D = Deaths.

Table 2.2 compares pulmonary tuberculosis death and all other types of tuberculosis deaths with epidemic deaths in Buenos Aires and Philadelphia. Because of a major smallpox epidemic in both Buenos Aires and Philadelphia in 1871–1872, tuberculosis deaths in these years were a smaller proportion of total death—twenty-six percent of epidemic deaths in Buenos Aires in 1872 and the following year fifty percent; and in Philadelphia eighty-three percent of epidemic deaths in 1871 and sixty-six percent in 1872. The development of a smallpox vaccine and the success of public health campaigns to encourage vaccination, led to decreased deaths. By 1913, in Philadelphia and 1916 in Buenos Aires, smallpox had declined to zero significance.

Diphtheria remained an important killer in both Buenos Aires and Philadelphia throughout the era. Deaths due to diphtheria increased steadily in both cities from 1869 to 1890 and were endemic in Philadelphia from 1890 to 1900. Diphtheria gradually decreased in Philadelphia and then declined rapidly from 230 deaths in 1928 to ten in 1938. Diphtheria remained a significant killer in Buenos Aires through 1938. From 1869 to 1894, scarlet fever caused a substantial number of deaths in Philadelphia but was insignificant in Buenos Aires except from 1895 to 1901. Whooping cough represented fewer deaths in Buenos Aires than Philadelphia. Typhoid fever was a more regular cause of death in Philadelphia than Buenos Aires. Except for a major measles outbreak in Buenos Aires in 1893, the disease did not reach epidemic proportions. Recurring epidemics caused more deaths in Buenos Aires than Philadelphia.

Francis Lawrence Flick and the Henry Phipps Institute

Both Philadelphia and Buenos Aires were home to globally recognized tuberculosis research and medical institutions. Francis Lawrence Flick (1856–1938) in Philadelphia and Emilio R. Coni (1855–1928) in Buenos Aires illustrate the commitment of individuals to preventing tuberculosis and treating tuberculosis patients. Flick directed the Henry Phipps Institute for the study, treatment and prevention of tuberculosis in center-city Philadelphia. Coni was associated with the Hospital Municipal Doctor Tornú, an urban sanatorium, located in Buenos Aires. Through institutions organized in their respective cities, Flick and Coni shaped their cities' and nations' tuberculosis programs and policies.[36]

Flick, an early supporter of the theory that tuberculosis is contagious, dominated the early history of Philadelphia's response to tuberculosis. He helped organize the Sixth International Congress of Tuberculosis in 1908 in Washington, D.C. He brought an exhibition, which was viewed by some 500,000 people, from the international congress to Philadelphia. Dr. Samuel G. Dixon (1851–1918), Pennsylvania's Commissioner of Health, viewed the founding of the Henry Phipps Institute in Philadelphia as one of the most important events in the campaign against tuberculosis. Many foreign guests, including Dr. Robert Koch, came to Philadelphia to see the Institute's tuberculosis programs.[37]

Henry Phipps, a business partner of Andrew Carnegie, provided the capital in 1903 to establish an institution to eradicate tuberculosis. Phipps recognized that the existing Philadelphia institutions that provided care for the tubercular were too small to serve the city's large infected population. He provided $54,000 to construct the main building in recognition of the need and out of respect for Flick. The Phipps Institute began operations in a rented building in 1903. It had three wards with a total of forty beds. The institute, divided into five sections, balanced its work between research and care. It supported a hospital with a small number of beds for patients, a dispensary with various clinics for out-patient treatment, a social service department that housed visiting nurses and did neighborhood studies, a laboratory with an X-ray machine and a research library focused on tuberculosis and other infectious diseases. Flick believed that an important means to prevent the spread of tuberculosis was the isolation of advanced tubercular patients. He also thought that private institutions rather than the state should care for tubercular patients. He clashed with Dixon over this concept.[38]

During its first complete year of operation, the institute treated 2,039 patients, of whom 1,458 were poor, in its hospital and dispensaries; forty percent of the patients were foreign-born. Of the patients whose ages were known, 587 were aged 20–30, 573 were aged 30–40, 346 were aged 40–50, 197 were over 50 and 50 were less than age 10. Of the 851 women, 360 were homemakers, while the others were factory workers, seamstresses, laundry workers or store employees. Most males were employed manual laborers; other male patients were tailors, clerks, cigar makers, salesmen, printers and shoemakers.[39] During its first years, the Institute staff focused on learning how to detect tuberculosis soon after it was contracted and increasing the knowledge of the disease. In 1904, physicians at the Institute treated patients with a serum developed in Italy, but it failed to provide the expected benefits. They continued to do research on new methods of treatment. At the request of a patient, in 1911, the institute performed the first U.S. thoracoplasty (the surgical removal of one or more ribs so as to collapse and rest a diseased lung).[40]

By 1908, the Phipps Institute had a staff of thirty-five and a worldwide reputation. Most patients suffered from tuberculosis of the lungs. Because the institute could not find enough nurses, it began its own educational program, successfully training recovered consumptives to serve as nurses. In 1908, after two years of training, and one-year working at a general hospital, six young women graduated and were certified registered nurses. The program discontinued in 1915 because of a lack of funds and because municipal and state hospitals had expanded their nursing programs to prepare women to care for the tubercular. Because the institute was affiliated with the Visiting Nurse Society and the Philadelphia Training School for Social Workers, it was instrumental in 1913 in starting a postgraduate course in public health for nurses.[41]

The Phipps Institute sought to educate its patients. It distributed leaflets in English, Yiddish and Italian that contained rules for preventing the spread of tuberculosis. The leaflets stressed that fresh air and rest were important. Convalescents were encouraged to live in tents on roofs and in yards. Patients learned to make tents in windows (so they could have their head outside the window but with a blanket awning around the window to keep the cold air from entering the room, so that other family members could sleep in the same room). Since diet was also important, nurses taught patients how to purchase, prepare and preserve food in window refrigerators. Patients also received tissues to cover their mouths when coughing and paper bags and sputum cups. Some patients learned to take their own temperature, to weight themselves, to take their pulse and to calculate the caloric value of foods. The instruction was particularly important for patients who did not wish to go to sanatoriums. The classes encouraged friendly competition over weight gain. Patients met every two weeks to hear lectures on health topics and to submit their personal records. Nurses and patients effectively led the small classes.[42]

In 1911, the Phipps Institute established an open-air school for children who had been exposed to tuberculosis. The Philadelphia Board of Education subsequently took over this school. In 1918, the Phipps Institute began to focus on children infected with tuberculosis. It used the open-air wards on the third floor of its main building for classes for tubercular children and also studied their diet and treatment. This endeavor attracted to the Institute a new director, Eugene Opie, a pathologist with a special interest in ending tuberculosis among Philadelphia's school children. He directed the institute from 1923 until 1932. By the third year, medical students at the University of Pennsylvania were required to obtain experience in tuberculosis dispensaries as well as to study the disease.[43]

The institute was concerned that only a few African Americans took advantage of its services, even though the district in which it was located was predominantly African American. Thus, in 1914, the institute hired an African-American nurse to see Black patients. After 1914, the proportion of African Americans rapidly increased; more Black patients were seen that year than in the previous nine. Whereas no Blacks previously went to weekly clinics, twenty-five to thirty now attended each week. With the hiring of African-American nurses, the Phipps was the first Philadelphia institute to successfully treat African Americans. The new hires' efforts also helped attract Blacks to other clinics; and by the end of 1914, the Pennsylvania Society for the Study of Tuberculosis hired two more African-American nurses to work in clinics. In 1921,

4,466 new African-American patients were diagnosed in the city's various hospitals and clinics; State Clinic No. 21 and the Phipps Institute served sixty-three percent of the African-American tubercular population. By the mid-1920s, the Phipps Institute joined with other charitable organizations to support tuberculosis clinics in other parts of the city that had large African-American populations.[44]

In 1910, the Institute affiliated with the University of Pennsylvania. In 1920, the Phipps family endowed the institution with $500,000 with the hope that funding from the endowment would support the Institute. From 1921 to 1926, the Carnegie Foundation provided an additional $25,000 each year.[45] During the 1930s and early 1940s, the international reputation of the Phipps Institute attracted many foreign visitors, who were impressed because the clinic provided both clinical services and supported cutting-edge research. In the 1930s, it did research on the BCG (Bacillus Calmette-Guerin) vaccination used to prevent tuberculosis. In 1928, Florence B. Seibert, who began working in the lab in 1924, crystallized the tuberculoprotein; and in 1941, the U.S. government made her Purified Protein Derivative (PPD) the standard for purified tuberculin used to test for tuberculosis infection. Antibiotic treatment for tuberculosis after 1945 decreased the relevance of the institute; in 1958, the Henry Phipps's building was sold and demolished, and the endowment distributed to research departments of public health at the University of Pennsylvania.[46]

Emilio R. Coni and the Hospital Tornú

Emilio R. Coni was a public health physician and liberal reformer who organized the Buenos Aires municipal health services. Just as Flick was instrumental in founding the Pennsylvania Society for the Prevention of Tuberculosis, Coni helped found the Argentine Anti-Tuberculosis League. Coni considered the establishment of Hospital Tornú as one of his most significant accomplishments. The Sanatorium and Hospital Municipal Doctor Tornú cared for the tubercular who lived and worked in Buenos Aires. When government officials agreed to build a tuberculosis hospital in an urban area, they signaled their agreement with international tuberculosis experts: it was unnecessary to locate a clinic on a mountain in order to cure tuberculosis.[47]

The Hospital Tornú began accepting patients in 1904. Until the creation of this facility, Buenos Aires' patients were treated in community hospitals—with the exception of advanced cases who entered the Hospital Muñiz, a facility treating patients with contagious diseases. The Tornú initially treated pulmonary tubercular patients who could not afford to go to the hilly northern province of Córdoba for treatment and did not have a family to care for them. The hospital location on urban transport routes encouraged families to visit patients. Coni directed the hospital.[48]

Within a year of its opening, the Tornú cared for 200 men and women in four pavilions, which were oriented so galleries were bathed in sun and protected from strong winds. The buildings had large halls, broad doorways that opened on a garden and wide windows that provided superior ventilation. Private and dispensary physicians recommended admitting patients in the early stages of the disease, who were likely to benefit from the regime of a healthy diet, rest and fresh air. Patients who appeared to be incurable continued to go to the Hospital Muñiz.[49] The demand for beds for the city's tuberculosis patients led the Buenos Aires Municipality to support the expansion of Hospital Tornú. By 1940, the hospital had a capacity of 900 beds. Among the pavilions added was one providing separate space for pregnant tubercular women and children. At birth, babies were isolated from their tubercular mothers. In the early 1940s, nurses vaccinated both the newborns and the children with BCG. Children received the same care that was given to adults.[50]

At the Hospital Tornú, physicians examined entering patients, took their medical histories and sent their saliva to the laboratory for analysis. Patients learned the rules of the sanatorium and were taught that consumption was curable if they followed the prescribed routine. After taking a warm bath, patients received items such as spittoons, soap, toothbrushes, mouth disinfectant, combs, table utensils, metal drinking cups, napkins and a napkin ring. They were also given items needed for living in the fresh air, including sheets and woolen blankets for room use and a rug to be used when seated on an exterior lounge chair, along with summer and winter hats and a cape to keep off the rain.[51]

The patients followed a strict schedule of diet, rest and fresh air, a regimen that was similar to that prescribed in the best European sanatoriums. Patients were weighed each Saturday, and their temperature was taken morning and night; urine was analyzed regularly and saliva was sent to the laboratory twice a month; showers and dry or wet rubs were given as prescribed by the doctor while warm baths were taken periodically. Patients were instructed to wash their mouths and brush their teeth after every meal. Food was abundant. It included beef, lamb and fish twice a week, rice, beans, string beans, lima beans, bread, potatoes, eggs, sugar and coffee. Each patient received two liters of pasteurized milk a day. Not surprisingly, the patients were prohibited from spitting on the floor and received three types of spittoons: a bag, one for the table at night, and one for the floor. They were advised to cough only when necessary. Coughing posed a problem, and patients were told to drink water or milk when their throats were irritated. Little medication was used for a cough because codeine and morphine have a bad effect on the stomach. Patients were taught to put a handkerchief to the mouth each time they coughed so as not to spread bacteria.[52]

To alleviate boredom and resentment against regulations, the Tornú was among the first institutions to provide a variety of activities for the residents and welfare support for resident families. The primary school instruction was offered for illiterates. The library had more than 250 books as well as newspapers and magazines. Dominoes, cards and croquet were available; and patients who knew musical instruments were encouraged to play them. Patients received visits from family and friends on Thursdays and Sundays. In order to minimize patient's worry, charity organizations assisted patient families with housing, clothes and food. Discussions on politics or religious matters that might upset the patients were prohibited, as was noisy conversation, singing, and shouting. Tobacco and alcohol were prohibited except as medicine. Patients who complained excessively or broke the rules were expelled.[53]

The Hospital Municipal Doctor Tornú regimen and services were similar to those in tuberculosis hospital-sanatoriums worldwide. The patient schedules and activities did not differ from what was found in other institutions in Buenos Aires or Philadelphia. What made the Tornú significant was its location on the outskirts of Buenos Aires and its recognition that high altitude was not necessary to treat tuberculosis patients. Because the hospital was conveniently located, public officials could more easily induce families to send their tubercular relatives to it. Since the Hospital Tornú was the premiere tuberculosis institution in the city, the ill were more willing to enter it. Its location also made it easy for students studying at the Facultad de Medicina to visit the institution frequently and to do research on the effects of particular regimens. Physicians focusing on tuberculosis implemented new procedures and willingly experimented and published results in medical journals.

After 1945, as was true in other tuberculosis hospitals, the Tornú refocused its operations. Although many of the pavilions of the Tornú were no longer needed and fell into disrepair, the main hospital was modernized and now provides a wide variety of services. The Hospital Municipal Doctor Tornú operates as a general hospital serving the local community and it still has physicians specialized in tuberculosis. With the growing number of tuberculosis patients, due to the recent worldwide increase in the disease, the demand for diagnosis and care have increased.[54]

A Comparison of Two Cities

Although Buenos Aires and Philadelphia implemented globally accepted policies, the two cities differed in important respects, specifically regarding climate and culture. Even though both Buenos Aires and Philadelphia have rainy springs, hot summers and pleasant autumns, Porteños rarely experienced either frost or snow. A warmer year-round climate allowed the Buenos Aires government to build public housing more cheaply than Philadelphia. Philadelphia's shorter summers and colder winters decreased the effect of some epidemics. Buenos Aires, a capital, had more political power nationally than Philadelphia. As a commercial city that was home to large government bureaucracies, Buenos Aires had a more diversified economy than Philadelphia in which the transport and industrial sectors predominated.

The different colonial traditions of Buenos Aires and Philadelphia explain other disparities. The colonial British government stressed local initiatives, and the young republic's emphasis on free enterprise encouraged private efforts to construct public housing and medical facilities. In contrast, the colonial Spanish policy supported government regulation and control which encouraged public construction of housing and hospitals. The cities also differed in their resident's preferences as to where to build the houses. Porteños preferred to live in the center of the city; they moved to the outskirts largely for cheaper housing and to be nearer the factories that were being built in greater Buenos Aires. Philadelphians viewed a move to the suburbs as a sign of upward mobility. By the 1930s, it was the poor and lower classes who lived in Philadelphia's urban historic center, whereas the wealthy and middle classes of Buenos Aires preferred to live near the historic center. In the 1940s, when the population of Buenos Aries surpassed that of Philadelphia, both cities faced new medical, social and economic problems due to increased populations.

Between 1870 and 1945, Buenos Aires and Philadelphia were vibrant and growing cities actually with more similarities than differences. Both provided the social, economic and political environment in which individuals confronted tuberculosis. Both offered new arrivals, economic opportunities and the chance to live with those of similar ethnicity near to the place where they worked. At the end of the nineteenth century, expanding port facilities and growing trade attracted immigrants from abroad and migrants from elsewhere in each city's country. In both cities, the large migrations outstripped available housing and social services. In the early twentieth century, the center cities modernized and extended their reach through tram and railroads systems going to the suburbs. Buenos Aires and Philadelphia further developed new cultural, educational and medical institutions to provide more effectively for their expanding populations. Public officials recognized the importance of creating a healthy environment for their residents and promoted the development of water and sewer systems to control epidemic and chronic diseases. Both cities gathered data on tuberculosis, epidemics and other diseases. They showcased their public health programs.

Both metropolises had internationally recognized institutions which offered tubercular patients up-to-date treatments and which attracted physicians who focused on tuberculosis. The cities supported significant philanthropic institutions committed to combating tuberculosis. The privately funded Henry Phipps Institute focused on research and innovative techniques, while the government supported Hospital Municipal Doctor Tornú cared for more patients. Both the Phipps Institute in

Philadelphia and the Hospital Tornú of Buenos Aires provided important services to an urban region—encouraging their respective cities to develop tuberculosis prevention and treatment programs. The Phipps was among the first U.S. institutions to use trained social workers, acquaint doctors and nurses with public health issues and establish a nursing school for women who had recovered from tuberculosis. Both the Phipps and the Tornú showed that tuberculosis patients could be treated and possibly cured within the city with a healthy diet, rest and fresh air. The commitment, efforts and historical significance of both these institutions in the treatment of tubercular patients laid the basis for broader prevention efforts. Although both institutions faced new challenges after 1945, they still exemplify the vibrant global institutions that sought to prevent and treat tuberculosis in an urban environment in the first half of the twentieth century. The Henry Phipps Institute was torn down as Pennsylvania's government-run and -subsidized sanatoriums and clinics, rather than private institutions, came to dominate the state's tuberculosis prevention and care efforts. In contrast, the modernized Hospital Municipal Doctor Tornú continues to operate and serve the Buenos Aires community.

Public and private institutions in Buenos Aires and Philadelphia confronted the challenge of both epidemics and tuberculosis. Whether epidemics in any given year were more significant than tuberculosis in contributing to the mortality rates of Buenos Aires and Philadelphia depended on two factors: first, the size of the epidemic and second, its effect on the tuberculosis population. When there was a major epidemic, tuberculosis deaths were a smaller percentage of all deaths in both cities. However, as epidemics were conquered, tuberculosis increasingly became the major killer. From 1893 to 1938, in Philadelphia and from 1903 to 1938 in Buenos Aires tuberculosis deaths surpassed deaths from epidemics. Beginning in 1907, tuberculosis deaths were more than double epidemic deaths in both cities. By 1933, tuberculosis was 1,168 percent of all deaths from epidemics in Buenos Aires and in the same year 1,744 percent of epidemic deaths in Philadelphia. With the decline of epidemics in both cities, other diseases surpassed tuberculosis as the major cause of death. By 1930, heart disease was the number one killer in Philadelphia.[55]

The second influence on tuberculosis mortality statistics was the degree to which an epidemic killed those with tuberculosis who were already very ill. Co-infection, the simultaneous infection of an individual by two or more viruses or bacteria that causes disease, influences mortality rates by the diseases.[56] According to Table 2.2, after epidemics of smallpox and scarlet fever in Buenos Aires and Philadelphia tuberculosis deaths increased, suggesting that the epidemics killed some tuberculosis patients and weakened others. In both Buenos Aires and Philadelphia, tuberculosis deaths had begun to decline before World War I. This decline was interrupted by increasing rates of death in Buenos Aires in 1914 and Philadelphia in 1916. In both cities, the 1918 influenza pandemic killed the physically weak with the result that later tuberculosis rates decreased rapidly.[57] Statistics provided the evidence of the prevalence of death in Buenos Aires and Philadelphia from 1869 to 1938. What data cannot do is reveal the emotional impact of the death of a father, mother or child; nor do the statistics illuminate the mental and physical toll on all individuals who resulted from the reality in which friends and family die young.

The difficulties Buenos Aires and Philadelphia faced in coping with expanding populations and efforts to expand public health services to deal with the tuberculosis crisis were similar to those confronted by other western cities. The similar social and economic developments of Buenos Aires and Philadelphia provided the basis for the implementation of comparable tuberculosis prevention programs. As will be seen in the next chapter, the public health officials of Buenos Aires and Philadelphia were committed to developing policies for preventing tuberculosis. The two cities faced similar challenges as they sought to implement global public health initiatives to keep their residents healthy.

Notes

1 James Bryce, *South America: Observations and Impressions* (New York: The Macmillan Company, 1923), 317–18.

2 George Barton, *Little Journeys around Old Philadelphia* (Philadelphia: The Peter Reilly Company, 1925), 17.

3 Six works are particularly significant for providing a general understanding of Buenos Aires: James Scobie, *Buenos Aires Plaza to Suburb, 1870–1910* (New York: Oxford University Press, 1974); Richard J. Walter, *Politics and Urban Growth in Buenos Aires, 1810–1942* (New York: Cambridge University Press, 1993); Stanley R. Ross and Thomas F. McGann, eds., *Buenos Aires: 400 Years* (Austin: University of Texas Press, 1982); José Luis Romero and Luis Alberto Romero, *Buenos Aires, Historia de cuatros siglos*, 2 vols. (Buenos Aires: Editorial Abril, 1983); Mario Rapoport and María Seoane, *Buenos Aires, historia de una ciudad: De la modernidad al siglo XXI: Sociedad, política, economía, y cultura (*Buenos Aires: Planeta-Fundación Banco Ciudad, 2007), 2 vols. and Diego Armus, *The Ailing City: Health, Tuberculosis, and Culture in Buenos Aires, 1870–1950* (Durham: Duke University Press, 2011).

4 The starting point for the history of Philadelphia is Russell F. Weigley, ed., *Philadelphia A 300-Year History* (New York: W.W. Norton & Co, 1982) with seventeen articles by various authors; a work that deals with class issues is John Henry Hepp IV, *The Middle-Class City: Transforming Space and Time in Philadelphia, 1876–1926* (Philadelphia: University of Pennsylvania Press, 2003).

5 To sample the diverse observers of Buenos Aires, see Frank Vincent, *Around and about South America: Twenty Months of Quest and Query* (New York: D. Appleton and Company, 1890), 151–58; (quote 153); Arthur Ruhl, *The Other Americans: The Cities, the Countries, and Especially the People of*

South America (New York: Charles Scribner's Sons, 1910), 207–53; Clayton Sedgwick Cooper, *Understanding South America* (New York: George H. Doran Company, 1918), 248–60; Frederick Augustus Sherwood, *Glimpses of South America* (New York: The Century Co., 1920), 255–352; Bryce, 315–48; and Sydney Clark, *All the Best in South America: East Coast* (New York: Dodd, Mead & Company, 1956; first edition 1940), 217–23.

6 Bryce, 320.

7 Emilio Daireaux, *Industrias y productos*: vol. 2 of *Vida y Costumbres in la Plata* (Buenos Aires: Félix Lojouane, 1888), 123–31, 138; Adrián Patroni, *Los Trabajadores en la Argentina* (Buenos Aires: Imprenta Litografía y Encuadernación, 1897), 127–29; Rafael E. J. Iglesia, "La vivienda opulenta en Buenos Aires, 1880–1900, hechos y testimonios," in *Primeras Jornadas de Historia de la Ciudad de Buenos Aires, "La Vivienda en Buenos Aires,"* (Buenos Aires: Municipalidad de la Ciudad d Buenos Aries, 1885), 135–39 (for statistics on the number of floors, 142); Oscar Yujnovsky, "Políticas de vivienda en la ciudad de Buenos Aires (1880–1914)," *Desarrollo Económico-Revista de Ciencias Sociales* 14, no. 5 (July–September 1974): 371–72.

8 Ricardo D. Salvatore, "Stature Growth in Industrializing Argentina: The Buenos Aires Industrial Belt 1916–1950," *Explorations in Economic History* 46, no. 1 (January 2009): 72–75. From 1937 to 1947, an influx of population from the hinterland increased the city's population by thirty-seven percent according to David Rock, *Argentina, 1516–1867: From Spanish Colonization to Alfonsín* (Berkeley: University of California Press, 1987), 235.

9 For the Population of Philadelphia, see "Tuberculosis Mortality among Residents of Fifty American Cities," *Tuberculosis Reference Statistical Yearbook*, 1947 (New York: Tuberculosis and Health Association 1948), 24; for population of Philadelphia; for the city of Buenos Aires, see http://demographia.com/db-ba1869.htm (22 March 2018); depending on the statistics utilized, the population of the city of Buenos Aires varies from being proximately equal to Philadelphia to two and a half times larger.

10 Oscar Yujnovsky, "Del conventillo a la 'villa miseria,'" in José Luis Romero and Luis Alberto Romero, *Buenos Aires de historia de cuatro siglos*, vol. 2, 451–64 (Buenos Aires: Editorial Abril 1983) discusses housing in Buenos Aries from 1880 to 1980. Guillermo Rawson, "Casas de Inquilinato," in *Escritos y Discursos del Doctor Guillermo Rawson*, ed. Alberto B. Martinez (Buenos Aires: Compañía Sud-Americana de Boletes de Banco, 1891), vol. 1, 113–14; Patroni, 130; Scobie, 147–56.

11 Jacinto Velásquez, "Mortalidad por tuberculosis," *Alianza de Higiene Social* 9 (1909): 10–11. Samuel Gache, *La tuberculose dans République Argentine* (Buenos Aires: Augustín Etchepareborda, 1899), 149–50, in examining the 1896 deaths by parishes notes that the most dense populations had the largest number of cases of tuberculosis: Balvanera with 70 and San Cristóbal with 71, while the wealthiest Cathedral Norte parish had only eight and the Cathedral Sud parish had only five. But Gache did not adjust for the size of the total population in each district. Vera Blinn Reber, "Blood, Coughs, and Fever: Tuberculosis and the Working Class of Buenos Aires, Argentina, 1884–1915," *Social History of Medicine* 12, no. 1 (April 1999): 81–82.

12 Scobie, 156; Yujnovsky, 348–49, 361–63; Margarita Gutman and Jorge Enrique Hardy, *Buenos Aires: Historia urbana del área metropolitana* (Madrid: Mapfre, 1992), 159–60.

13 Juan A. Alsina, *El obrero en la República Argentina* (Buenos Aires: Imprenta, Calle de Mexico, 1905), 222; Rawson I: 161–66; James A. Baer,

"Buenos Aires and the Decline of the Liberal State in Argentina," in *Cities of Hope and Despair: People, Protests and Progress in Urbanizing Latin America, 1870–1930*, eds. Ronn Pineo and James A. Baer (Boulder: Westview Press, 1998), 130–34; Yujnovsky, 341–46; Scobie, 53, 152.

14 Yujnovsky, "Del conventillo a la 'villa miseria,'" 453 (for the percent of people living in tenements); Walter, 19; Salvatore, 2, 5–6.

15 "Mortalidad por enfermedades infecciosas en la ciudad de Buenos Aires durante los años 1895 y 1896," *Anales del Departamento Nacional de Higiene* 7, nos. 1 & 2 (January 1897): 21–23. Buenos Aires (city), *Anuario estadístico de la ciudad de Buenos Aires* (Buenos Aires: Compañía Sud-Americana de Billetes de Banco, 1900), 217. Samuel Gache, *Les logements ouvriers à Buenos Ayres* (Paris: G. Steinhell), 2 suggests that there were twenty hospitals in Buenos Aires in 1898, whereas "Mortalidad por enfermedades," *Anales del Departamento Nacional de Higiene* 6, no. 25 (1 July 1896): 403–11 lists fourteen hospitals for 1895 and "Mortalidad por enfermedades," *Anales del Departamento Nacional de Higiene* 6, no. 34 (8 September 1896): 611 lists sixteen hospitals that took tuberculosis patients in 1896. Benjamin Bryce, *To Belong in Buenos Aires: Germans, Argentines, and the Rise of a Pluralist Society* (Stanford: Stanford University Press, 2018), 31.

16 Scobie, 85–86; José C. Moya, *Cousins and Strangers: Spanish Immigrants in Buenos Aires, 1850–1930* (Berkeley: University of California Press, 1998), 149.

17 Walter, 15, 17, 236; Rock, 233; Salvatore, 3.

18 Augusto Bunge, "Las conquistas de la higiene social; Los peligros de la industria: II El ambiente del trabajo," *Anales del Departamento Nacional de Higiene* 16, no. 7 (July 1909): 260–70, 324–27.

19 Augusto Bunge, "El trabajo industrial en Buenos Aires: Informe presentado al Departamento Nacional de Higiene," *Anales del Departamento Nacional de Higiene* 11, no. 8 (August 1904): 339–42.

20 Alejandro Bunge, "Costo de la vida en la Argentina, de 1910 a 1917," *Revista de Economía Argentina* (1918): 3, 41–52, 54 for statistics; also see Roberto Cortés, *El progreso argentino, 1880–1914* (Buenos Aires: Sudamericana, 1979), which has excellent tables providing cost of living information about salaries and the cost of land and food, 257–60, 280–85; "Variaciones del salario en la ciudad de Buenos Aires," *Boletiín del Departamento Nacional de Trabajo* 19 (31 December 1911): 807–11; Julio Lezana, "Elevando los informes parciales sobre investigación de la condición económica de las clases obreras," *Boletín Departamento Nacional del Trabajo* 21 (30 November 1919): 302–3, has excellent data on workers' expenses. For tuberculosis deaths, see Nicolás Lozano, "Estadística de la mortalidad por tuberculosis en la República Argentina en el decenio de 1911–1920," *La Semana Médica* 29, no. 10 (9 March 1922): 372.

21 Walter, 235–55, provides an excellent description of Buenos Aires in the 1940s (statistics, 234–35).

22 Mary Maples Dunn and Richard S. Dunn, "The Founding, 1681–1701," in *Philadelphia: A 300-Year History*, ed. Russell Weigley (New York: W.W. Norton & Company, 1982), 7; Carolyn Adams et al., *Philadelphia: Neighborhoods, Divisions, and Conflict in a Postindustrial City* (Philadelphia: Temple University Press, 1991), 5.

23 Roger D. Simon, *Philadelphia: A Brief History* (University Park: Pennsylvania Historical Association, 2003), 38, 43; John F. Sutherland, "Housing the Poor in the City of Homes: Philadelphia at the Turn of the Century," in *The Peoples of Philadelphia: A History of Ethnic Groups and Lower Class Life,*

1790–1940, eds. Allen F. Davis and Mark H. Haller (Philadelphia: Temple University Press, 1973), 175–76, 180. Jerome P. Bjelopera, *City of Clerks: Office and Sales Workers in Philadelphia 1870–1920* (Chicago: University of Illinois Press, 2005), 144.

24 Nathaniel Burt and Wallace E. Davies, "The Iron Age 1876–1905," *Philadelphia: A 300-Year History*, ed. Russell Weigley (New York: W.W. Norton & Company, 1982), 483.

25 Carolyn Adams et al., 7. Sutherland, 184–86.

26 Burt and Davies, 495–96.

27 Hepp, 1, 177–79; Simon, 57–58. Sutherland 177–78, 181–82. Table 3.1: Comparison of White and Black TB Pulmonary Deaths in Philadelphia.

28 Hepp, 29–35. Burt and Davies, 477–79, 484–85; Walter, 37–42, 85–87, 142, 154, 190–01; Lloyd M. Abernethy, "Progressivism 1905–1919," in *Philadelphia: 300-Year History*, ed. Russell F. Weigley (New York: W.W. Norton & Company, 1982), 525–26; Arthur P. Dudden "The City Embraces 'Normalcy' in 1919–1929," in *Philadelphia: 300-Year History*, ed. Russell F. Weigley (New York: W.W. Norton & Company, 1982), 599–600.

29 Sam B. Warner, *The Private City; Philadelphia in Three Periods of Its Growth* (Philadelphia: University of Pennsylvania Press, 1968), 171; Carolyn Adams et al., *Philadelphia: Neighborhoods, Divisions*, 16–19.

30 Burt and Davies, 479–83. Abernethy, 532–33, 558–59.

31 Caroline Golab, "The Immigrant and the City: Poles, Italians and Jews in Philadelphia, 1870–1920," in *Peoples of Philadelphia: A History of Ethnic Groups and Lower-Class Life, 1790–1940*, eds. Allen F. Davis and Mark H. Haller (Philadelphia: Temple University Press, 1973), 212–13.

32 Burt and Davies, 499–501; Simon, 63; the date of the founding of the University of Pennsylvania is disputed by historians and other universities. See www.google.com/#q=http:%2F%2Fen.wikipedia.org%2Fwiki%2FUniversity_of_Pennsylvania (22 March 2018) notes one and two.

33 Joseph M. Spellissy, *Founders' Week Memorial Volume: Containing an Account of the Two Hundred and Twenty-Fifth Anniversary of the Founding of the City of Philadelphia, and Histories of Its Principal Scientific Institutions, Medical Colleges, Hospitals, etc.*, ed. Frederick P. Henry (Philadelphia: City of Philadelphia, 1909) is the primary source for identifying Philadelphia hospitals; John Frances Marion, *Philadelphia Medica: Being a Guide to the City's Historical Places of Health Interest* (SmithKline Corporation, 1975), 89–90.

34 Simon, 94–95, 97, 102–3; Margaret B. Tinkcom "Depression and War 1919–1946," *Philadelphia: A 300-Year History*, ed. Russell F. Weigley (New York: W.W. Norton & Company, 1981), 647–48; CPP, Joseph Walsh papers (hereafter JWP) "Tuberculosis Institutions," (1932), 1925–1936, vol. 6.

35 All Calculations are based on the data provided by Table 2.1: Comparative Demographics.

36 CPP, Lawrence Francis Flick, Collected Reprints (hereafter FCR), 'The Strittmatter Award, 1933 to Dr. Lawrence Flick', privately printed for The Philadelphia County Medical Society, 22 March 1933 for a resume and for Coni see Donna J. Guy, "Emilio and Gabriela Coni: Reformers, Public Health, and Working Women," in *The Human Tradition in the Human Tradition of Latin America: The Nineteenth Century*, eds. Judy Ewell and W. H. Beezley (Wilmington, DE: Scholarly Resources, 1989), 233–48. Both men were sons of French immigrants.

37 Samuel Gibson Dixon, "The Prevention of Tuberculosis," read before the section of the State Medicine of the British Medical Association at Toronto, Canada, 21 August 1906: 8; J. Woodrow Savacool, "Philadelphia and the White Plague," *Transactions and Studies of the College of Physicians ser.* 5, 8, no. 3 (1986): 165.
38 David McBride, "Henry Phipps Institute, 1903–1937: Pioneering Tuberculosis Work with an Urban Minority," *Bulletin of the History of Medicine* 61, no. 1 (1987): 80–81; Lawrence Francis Flick, "Henry Phipps Institute for the Study, Treatment and Prevention of Tuberculosis," *Philadelphia Medical Journal* (31 January 1903): 208–9; Frank A. Craig, *Early Days at Phipps* (Philadelphia: University of Pennsylvania, 1952), 4, 7, 37; Savacool, 159.
39 Lawrence F. Flick, "The Work of the First Year," *First Annual Report of the Henry Phipps Institute for the Study, Treatment, and Prevention of Tuberculosis* (Philadelphia: Henry Phipps Institute, 1905), 11, 17.
40 Craig, *Early Days at Phipps*, 24–26.
41 CPP, JWP, vol. 2, Phipps Institute, 1905–1910, "Official Address, 1908"; Craig, 20–21; Savacool, 161.
42 Craig, 15–17, 22; Michael E. Teller, *The Tuberculosis Movement: A Public Health Campaign in the Progressive Era* (New York: Greenwood Press, 1988), 80–81.
43 Craig, *Early Days at Phipps*, 25; University of Pennsylvania (hereafter UP) University Archives and Records Center (hereafter GA), Phipps Institute (hereafter AGPI) 1918, "Report of the Advisory Council of the Henry Phipps Institute at its Meeting on Saturday, 9 November 1918; American Philosophical Society (hereafter APS), Eugene Opie Papers (hereafter OP), biography; UP, GA, Alfred Newton Richard Papers(hereafter ANRP), UPT 50/R514 Organizations; UP, GA, AGPI, Third Party Correspondence, 1934–1935, Box 15, ff 17., pp. 1–4.
44 Pennsylvania Society for the Prevention of Tuberculosis "Work among the Negroes of Pennsylvania," *Annual Report 1916* (Philadelphia, 1916): 10; McBride, "Henry Phipps Institute," 86; Craig, *Early Days at Phipps*, 27–28; David McBride, *Integrating the City of Medicine: Blacks in Philadelphia Health Care, 1910–1965* (Philadelphia: Temple University Press, 1988), 42, 50, 66–68.
45 "Phipps Institute," *Old Penn* (Weekly Review of the University of Pennsylvania), 8: 15 (22 January 1910): 2; McBride, "Henry Phipps Institute," 81, 90; UP, GA, AGPI, 1910, no. 2 "Report of the Committee Appointed by the Provost to Consider Plans for the Future Operation of the Phipps Institute," 4.
46 Eva S. Leake, "The Henry Phipps Institute: Recollections of a Foreign Research Fellow," *Transactions & Studies of the College of Physicians of Philadelphia* 3, no. 4 (December 1981): 257, 259–62.
47 Emilio R. Coni, "La campaña contra la tuberculosis en la República Argentina," *La Semana Médica* 16, no. 41 (14 October 1909): 1447.
48 "Hospital para tuberculosos," *La Semana Medica* 11, no. 41 (13 October 1904): 1110; Coni, "La campaña contra la tuberculosis" (14 October 1909): 1447; Alberto B. Martínez, *Censo general de población edificaciones, comercio e industrias de la ciudad Buenos Aires, levantado en los días 11 y 18 septiembre de 1904* (Buenos Aires: Cía. Sudamericana de Billetes de Banco, 1906), 319–20.
49 Coni, 1437–1449, provided a detailed description of the structure. "Liga Argentina contra la tuberculosis: Informe, anual de su presidente correspondiente al año 1907," *Alianza de Higiene Social* 7 (1907–1908): 333;

Emilio R. Coni, *Higiene Social: asistencia y previsión social Buenos Aires caritativo y previsor* (Buenos Aires: Imprenta de Emilio Spinella Ed. 1918), 432–35; "Sanatorio Municipal Doctor Tornú," *Lucha Antituberculosa* 4, no. 12 (12 May 1905): 531–35; "Hospital para tuberculosos," 1110. Manuel Schneier, "Hospital Tornú," *Mundo Hospitalario* 27 (November 1941): 55–56; Martínez, *Censo general,* 319.

50 Schneier, 55–56.

51 Coni, 1437; "Sanatorio Municipal Doctor Tornú," 533–35; Emilio R. Coni, "La Lucha antituberculosa en la República Argentina," *La Lucha Antituberculosa* 5, nos. 4–8 (1905): 172–74.

52 Coni, 170–78; Coni, 1449, provides weekly amounts of various foods served patients. "Sanatorio Municipal Doctor Tornú," 536; Martínez, *Censo general*, 319–20.

53 Coni, "La Lucha antituberculosa en la República," 172–79; "La asistencia de los tuberculosos pobres en Buenos Aires," *La Lucha Antituberculosa* 5, no. 3 (1905): 85–87; Alberto Martinez, *Censo general*, 320; "En el Hospital Tornú: Un caso Grave," *La Vanguardia*, 28 August 1914, p. 2.

54 The author's visit to Hospital Dr. Enrique Tornú, November 1995.

55 Philadelphia, *Annual Message of Mayor of the City of Philadelphia with Annual Report of the Bureau of Health for 1930* (Philadelphia 1930), 300; Table 2.2: Comparison of Number of Deaths due to Epidemic Diseases.

56 Kathryn Lougheed, *Catching Breath: The Making and Unmaking of Tuberculosis* (London: Bloomsburg Sigma, 2017), 106–7.

57 "A Note on the Course of Pulmonary Tuberculosis Mortality since 1914," *Public Health Reports (1896–1970)* 36, no. 21 (27 May 1921): 1181 compares U.S., Great Britain and Spain and find a similar pattern.

3 Immigrants, Migrants and Public Health Policies in Buenos Aires and Philadelphia

> Santiago Marchinelli, twenty-four years of age, an Italian living in Buenos Aires, prematurely grey, appears robust but weak with little appetite ... His paternal grandfather, an uncle, and an aunt had all died of tuberculosis and his father and sister were tubercular. When a child, he had been sickly, often coughing. In 1886, he had bloody mucus (hemoptysis) for ten months... he was always ill with a cough and light hemoptysis until May 1891 when he entered the hospital for a five-month stay... but after two months with a family in the country, his health first improved and then deteriorated, and he returned to hospital.[1]

> F.M. Kirby of Wilkes Barre, Pennsylvania wrote Lawrence Flick on 27 August 1915. He had several colored house servants, one who was Ed Rasper. In the previous year, he developed rheumatism and was sent to Hot Springs, Arkansas; he returned much better, but was again stricken a few months later, so he was sent back. Kirby received a letter in which Ed stated that he had TB and wanted to return to die. Kirby wanted to know whether Ed could be admitted to the White Haven Sanatorium.[2]

An Italian immigrant in Buenos Aires and an African American in Philadelphia displayed the medical symptoms of tuberculosis and faced treatment choices. Although tubercular individuals had unique experiences, their class and ethnicity contributed to their specific problems. The working poor—among them African Americans in Philadelphia and recent immigrants in Buenos Aires—encountered middle-class prejudices in seeking to obtain treatment. At the same time, the substandard working and living conditions that immigrants and migrants faced contributed significantly to their contracting tuberculosis.

In the early nineteenth century, public health specialists in most industrializing urban areas, including Buenos Aires and Philadelphia, were becoming more concerned about the increasing incidences of tuberculosis. Because elite citizens and national governments frequently believed that immigrants and the poor spread tuberculosis, policies aimed at preventing it often targeted the working class and the poor. Public health officials sought to improve public health through disinfection policies, hygienic measures and changes in the morals of the poor. The diverse ethnicities and large numbers of immigrants in both Buenos Aires and Philadelphia added to the public health concerns. The growing international consensus on the nature and treatment of tuberculosis shaped the development of similar public policies in the two cities, despite the thousands of miles that separated them.

Porteño Attitudes toward Immigrants

During much of the nineteenth century, the Buenos Aires population was primarily divided into two classes: the upper class of rural and city landowners, bankers, merchants and investors, which held most of the wealth of the community, and a working class of semiskilled and day laborers. From the late nineteenth century until the start of World War I, immigrants contributed to the country's economic expansion, demographic growth, social diversity and the rise of a middle class of white-collar workers, petty manufacturers and shopkeepers. In turn, Argentina offered foreigners economic and social mobility. In Buenos Aires, wages for skilled and semi-skilled manual laborers were double and triple those in Italy, Spain and France. By 1909, foreigners in Buenos Aires dominated the ownership of real estate, industry and commerce. Recognizing the value of immigrants, Argentina actively recruited them and initially offered them social services. Those who traveled second- and third-class on ships stayed free at government expense at the immigrant hotel. At the same time, Argentine nationals were concerned about the health of immigrants, worrying in particular that they might bring contagious diseases with them. Physicians examined foreigners to ensure they were healthy before immigrants could enter the country.[3]

The censuses of 1909 and 1914 indicated that foreigners comprised between thirty-five and sixty-six percent of the population of Buenos Aires. Although foreigners made up three-fourths of the city's working class, Buenos Aires had the least segregated ethnic residences of any major city in the Americas. No single foreign nationality or particular village dominated a district or even a few blocks. It was normal for people of different nationalities to live in the same block. But in spite of the mixed ethnic communities, there was little intermarriage between members of different nationalities, and there were also few social interactions among them. When foreign immigration began to decline in the 1920s, internal migration augmented the city's growth. After World War II, foreign immigrants continued to arrive, but never in the numbers of the pre-1914 era. Argentine and Latin American migrants joined the half million new European immigrants who came to Buenos Aires immediately after World War II. By the 1950s, three-fourths of the Buenos Aires population was Argentine-born.[4]

The high cost of living created a difficult environment for the working class. Real wages fell during the recession years of 1874–1878 and 1890–1893 leading to unemployment and increased emigration. Declining wages, high living costs and the restricted nature of the Argentine political system attracted workers to anarchism and syndicalism. While anarchism first appeared in the 1880s among Italian and Spanish immigrants, the movement's appeal grew after 1899, when wages declined and rents increased. Argentine authorities sought to prevent immigrants from participating in civil conflicts, and city laws prevented them from taking part in the political system. Although some immigrants joined the syndicalist movements, they rarely chose to become citizens. The 1869 Argentine citizenship law entitled foreigners to become citizens and vote after residing in the country for two years. But because foreigners were free to move around the country, marry, own property and avoid military service, they saw little civil or political advantage in citizenship. In 1895, only 0.2 percent of the foreign-born population of Buenos Aires was naturalized; by 1914, the number had increased to only 2.3 percent.[5]

Argentines were ambivalent about foreigners and what was foreign. The elite read French literature, went to Italian operas, studied German science and bought English products, but they often distrusted lower-class immigrants. Nevertheless, the upper class supported immigration and viewed immigrants as hard workers. In contrast, lower-class Porteños, who competed with foreigners for services and jobs, tended to denigrate the new arrivals and were often anti-immigrant. The Buenos Aires Afro-Argentine press often expressed anti-immigration sentiments. Two groups in particular suffered from discrimination: Afro-Argentines and Jews. At the same time, Argentines did not see themselves as racist and discriminatory. They defined racism as hostility towards members of a culture or race different from their own. Because Porteños did not regard themselves as hostile, they did not view themselves as racist.[6]

Italians in Buenos Aires

Italians comprised the largest ethnic group in Buenos Aires. The first Italians settled in La Boca, the port area of Buenos Aires. By the 1870s, depressed crop prices in Europe and the development of farming colonies in Argentina encouraged rural immigrants from southern Italy to go to Buenos Aires. Of the 725,000 Italians who immigrated to Argentina between 1876 and 1896, seventy-three percent were farmers and another ten percent came from rural areas. By 1895, Italians represented fifty-three percent of all foreigners in Buenos Aires and lived throughout the city; as a result, at least nineteen percent of its inhabitants of all but one of the city's districts were Italians. In 1914, Italians comprised thirty-nine percent of the city's population.[7]

From 1880 to 1910, seventy-one percent of the Italian immigrants worked in blue-collar jobs. Women worked primarily in personal services and the clothing industry and held few white-collar jobs. Both Italian men and women, who overwhelmingly occupied skilled and unskilled jobs in industry and who hoped to ensure the passage of beneficial labor legislation, participated in strikes and joined the labor movement. Many Italian immigrants started their own businesses. At the same time, their large numbers make them the focus of elite anti-tuberculosis policies.[8] By the 1870s, Italians had discarded loyalties to their regions of origin in Italy and instead supported institutions that aided their entire community. Italian-language newspapers greatly expanded from 1890 to 1910 and helped unify the Italian community, while mutual aid societies—which provided insurance for Italians facing economic difficulties—supported families. By 1910, there were approximately seventy-five mutual aid societies in Buenos Aires with 52,000 members, of which seventeen percent were women. The inadequacy of medical care persuaded the Italian community in 1853 to build a hospital. By 1919, the hospital included isolation wards for individuals with infectious diseases. It analyzed saliva at no charge so as to diagnose tuberculosis.[9]

Family was important to Italians. Although up to forty percent of the Italian immigrant population returned to Italy before 1900, those who remained adjusted to life in Argentina. Italians who chose to reside permanently in Buenos Aires sent little money back to Italy, but instead invested their savings in homes, mutual aid societies, schools and businesses. In 1872, prominent Italian businessmen founded the Banco de Italia y Río de la Plata, which provided financial support for the community and strengthened the Italian influence. In spite of their growing economic power, Italian immigrants rarely participated directly in the political system (which before 1912 depended on a small Argentine elite). Although most Italians were Catholic, the limited number of priests, the anticlerical attitude of some community leaders, and Argentine government restrictions on church involvement in politics limited the ability of the Italian parishes to shape public policies. Italians did, however, create pressure groups. They also worked with their labor unions through petitions and demonstrations to influence political decisions and health policies.[10]

Spanish Immigrants

Spaniards came to Buenos Aires in increasing numbers during the first decade of the twentieth century and became a significant immigrant community after the Italians did. Only in 1914 did Spaniards—who numbered 306,850—represent nineteen percent of the population of Buenos Aires and thirty-eight percent of the foreign-born population. Ninety-two percent of the Spanish immigrants were unskilled or semi-skilled. In contrast to Italian women who rarely worked as servants, Spanish women in Buenos Aires were concentrated in domestic services and were often falsely blamed for the spread of tuberculosis to elite families. Because of their late arrival, Spaniards were slower than others to own their own homes. In 1909, only 8.2 percent of Buenos Aires homes were owned by Spaniards. By contrast, 14.5 percent of homes were owned by Italians and nineteen percent were owned by the French.[11]

In 1852, Spanish immigrants published their first newspaper and established their first social club. The Sociedad Española de Beneficencia was founded in 1857. Its main function was to provide free medical care for destitute compatriots and to run the Spanish hospital, which by 1919 could serve 250 patients. At the turn of the century, the Sociedad was the wealthiest private voluntary association in Argentina. As Spanish immigration increased, the number of associations that aided the Spanish community grew: there were only eight such associations in 1864, compared to 237 in 1925. The number of publications grew from two in 1864 to thirteen in 1914. The Banco Español y del Rio de la Plata, founded by immigrant merchants in the 1870s, became by 1914 the largest private bank in South America.[12]

In common with other immigrant communities, the Spanish established mutual aid societies which by 1894 were open to all economic classes and welcomed women as well as men. The oldest Spanish mutual aid society, AESM, with 33,000 members in 1920, became the largest in Argentina. By 1920, nearly 100,000 Spaniards belonged to mutual aid societies, which provided for disability care, visits to physicians, medical treatment and burial services. More working-class immigrants joined mutual aid societies than labor unions. Although immigrants tended to prefer ethnic associations to radical labor organizations, by 1902, twenty-three percent of Porteño anarchists were Spaniards. At that time, Spaniards represented only eleven percent of the city's population. Like other immigrants and in spite of a common language and history with Argentina, recent Spanish immigrants did not participate in Buenos Aires politics; and only four percent became Argentine citizens.[13]

The Jewish Population of Buenos Aires

The Jewish population of Buenos Aires represented Argentina's third largest immigrant group. Immigrants from Eastern Europe and Russia comprised over eighty percent of the total Jewish population. Immigrants clustered first near the city's core and port area but eventually moved into the northern and western parts of the city, where they had their businesses, synagogues and religious organizations. In 1936, the Jewish population rose to 120,195 or five percent of the city's population; by 1947, it increased to more than 150,000. In that year, two-thirds of the nation's Jewish population lived in Buenos Aires. Although

Jewish families dispersed throughout the city, they remained six times more segregated than other migrant communities.[14] At the beginning of the twentieth century, more than half the Jewish immigrants were in the working class and suffered poor working conditions. They worked in petty commerce and dominated the production of cheap furniture and clothing. Those who labored in sub-cellars, in the intense oven-heat of bakeries and in the garment industry's poorly ventilated buildings often supported a militant labor movement. During the Semana Trágica, the week of 7 January 1919 in which an initial general strike turned violent, the police and army sent to restore order targeted foreign workers and, in particular, the Jewish population and organizations; Jews were blamed unfairly both for the labor unrest and spreading disease. However, increasingly Jews entered the middle class; they became physicians, pharmacists and engineers and benefited from increased wages of labor during the 1940s.[15]

Like other immigrant groups, Jewish organizations provided support to community members. The oldest, wealthiest and most important Jewish organization was the Chevra Kadisha Ashkenazi, which was established in 1895 to ensure that Jews could have traditional burials. Synagogues had limited significance in the late nineteenth century when Jewish shops mostly remained open on Saturdays and Jews in Buenos Aires appeared indifferent to Jewish observance. Jews coming from the eastern regions of Europe and North Africa brought different traditions with them; as a result, the number of synagogues increased from one in the 1870s to half a dozen by the 1900s and (remarkably) 120 by the 1930s. The Zionist movement in Buenos Aires grew only slowly with the creation of the state of Israel, as most Argentine Jews remained ambivalent about it. Hebrew was spoken by only a few of the educated elite, while the general Jewish public spoke Yiddish. Buenos Aires in the 1930s became a center of Yiddish theater.[16]

Argentine Jews donated money, clothing and food through an increasing number of associations to help poor and sick community members. The first pavilion of Hospital Israelita was inaugurated in 1921, and in 1928, a second pavilion increased the number of beds from 65 to 189. However, the pavilions had no space in which tubercular patients could be isolated. By 1930, Jews in Argentina also supported two orphanages and an old-age home.[17] Although overt discrimination fluctuated, Jews faced more prejudice than other immigrants. Argentine students read textbooks that denigrated Jews. Some Catholic groups disseminated anti-Semitic propaganda. Anti-Jewish sentiment in the early twentieth century was particularly directed at Jewish worker organizations since the Argentine elite thought that Jewish radicals promoted class conflict. As a result, some Jews in Buenos Aires hid their ethnic origin; the community also de-emphasized its religious and cultural heritage and exerted no political influence.[18]

French, German and British Immigrants

The French, German and British immigrants, similar to the Italians and Spanish, formed cohesive cultural communities in Buenos Aires. Of the three, the French immigrants represented the largest group. Although French immigrants arrived in Buenos Aires from 1857 to 1925, the height of immigration, 1885–1891, was when large numbers of male working class came from France.[19] Although class determined where the French lived in Buenos Aires, they initially concentrated in districts in the center and north of the city. Similar to other immigrant communities, the French elite helped working-class immigrants adapt to the city. The French community founded the French hospital in 1845, the second hospital of an immigrant community in Buenos Aires. Mutual aid societies, among the most important French associations, provided its members with financial, educational and legal support. The French elite founded Club Français in 1866, just as the Italians (Circolo Italiano), Germans (Club Alemán) and the British (The English Club) founded their own associations. The celebration of festivals, particularly Bastille Day, unified the community, and by linking the July 14th celebration to Argentine independence, Franco-Argentine citizens sought to become a part of Buenos Aires life. The French press united the immigrant community. By the 1860s, there were thirteen French newspapers; the best known was *Le Courrier de la Plata*, which existed for eighty-one years.[20]

The French community differed from other foreign communities in its efforts to expand French cultural influence in Argentina. For example, French schools catered not only to children of French immigrants but also sought to attract Porteño children and to promote the French language and culture. French became the Porteño's second language; bookstores in the city sold classic and contemporary French literature. As early as the 1820s, French residents were teaching the language and administrating schools. By the end of the century, Argentine students learned French in high school and studied French literature at university. In 1893, the first Alliance Française, a French government agency, opened in Buenos Aires. Because many Porteños viewed Paris as the capital of the civilized world, they sought to make Buenos Aires in its image. Argentine intellectuals, architects and engineers studied in Paris; their education influenced their ideas about how to reform Argentine society. Although French remained a second language for the Porteño elite, the arrival of large numbers of Spanish and Italian immigrants at the end of the nineteenth century decreased the French influence in Buenos Aires.[21]

Benjamin Bryce, in his monograph, *To Belong in Buenos Aires,* argues that affluent German immigrants used their positions and wealth to promote an idealized community in which healthy men financially supported their families through work and contributed to the greater Buenos

Aires community. Germans owned bakeries, bookstores, restaurants, retail shops, import-export companies and served as directors of diverse companies. These affluent Germans supported a hospital, charity institutions, bilingual schools and mutual aid societies. These institutions provided a support system for working-class German immigrants.[22]

The German hospital, similar to other ethnic-run hospitals of Buenos Aires sought to provide health care to two groups of patients: paying customers of all ethnicities and poor German-speakers. Campaigns were carried out to raise contributions to offer free treatment to German-speaking, working-class patients. Similar to other elite Porteño health institutions, men controlled the organizations, but women contributed their labor and fundraising abilities. In 1896, they created the German Women's Home charity, the only German organization completely focused on working-class women. Like similar organizations of Porteña woman, the German Women's Home charity sought to improve the sexual morality of working-class women. These elite women desired to assure the upright standing of working-class women, so they would provide a positive view of the German community to the larger Buenos Aires community.[23]

There were more British nationals than Germans in Argentina from 1895 through 1914, but the most significant British immigrant influence was during the nineteenth century.[24] In 1806, new commercial opportunities attracted merchants to Buenos Aires. British merchants were self-sufficient and cohesive; they focused on preserving British values and commercial success, not on exporting culture. The British Friendly Society of Buenos Aires helped immigrants adapt to city life. British immigrants founded English language Anglican, Presbyterian and Methodist churches and supported a boy's and a girl's school under the auspices of the Church of England. In 1843, British residents agreed to establish a hospital to serve the community. Investors, resident in England, founded The Bank of London and River Plate in 1865. Britons invested in Argentine financial institutions, shipping, railroads, extractive industries, meat preservation and agriculture. Before 1914, Great Britain was for investment and capital what France was for culture. After 1900, investment capital from France and Germany competed with British funds.[25]

Discrimination Against Afro-Argentines and Rural Migrants

In 1887, Afro-Argentines numbered only 8,005 or 1.8 percent of the population; by 1970, there were not more than three or four thousand Afro-Argentines in a city of eight million. Traditionally, Afro-Argentines worked as porters, petty vendors and domestic servants, but during the decades between 1880 and 1910 Buenos Aires' dependence on their manual labor declined, as Italians willingly performed such work for less pay. With the loss of positions in manual labor, a few

Afro-Argentines moved into government work to serve as orderlies and secretaries. Afro-Argentines often faced conflicts with immigrants over housing. By the 1870s, Afro-Argentines were leaving neighborhoods in the center city because of rising rents and animosity and were moving to outlying areas of the city.[26]

Although from 1850 to 1900, an Afro-Argentine press sought to unify the community, politics, class and culture divided it. In the 1860s and 1870s, Afro-Argentine mutual aid societies—which provided funds for expenses caused by illnesses and deaths—declined, as young Afro-Argentines sought to distance themselves from their African origins. Although mulattoes viewed themselves as members of the Buenos Aires white-collar class, white Porteños saw them as impoverished Afro-Argentines. Because of community disunity and their small numbers, Afro-Argentines founded no hospitals. By the end of the nineteenth-century, discrimination led the Afro-Argentine middle class to join the working class in seeking to improve wages and working conditions.[27]

Rural workers from Argentina's interior provinces and from other Latin American countries were the last group to arrive in Buenos Aires in large numbers. Between 1914 and 1935, migrants from the hinterland contributed five percent to the growth of greater Buenos Aires. On average, 70,000 such migrants came to Buenos Aires per year between 1937 and 1943, but that number increased to 117,000 between 1943 and 1947. Newly arriving migrants faced discrimination from earlier arrivals. They also occupied the poorest paid and lowest status jobs in domestic service and construction. When they obtained jobs in industry, migrants from the interior became the backbone of union membership during Juan Peron's presidency (1946–1955, 1973–1974); union membership quadrupled between 1945 and 1949. As the interior farming districts became more impoverished, migration to Buenos Aires increased, but urban manufacturing could not provide jobs for all the migrants. Facing high unemployment and underemployment, many migrants lived in shanty towns situated around the capital. Porteños looked down on Indians and mestizos from the interior, likening them to Afro-Argentines. The elite and the middle class blamed the new groups for contributing to the public health issues confronting the city.[28]

Immigration and Porteño Government Health Services

The arrival of large numbers of immigrants and migrants challenged the Buenos Aires municipal government. Only slowly did the city provide the needed water and sewage services and deal with the unhealthy working and living conditions. The limited political influence of immigrant groups ensured that native-born Porteños shaped Buenos Aires' public conversation and defined tuberculosis policies affecting foreigners and migrants. Much of the public discourse in Buenos Aires between 1870 and 1945 focused on two themes: What sorts of immigrants were desirable? How could the national character be improved?

The Argentine upper class was concerned that the increased number of immigrants and the lack of laws regulating their behavior contributed to the spread of contagious diseases and dangerous ideas, and to the growth of a criminal class. They thought that their homes suffered from what historians have defined as "moral contagion": a working-class immorality reflected in alcoholism, prostitution, suicide and anarchism. The elite incorrectly alleged that maids and gardeners introduced ignorance and bad habits to their homes. The upper class also believed that neither the rich nor the poor could avoid physical and moral contagion: filthy streets, inadequate sewers and over-crowded slums that produced tuberculosis, syphilis and madness. Only by improving the urban environment and individual morality could the good health of citizens be assured. Health experts thought that the city needed to be reorganized: they perceived that parts of the city amounted to a "degenerate space" that supported immorality and crime. Public health officials also believed that tuberculosis could be overcome only by improving the living and working conditions of the lower classes and conquering both physical and moral contagion. Earlier epidemics supported elite fears about contagious disease. On the other hand, the idea of moral contagion was nebulous and reflected elite prejudices against immigrants and the working class.[29]

Emilio Coni provided the necessary medical leadership in Buenos Aires to confront the new urban public health challenges. When in 1892, the municipality of Buenos Aires divided the Asistencia Pública into two divisions (Asistencia Pública and the Administración Sanitaria), it created a centralized authority to administer public assistance programs and to regulate health practices. Between 1895 and 1915, the municipality implemented a series of reforms that sought to improve the sanitary conditions of the city and thereby to prevent the spread of tuberculosis. These regulations dealt with the services offered by public hospitals and clinics, care for children and pregnant women, disinfection of the homes of contagious patients, and the conditions under which meat and milk were handled and served.[30]

Buenos Aires passed legislation in 1892 reflecting the assumption that tuberculosis was contagious. The Asistencia Pública sought to prevent the spread of tuberculosis by requiring physicians to report new tuberculosis cases within twenty-four hours of their identification, so that the apartment buildings in which the patients lived could be disinfected and the sick isolated. Families were to bring those with pulmonary tuberculosis to the Hospital Muñiz, where patients with contagious diseases were isolated in special rooms. In 1888, the Buenos Aires government began to disinfect the homes of those dying of contagious disease, but it was hampered by a shortage of personnel. With additional hires and the purchase of new steam equipment for fumigation, the services expanded two years later. In 1892, the Buenos Aires government began requiring that houses be disinfected if individuals had died of yellow fever, smallpox or tuberculosis. Public health officials also recommended that chloride be used to wash doors, walls and floor. The rooms were fumigated with sulfur, and the walls were repainted. These municipal regulations were, however, usually ignored for several reasons: diagnosis was unreliable, families did not wish to leave their lodgings, and landlords did not want to submit to the inconvenience and expense of disinfection (even though they risked incurring a fine if they knowingly rented an infected room). Thus, the number of those dying of tuberculosis far exceeded the number of rooms being disinfected.[31]

The Argentine Anti-Tuberculosis League increased efforts to combat tuberculosis by supporting municipal passage of new sanitation laws. The league worked to make the public aware of contagion and increased public concern for the sick and their families. Disinfection came to be applied not only to homes but also to public spaces such as trams, railway carriages, coaches and theaters. Libraries were to disinfect their books, and banks were to decontaminate their notes. Ordinances prohibited those with tuberculosis from selling food or working in restaurants. The municipal legislation also prohibited spitting on the streets and in public places. All public places—including hospitals, schools, restaurants, hotels, factories, churches and theaters—were to have spittoons. Factory owners were to provide workers with their own drinking cups and to improve the sanitation in working places by disinfecting latrines and washrooms, installing ventilators to limit dust, and making certain that workers did not wear clothes that touched the ground and might pick up dust containing tubercular bacilli. The social drinking of mate (dried leaves from a yerba mate plant found in Argentina, Paraguay and Brazil that has similarities in preparation and social use to Asia teas) provided a unique challenge to Argentine medical officials. The communal sharing of the mate gourd with a bombilla (a straw filter) could potentially transmit the tuberculosis bacteria. The failure of public officials to directly condemn mate use may reflect two factors: first, tuberculosis was viewed as an immigrant disease and second, health officials sought to improve the morals of the working class and focused on decreased alcohol consumption and improved personal hygiene.[32]

The medical professionals believed that the cheapness of beef in Argentina helped prevent tuberculosis, because it enabled the poor to eat it on a regular basis. Beef is, of course, rich in protein, which is crucial for building up resistance to disease; its consumption probably lowered tuberculosis mortality rates in the city. Unfortunately, food was often of poor quality and impurity. Meat, bread, milk and wine were often adulterated. As early as 1896, the municipal council of Buenos Aires banned free-roaming cows and required all cows in the city to be inoculated with tuberculin. But ten years later, less than a third of the cows had been tested for tuberculosis. Beginning in 1907, milk sold in Buenos Aires was to be sterilized or pasteurized. By 1909, the city's six municipal dispensaries and charity dispensaries provided children with free or low-priced sterilized milk. However, the municipal government enforced regulations haphazardly so that those on limited budgets continued to buy poor-quality food.[33]

Although during the twentieth century the municipal and national governments were primarily responsible for public health efforts and social welfare assistance in Buenos Aires, two semiprivate organizations increased the aid to the urban poor and sought to change working-class values. The national government funded welfare for the poor through the Sociedad de Beneficencia, a secular charity founded by the Argentine government in 1823. The Roman Catholic Church organized the Conferencias de Señoras de San Vicente de Paul, which was initially operated by Catholic women and focused on teaching middle-class values to the lower classes.

The elite women who operated the Sociedad de Beneficencia developed criteria for determining who should and should not obtain the aid. Although the Sociedad provided some cash to the needy, few individuals received direct help; instead, most of the funding went to hospitals and asylums. By 1905, elite Porteño women operated at least twelve hospitals and orphanages. In addition, the Sociedad women provided shelters for women and children, staffed soup kitchens for pregnant women and workers, and operated schools for children. They raised funds from private groups and organizations and also received funds from the national lottery. The Sociedad succeeded in incorporating women into public life through their involvement in the care of the poor. The Sociedad believed that tubercular women were among those most in need of reforming and deserved charity. It was, therefore, instrumental in raising funds for the construction of pavilions for tubercular patients in existing hospitals and building new tubercular hospitals for women and children.[34]

The Conferencias de Señoras de San Vicente de Paul, which involved Catholic women was more inclusive than the Sociedad de Beneficencia because it encouraged women of all classes to provide leadership and service. Through cooperation with the state government, the Señoras regularly contributed funds and goods and helped workers obtain low-cost housing. Recognizing that women might work outside the home to support their families, the Señoras taught principles of good home management, so that women could both improve their home life and work as domestics rather than go into prostitution. Lodgings for single women, workshops teaching women how to apply for jobs and to develop their talents, and efforts to make the workplace safe for women recognized the needs of lower-class women. By visiting homes, the Señoras sought to teach the poor how to live healthy lives. In its first twenty-five years of existence (1889–1914), the Señoras made 2,009,125 home visits and assisted 120,351 families. However, in spite of their efforts, their services were too limited to meet all the needs of the large female immigrant population. At the same time, the male hierarchy of the Catholic Church, recognized the successes of the Conferencias de Señoras de San Vicente de Paul. By 1930, it took over its programs.[35]

Buenos Aires' charity institutions served two broad functions. They ensured the integration and supervision of the women who received aid, and they enabled women to raise money for social causes and to work with the poor. Children were a particular focus; the charitable organizations believed that teaching children would benefit both society and the children themselves.[36] In addition, the municipal government created new organizations, such as the Patronato de la Infancia, to demonstrate that women could play important roles in aiding children. Society encouraged women's good works, and the models of the charitable woman appeared frequently in popular middle-class literature. Schools and teachers were also converted into agents of change. Even the poor contributed by providing funds for orphans and abandoned children. Home visits were seen as a means of social control. Public health officials thought that by shaping the values of immigrants, improving their living conditions and ending prostitution, the poor would learn social discipline and societal stability would be maintained.[37] Officials' expectations were unrealistic because values are difficult to change, improving living conditions required increased income and women with no skills in a difficult labor market have few employment options.

By 1914, the Buenos Aires municipal government provided many residents with water, sewerage, lighting, garbage collection, police protection and schools. The increased availability of affordable housing in greater Buenos Aires improved the living conditions for migrants and immigrants. Disinfection regulations and anti-spitting laws seemed to persuade the middle class that efforts were being made to prevent the poor and immigrants from spreading infection. The increased amount of green space in the center of the city beautified Buenos Aires and encouraged the middle class to continue to reside in it. Yet, in spite of the efforts of the Buenos Aires's public health department, the city was dependent on private charities to provide additional services to the urban poor.

Immigration to Philadelphia

The immigrant population of Philadelphia reached its peak in 1870 when twenty-eight percent of Philadelphians were immigrants. The figure receded slightly to twenty-five percent by 1910. At that time more than forty percent of New York City's and Chicago's population—and fifty percent of Buenos Aires' population—consisted of immigrants.

After 1880, the number of immigrants from Great Britain and Northern Europe decreased and more immigrants came from Russia and Italy. From 1870 to 1910, the population of Philadelphia more than doubled, due primarily to migrants from elsewhere in the U.S. and immigrants.[38] The African-American population also expanded in the twentieth century. By 1910, African Americans, coming primarily from the rural south, made up 5.6 percent of the city's population. As the middle class grew, center-city Philadelphia became the place to work, to shop and to be entertained.[39]

By 1920—when there were 400,744 foreign-born Philadelphians—the largest ethnic groups were as follows: 95,744 Russians; 64,590 Irish; 63,723 Italians; 39,766 Germans; 31,112 Poles; and 30,886 English. The immigrants who arrived most recently were Jews, Italians and Poles. Nevertheless, Philadelphia's immigrant population was proportionally smaller than the immigrant population of most other large U.S. cities.[40] Specific foreign groups settled in particular cities and districts within those cities. For example, early in the twentieth century, some groups such as the Poles and Italians competed for factory jobs; when Italians secured more of those jobs in Philadelphia, many Poles began to go elsewhere. Between 1910 and 1920, seventy percent of foreign-born Italians lived in four adjacent districts in South Philadelphia and nearly fifty percent of the Russian-Jewish population lived in the same districts. As in Buenos Aires, neighborhoods contained residents of diverse ethnicities.[41]

German Immigrants in Philadelphia

The posting of signs in both German and English in late eighteenth-century Philadelphia demonstrates the significance of German migration during the colonial period. Like other immigrant communities, Germans established social clubs that welcomed immigrants from a particular German region and founded mutual-aid societies to increase their economic security. Several German language newspapers existed. But the German immigrants were also divided by ethnic, religious, regional and social differences. For example, the split between Catholics and Protestants explained why the German community supported two different hospitals. In 1860, the Pennsylvania state legislature—assisted by private donors—supported the founding of the German Hospital. The hospital accepted tuberculosis patients of all nationalities and races. In the same year, Franciscan nuns opened St. Francis Hospital to serve German Catholics. St Mary's hospital, which replaced St. Francis in 1866, accepted poor consumptive patients of other faiths because it faced financial challenges with the decline of German Catholics. In the first half of the twentieth-century, Germans represented between one and five percent of Philadelphia's population.[42]

The Jewish Population of Philadelphia

Seventy percent of the Jews who came to Pennsylvania settled in Philadelphia. They founded synagogues, charitable associations, mutual-aid societies, medical organizations, orphanages, educational institutions, social clubs and newspapers. As early as 1866, Jewish philanthropists founded a general hospital and the Lucien Moss Home for incurables that primarily housed consumptive patients. The community continued to expand its hospitals; in 1902, it received funds from the Commonwealth of Pennsylvania to care for patients with contagious diseases. Jewish immigrants were divided by ethnicity and class. Before 1870, Yiddish-speaking men and women from Russia and Poland settled in the port area and kept aloof from German-speaking Jews. Subsequent immigrants from Russia and Eastern Europe settled in South Philadelphia and contributed to the overcrowding of the area and the resulting housing shortage. By 1930, there were more Jewish immigrants than Italian immigrants, and affluent Jews were moving to better housing in West Philadelphia.[43]

The Irish and Italians in Philadelphia

A great influx of rural Irish came to Philadelphia after the potato famine of 1846–1847. By 1870, Philadelphia had more Irish immigrants (who represented 14.35 percent of all immigrants) than Germans immigrants (who represented only 7.53 percent of all immigrants). The Irish represented the largest foreign-born group in Philadelphia; in 1880, one-half of the city's population was Irish of descent and one-third in 1900. The population growth of the Irish community correlated with the city's physical expansion and industrialization. Philadelphia offered Irish immigrants greater job opportunities, longer lives and a higher standing of living than other U.S. cities. Irish immigrants supported the expansion of Catholic schools, orphanages and medical institutions. In 1849, St. Joseph's Hospital opened to serve primarily Irish immigrants. By 1909, it had 170 beds and a training school for nurses. Although it installed an X-ray machine in 1898, St. Joseph's accepted few tuberculosis patients because it had no isolation ward. In 1918, the Sisters of Mercy from Ireland founded the Misericordia Hospital (Mercy Philadelphia) to serve patients of all faiths. The Irish comprised over ten percent of immigrants throughout the 1890s, but their percentage began to decline by the start of the twentieth century; in the 1940s, only a bit more than one percent of the Philadelphians were born in Ireland.[44]

Between 1890 and 1920, more Italians migrated to Philadelphia than during any other period. They initially settled in South Philadelphia, where several families often lived in a single building, partitioned into one- or two-room apartments with each family doing its own cooking.

The Italian concentration in a few neighborhoods, high birthrates and citizenship increased their influence in Philadelphia out of proportion to their numbers. In 1888, the Sisters of St. Francis, who had managed St. Mary's Hospital, opened St. Agnes Hospital in South Philadelphia for Italian immigrants. Ten years later, St. Agnes accommodated 200 patients. In 1899, the two wards reserved for tuberculosis cases accommodated twenty-eight patients. Giuseppe Fabiani founded the Fabiani Italian Hospital in 1904 to further meet the needs of the Italian community. Due to high birth rates, children of Italian parentage from 1914 to 1917 replaced Russian Jews as the largest immigrant group in Philadelphia. Housing in South Philadelphia worsened and medical needs increased as Poles, Slavs and Lithuanians crowded into Italian districts.[45]

African Americans Face Discrimination

Although Philadelphia had the largest African-American population outside the slave states before the Civil War, it was during the twentieth century that Blacks came to Philadelphia in large numbers. Table 3.1 indicates that the African-American population grew from 5.15 percent of the city's population (70,724) in 1903 to 14.04 percent of the population (288,305) in 1938. Before World War I, African Americans lived throughout the city and in areas in which more than half the population was White. But by the 1920s, African Americans—more than other ethnic groups—came to be segregated in Black neighborhoods. By 1930, eighty percent of the African-American population lived in Black neighborhoods in South and West Philadelphia. By 1950, 376,041 Philadelphians (comprising of 18.15 percent of the city's population of 2,071,605) were African Americans.[46]

African Americans were a cheap source of labor and they faced strong racial prejudice when they competed with European immigrants for unskilled jobs. In 1915, African Americans did twenty percent of the work in brick, stone paving and road construction; thirteen percent in general building construction; and ten percent in railway construction. Because African Americans had limited economic and social mobility, in the 1890s, forty percent of them were employed as manual laborers, while only two percent were professionals. African-American nurses found opportunities working in public health. African-American men found one of the few professional opportunities available to them in the ministry of Black churches.[47]

Table 3.1 compares the White and Black populations in Philadelphia between 1903 and 1938 by total deaths and tubercular pulmonary deaths. In the first third of the twentieth century, pulmonary tuberculosis was one of the top three causes of death among African-American Philadelphians. Table 3.1 indicates that between 1903 and 1938, African-American pulmonary tuberculosis deaths varied from 22.9 percent of

Table 3.1 Comparison of White and Black TB Pulmonary Deaths in Philadelphia, 1903–1938

Year	Tot Pop	Tot Death	W Pop	White Population			Black Population						Total Pul Deaths	Rate W	Rate B	B TB rate to W Pop
				Deaths	TB D	TB %D	B Pop	%Tot Pop	Deaths	TB D	TB%D			Per 100,000 Pop		
1903	1,374,414	25,947	1,303,690	24,510	2,760	11.3%	70,724	5.15%	1,437	293	20.4%		3,053	208.09	414.29	2.0
1904	1,399,268	25,976	1,326,371	24,478	2,777	11.3%	72,897	5.21%	1,498	340	22.7%		3,117	205.70	466.41	2.3
1905	1,425,122	24,807	1,350,052	23,228	2,526	10.9%	75,070	5.27%	1,579	312	19.8%		2,838	187.10	415.61	2.2
1906	1,450,976	27,768	1,373,733	25,337	2,804	11.1%	77,243	5.32%	2,431	357	14.7%		3,161	204.12	462.18	2.3
1907	1,476,830	27,750	1,397,414	25,456	2,776	10.9%	79,416	5.38%	2,294	381	16.6%		3,157	198.65	479.75	2.4
1908	1,502,685	26,304	1,421,096	24,298	2,638	10.9%	81,589	5.43%	2,006	430	21.4%		3,068	185.63	527.03	2.8
1909	1,528,540	25,029	1,444,778	22,914	2,485	10.8%	83,762	5.48%	2,115	378	17.9%		2,863	172.00	451.28	2.6
1910	1,554,902	27,045	1,468,195	24,740	2,544	10.3%	86,707	5.58%	2,305	329	14.3%		2,873	173.27	379.44	2.2
1911	1,583,190	26,276	1,491,350	24,251	2,674	11.0%	91,840	5.80%	2,025	286	14.1%		2,960	179.30	311.41	1.7
1912	1,611,478	25,660	1,514,505	23,952	2,435	10.2%	96,973	6.02%	1,708	219	12.8%		2,654	160.78	225.84	1.4
1913	1,639,766	25,612	1,537,660	23,405	2,278	9.7%	102,106	6.23%	2,207	414	18.8%		2,692	148.15	405.46	2.7
1914	1,668,054	26,918	1,560,815	24,624	2,289	9.3%	107,239	6.43%	2,294	395	17.2%		2,684	146.65	368.34	2.5
1915	1,696,342	26,287	1,583,971	23,952	2,318	9.7%	112,371	6.62%	2,335	436	18.7%		2,754	146.34	388.00	2.7
1916	1,724,498	27,621	1,607,127	25,193	2,456	9.7%	117,371	6.81%	2,428	557	22.9%		3,013	152.82	474.56	3.1
1917	1,753,058	29,681	1,630,423	26,505	2,509	9.5%	122,635	7.00%	3,176	510	16.1%		3,019	153.89	415.87	2.7
1918	1,781,346	42,643	1,653,579	38,689	2,762	7.1%	127,767	7.17%	3,954	588	14.9%		3,350	167.03	460.21	2.8
1919	1,809,635	26,046	1,676,735	23,353	2,110	9.0%	132,900	7.34%	2,693	472	17.5%		2,582	125.84	355.15	2.8
1920	1,829,983	26,516	1,691,582	23,674	1,791	7.6%	138,401	7.56%	2,842	428	15.1%		2,219	105.88	309.25	2.9
1921	1,842,391	23,704	1,695,662	21,477	1,531	7.1%	146,729	7.96%	2,227	381	17.1%		1,912	90.29	259.66	2.9

1922	1,854,799	25,103	1,699,742	22,456	1,507	6.7%	155,057	8.36%	2,647	386	14.6%	1,893	88.66	248.94	2.8
1923	1,867,207	26,654	1,703,822	23,409	1,444	6.2%	163,385	8.75%	3,245	423	13.0%	1,867	84.75	258.90	3.1
1924	1,879,615	24,980	1,707,902	21,880	1,334	6.1%	171,713	9.14%	3,100	443	14.3%	1,777	78.11	257.99	3.3
1925	1,892,023	26,061	1,711,982	22,465	1,327	5.9%	180,041	9.52%	3,596	454	12.6%	1,781	77.51	252.16	3.3
1926	1,904,431	27,692	1,716,062	23,764	1,247	5.2%	188,369	9.89%	3,928	492	12.5%	1,739	72.67	261.19	3.6
1927	1,916,839	24,801	1,720,142	21,081	1,024	4.9%	196,697	10.26%	3,720	484	13.0%	1,508	59.53	246.06	4.1
1928	1,929,247	26,930	1,724,222	22,983	1,153	5.0%	205,025	10.63%	3,947	454	11.5%	1,607	66.87	221.44	3.3
1929	1,941,655	25,346	1,728,302	21,660	995	4.6%	213,353	10.99%	3,686	456	12.4%	1,451	57.57	213.73	3.7
1930	1,954,063	24,541	1,732,382	20,962	910	4.3%	221,681	11.34%	3,579	486	13.6%	1,396	52.53	219.23	4.2
1931	1,966,471	25,214	1,736,462	21,552	925	4.3%	230,009	11.70%	3,662	480	13.1%	1,405	53.27	208.69	3.9
1932	1,978,879	23,777	1,740,542	20,370	790	3.9%	238,337	12.04%	3,407	444	13.0%	1,234	45.39	186.29	4.1
1933	1,991,287	23,916	1,744,622	20,473	825	4.0%	246,665	12.39%	3,443	413	12.0%	1,238	47.29	167.43	3.5
1934	2,003,695	24,984	1,748,702	21,378	831	3.9%	254,993	12.73%	3,606	427	11.8%	1,258	47.52	167.46	3.5
1935	2,016,103	24,168	1,752,782	20,686	690	3.3%	263,321	13.06%	3,482	380	10.9%	1,070	39.37	144.31	3.7
1936	2,028,511	25,015	1,756,862	21,362	768	3.6%	271,649	13.39%	3,653	426	11.7%	1,194	43.71	156.82	3.6
1937	2,040,919	25,239	1,760,942	21,604	773	3.6%	279,977	13.72%	3,635	417	11.5%	1,190	43.90	148.94	3.4
1938	2,053,327	24,309	1,765,022	20,618	643	3.1%	288,305	14.04%	3,691	461	12.5%	1,104	36.43	159.90	4.4

Abbreviations: Tot = Total; Pop = Population; W = White; B = Black; D = Death; Pul = Pulmonary TB.
Sources: Philadelphia, Annual Message of the Mayor of City, 1912, 3:109; 1920:582; 1938:450.

African-American total deaths (474.56 per 100,000 population) in 1916 to a low of 10.9 percent of deaths (144.31 per 100,000 population) in 1935. Although the percentage of African-American tuberculosis deaths decreased, Black deaths started at a higher percent than White tuberculosis deaths and declined more slowly. White tuberculosis deaths were never higher than 11.3 percent of deaths in 1903, and by 1938, they were 3.1 percent of Caucasian deaths; in 1938, African-American tuberculosis deaths were 12.5 percent of deaths, which was higher than White deaths in 1903. In 1938, an African-American was 4.4 times more likely to die of tuberculosis than a Caucasian.

The high tuberculosis death rate of African Americans was due to restricted job opportunities, poor housing, and initially limited access to health facilities. The African-American jobless rate in 1932 of fifty-six percent—even larger than the forty percent rate for Whites—devastated the community and contributed to the increased incidence of tuberculosis, since Black families could afford little health care. Because the city failed to expand public health facilities, African Americans who had migrated to improve their lives were more likely to die from tuberculosis in Philadelphia than in Birmingham or Memphis. In spite of the high frequency of tuberculosis among African Americans, in the early part of the century, hospitals and sanatoriums excluded them. In 1923, only twelve of the twenty-nine Pennsylvania tuberculosis institutions admitted African Americans. In Philadelphia, Rush Hospital, the Henry Phipps Institute, Philadelphia General Hospital, Jefferson Hospital and Frederick Douglass Memorial Hospital cared for African Americans. White Haven Sanatorium and Pennsylvania state sanatoriums—including Mont Alto which initially segregated by race—accepted few African Americans.[48]

Nathan F. Mossell, the University of Pennsylvania's first African-American medical graduate, recognized the need for a hospital that would serve African Americans. In 1895, with financial support from the state and Philadelphia communities, Mossell opened the fifteen-bed Frederick Douglass Memorial Hospital and Training School, the second hospital started and managed by African Americans in the United States. From the beginning, the hospital faced financial challenges. Many African-American patients were not accustomed to receiving care in hospitals and often were too poor to pay $5 a week for care. A power struggle at Douglass Memorial between Mossell and some of the hospital's physicians led to the establishment of a second African-American hospital in Philadelphia, in 1907, the Mercy Hospital and School for Nurses. The Mercy Hospital was more successful in attracting financial support because its managers were less committed to integration and more accommodating to white society than Mossell. In 1948, the two hospitals merged and in 1973, Mercy Douglas Hospital closed. Jefferson Hospital, which hired an African-American physician and later added African-American nurses, attracted black patients after 1910. When all

Philadelphia hospitals came to admit African-American patients—in the wake of a 1922 Pennsylvania Supreme Court decision that denied public funding to sectarian institutions and prorated state funding going to hospitals according to the number of days of free care that they provided to the impoverished—the Douglass and Mercy Hospitals had difficulty attracting patients.[49]

Tuberculosis Prevention Efforts in Philadelphia

The arrival of large numbers of immigrants impelled Philadelphia's public health authorities to address infectious diseases such as tuberculosis. They, therefore, attempted to create a healthier urban environment and to shape the morality of Philadelphia's immigrants and African Americans. Both private organizations and public institutions contributed to efforts to prevent and treat tuberculosis. Like their counterparts in Buenos Aires, the Philadelphian middle and upper classes blamed the poor for the city's diseases and epidemics. The city reorganized its public health department and professionals directed tuberculosis prevention programs aimed at immigrants and African Americans.

In 1786, Philadelphia established the first dispensary in the U.S. to care for sick indigents. Part-time physicians provided free service to the poor but also used them to train medical students. By the 1870s, the Guardians of the Poor, established by the city in the eighteenth century to provide for the destitute, managed the Philadelphia Hospital and Almshouse and provided groceries, fuel and medicine for the most needy. In 1887, its functions were transferred to the Philadelphia Department of Charity and Corrections, which emphasized crime control rather than medical services for the poor. In 1903, Philadelphia created the Department of Public Health, which was divided into two large agencies: the Bureau of Health and the Bureau of Hospitals. Between 1920 and 1951, the Bureau of Health included a division that inspected schools; the housing and sanitation division responsible for assessing housing, sanitation, and agricultural produce; and the child hygiene division in-charge of the public health clinics for children. The Bureau of Hospitals was responsible for the city-run health facilities, including Philadelphia General Hospital. Although Philadelphia, in the colonial period, developed a reputation for effective health care for the poor, by the end of the nineteenth century, the city had failed to keep up with the more progressive policies of other urban areas.[50]

By the early 1890s—when the health departments of New York City and Buenos Aires initiated policies to prevent and control tuberculosis and led the way in requiring notification of tuberculosis cases and institution disinfection policies—Philadelphia had reduced its financial commitment to public health. Although both Herman Briggs in New York City and Lawrence Flick and the Philadelphia County Medical Society recommended in 1893 that tuberculosis patients be registered, only New York implemented the policy. The Philadelphia Department of Public Health—which was unprepared to promote a tuberculosis prevention program and faced strong opposition from prominent members of the Philadelphia medical establishment—did not require registration until 1904. Perhaps because Philadelphia's immigrant population was smaller than New York's, Philadelphia's upper class may have worried less about the threat to public health that immigrants were thought to pose.[51]

In the early years of the twentieth century, Philadelphia's sanitarians (urban reformers and engineers) and public health officials (primarily doctors) disagreed on how to improve the environment, promote public health and whether an effective campaign against tuberculosis should focus on the bacterial causes or attack poverty. The urban reformers blamed the industrial environment and pointed out that Pennsylvania's lightly populated northern counties had pure air and few tuberculosis cases—whereas Philadelphia's densely populated industrial environment produced poor air quality and many tuberculosis cases. The public health community believed that the poor and working classes should change their behavior by improving their hygiene and adopting self-help measures. If the poor and working classes did so, public health officials believed, the urban environment would improve and diseases would decrease. Middle-class officials assumed that germs and dirt were prevalent in the slums because of the ignorance of the residents, their inadequate language skills and their ethnicity or race. Thus—in the absence of evidence—Philadelphia public health officials in the first half of the twentieth century generally blamed the spread of tuberculosis on the behavior of immigrants and the poor but not the industrial conditions in which they lived and worked.[52]

The Philadelphia Department of Public Health eventually followed international prevention efforts. In particular, it recommended the registration and isolation of the tubercular, the disinfection of all items affected by tubercular sputum and an educational campaign to teach healthy living to the poor. But these efforts faced several challenges. To begin with, the measures assumed that the ill would visit clinics, where physicians would correctly diagnose and report the incidence of tuberculosis. In addition, landlords had to be trusted to report the death of tubercular tenants. Furthermore, disinfection required that walls, floors, furniture and rugs be treated with cleansers such as bleach, carbolic acid, citric acid mercury or tartaric acid mercury solution. The laws forbidding spitting on the streets had to be enforced by the police. One measure, though, was successful: the requirement that the city's milk be pasteurized.[53]

Public health nurses, often graduates of premier nursing schools and funded by both government and private agencies, were at the forefront of efforts to provide health care for the working class. Nurses worked long hours visiting the sick in their homes in the mornings and evenings and laboring in public dispensaries in the afternoons. With cultural backgrounds often different from their patients', they sought to decrease contagion and to teach the immigrant poor how to care for sick relatives—and, more broadly, how and why to adopt middle-class values and to improve their hygiene. By 1912, there were some 3,000 public health nurses in the U.S., with over ninety percent working with organizations, focused on tuberculosis. City officials viewed public health nursing as a primary educational tool in preventing the spread of tuberculosis.[54]

Although the federal government and state and local governments passed regulations to prevent tuberculosis, few were enforced. The Philadelphia Department of Public Health failed adequately to implement prevention policies. For example, there were never enough inspectors to enforce disinfection regulations. Most individuals were unwilling to report those who failed to disinfect the property of the tubercular dead or to inform on workers who spat on the sidewalk. Immigrants often did not maintain the standards of cleanliness that the middle class demanded, and they seldom took the regulations seriously. Rules requiring the disinfection of the rooms of those who died of tuberculosis or fining spitters (whether or not they were enforced) seemed to satisfy Philadelphians that efforts were being made to prevent tuberculosis.[55]

When a reform movement to upgrade the condition of immigrant housing collapsed in 1893, public officials instead continued token efforts to expand the sewage system, pave cobblestone streets and flush and disinfect the alleyways. In the first quarter of the twentieth century, the Department of Housing and Sanitation could seldom deal with overcrowding in poor and working-class neighborhoods—even when mortality rates from scarlet fever, whooping cough, influenza and tuberculosis were on the rise.[56] Although the Department of Public Health and Charities had the power to promote sanitation improvements and housing reforms, it spent little time on these issues, because it did not want to alienate private contractors and property owners who wielded political power. It was easier for the authorities to make individuals responsible for sanitation than to ask hostile politicians and businessmen to provide more funding. The department generally ignored warnings from reformers linking tenement conditions, leaky sewer systems and the lack of fresh water to the spread of disease. However, the city's health department did work with volunteer agencies to establish clinics for tuberculosis diagnosis and health education.[57]

The failure of the city's public health implementation policies in the early part of the twentieth century meant that individuals—working through private organizations such as the Pennsylvania Society for the Prevention of Tuberculosis, the Phipps Institute and the White Haven Sanatorium—took the lead in supporting programs for the indigent and promoting the campaign against tuberculosis in Philadelphia. Henry R. M. Landis (1872–1937)—a tuberculosis physician and researcher at the Henry Phipps Institute—and Lawrence Flick oversaw prevention programs and the effort to improve the living and working conditions of the poor, so as to defeat tuberculosis. In 1913, Landis became president of the Whittier Center, a voluntary organization of Whites focusing on issues of concern to the Black community; he supported the development of the Phipps Institute's program to serve African Americans. Landis believed that there were three means to decrease tuberculosis: physicians needed to learn how to diagnose it; public health programs needed to improve working conditions in the "dusty trades" in which infection from tuberculosis was highest; and more clinics for African-Americans needed to be opened, because Philadelphia's Black population had more than quadrupled from 1903 to 1938.[58]

In 1915, Landis gave crucial support to Dr. Henry M. Minton, an African-American graduate of the Philadelphia College of Pharmacy and Jefferson Medical College. Minton obtained a part-time appointment at the Phipps Institute. He understood that Blacks needed to learn how to improve their hygiene and diet, and that tuberculosis patients in the early stages needed to be referred to clinics and that those in the later stages needed to be hospitalized. Between 1903 and 1938, African Americans died of pulmonary tuberculosis at a rate that was often more than double the rate for Whites. Landis believed that Black nurses and physicians could treat African Americans more effectively than Whites could; but he also wrongly believed that African-Americans domestic servants were responsible for outbreaks of tuberculosis among the elite. At that time, it was thought that African Americans were more susceptible to tuberculosis than Whites because of their race. That belief was refuted by Charles A. Lewis, a 1910 graduate of the University of Pennsylvania Medical School, who conducted a survey of South Philadelphia under the auspices of the Henry Phipps Institute between 1911 and 1912. The survey showed that social factors, not the race, made African Americans more susceptible to tuberculosis.[59]

By 1914, the city had increased its efforts to persuade African Americans to use public health facilities, in spite of its continuing discriminatory practices. Municipal officials were convinced that overcrowded housing increased the risks of transmitting tuberculosis to neighbors and family members and that the disease endangered the city's health. The two hospitals in Philadelphia for African Americans had only a limited impact in educating and treating Blacks. Greater success came when the Whittier Center (in co-operation with the Phipps Institute) hired African-American visiting nurses to work with the Black population. African-American nurses successfully instructed patients on home care and succeeded in getting advanced patients into hospitals and Pennsylvania state sanatoriums. The success of African-American health professionals helped stem the view that Blacks were incapable of following responsible medical practice. It also showed that tuberculosis stemmed from social rather than racial factors. African-American clinics associated with the Phipps Institute functioned through the Great Depression. Most neighborhood clinics were phased out during World War II when hospitals increased their range of medical services and Blacks gained access to public health facilities.[60]

The evolution of prevention efforts affects both the foreign and native-born individuals with tuberculosis. Table 3.2 provides information on the respiratory tuberculosis deaths of Argentine and foreign residents during the height of immigration to Buenos Aires. Usually, there was a correlation between the number of immigrants and the number of tubercular deaths. More Italians and Spanish died of tuberculosis than did the French, British and Germans. The Spanish immigrants were the exception. The Spanish population in Buenos Aires was one-fourth the size of the Italian one, yet between 1899 and 1911, in six of the thirteen years, more Spanish died of tuberculosis than Italians. There may have been more undercounting of Italian deaths as they were spread throughout the city and more difficult to count; the Spanish immigrants were concentrated in a few neighborhoods. However, the primary explanation is that the Spanish immigrants were late arrivals to Buenos Aires, lived in the city's most dilapidated housing and occupied the worse jobs—men in unskilled labor and women as domestics. Unlike poor Italian immigrants who lived in the La Boca area who had access to protein, the Spanish immigrants also suffered from a poor diet. The smaller number of tuberculosis deaths among the British in comparison with the Germans was also a reflection of neighborhood and class. The British lived in less crowded neighborhoods and worked in the business and professional sectors which had fewer cases of tuberculosis.[61]

In an examination of female gender, between 1899 and 1911, more Argentine women than men died of pulmonary tuberculosis; Porteñas were 103.21–132.03 percent of male deaths. This was most likely due to the high mortality of women of child-bearing ages (fifteen to twenty-nine). In the years 1908 and 1909, foreign women died in smaller numbers than men for every national group except the Uruguayans. Factoring in the two to one ratio of men to women, foreign females were from 67.15 to 101.42 percent of male deaths. In effect, foreign female tubercular deaths were a third lower than Porteña females. It is unclear why this is the case; undercounting may be a factor.

Porteños argued over whether foreigners were more likely than native-born to spread disease—specifically pulmonary tuberculosis. Argentine medical professionals speculated as to whether foreigners were more likely to die of pulmonary tuberculosis than Porteños. Both issues are difficult to answer. Buenos Aires statistical yearbooks provided the pulmonary tuberculosis deaths of members of the largest foreign

Table 3.2 Buenos Aires Pulmonary TB Deaths by Place of Birth, 1899–1911

Year	*Arg*			*Italy*			*Spain*			*France*			*UK*			*Germany*			*Uruguay*			*Miscellaneous*			*Total Foreign*			*Total TB D*	*FNG % of TB D*		
	F	*M*	*T*	*F*	*M*	*T*	*F*	*M*	*T*	*F*	*M*	*T*	*F*	*M*	*T*	*F*	*M*	*T*	*F*	*M*	*T*	*F*	*M*	*T*	*F*	*M*	*T*		*F*	*M*	*T*
1899	306	273	579	76	163	239	46	243	289	23	42	65	4	7	11	8	10	18	0	0	0	34	56	90	191	521	712	1291	14.8	40.4	55.2
1900	381	354	735	83	191	274	41	159	200	14	46	60	5	3	8	1	6	7	0	0	0	50	66	116	194	471	665	1400	13.9	33.6	47.5
1901	451	429	880	113	200	313	61	174	235	15	48	63	3	7	10	5	3	8	33	46	79	31	56	87	261	534	795	1675	15.6	31.9	47.5
1902	440	399	839	108	197	305	64	170	234	28	58	86	7	9	16	3	5	8	26	35	61	19	51	70	255	525	780	1619	15.8	32.4	48.2
1903	507	384	891	124	199	323	64	170	234	22	44	66	5	5	10	1	10	11	32	34	66	30	58	88	278	520	798	1689	16.5	30.8	47.2
1904	514	439	953	111	185	296	70	200	270	26	54	80	2	4	6	7	2	9	25	42	67	22	68	90	263	555	818	1771	14.9	31.3	46.2
1905	602	476	1078	121	211	332	72	189	261	25	40	65	3	9	12	2	2	4	41	33	74	23	65	88	287	549	836	1914	15	28.7	43.7
1906	614	501	1115	103	211	314	74	223	297	21	48	69	1	10	11	4	9	13	38	32	70	36	86	122	277	619	896	2011	13.8	30.8	44.6
1907	590	546	1136	128	212	340	87	270	357	17	31	48	6	6	12	5	20	25	45	49	94	33	70	103	321	658	979	2115	15.2	31.1	46.3
1908	575	536	1111	103	234	337	88	261	349	22	46	68	7	1	8	3	8	11	45	42	87	37	73	110	305	665	970	2081	14.7	32	46.6
1909	528	504	1032	101	206	307	92	267	359	15	24	39	2	9	11	4	13	17	48	37	85	34	80	114	296	636	932	1964	15.1	32.4	47.5
1910	579	561	1140	71	218	289	91	315	406	10	27	37	0	10	10	2	12	14	39	42	81	39	104	143	252	728	980	2120	11.9	34.3	46.2
1911	644	595	1239	108	212	320	129	327	456	18	26	44	1	6	7	2	9	11	33	41	74	46	107	153	337	728	1065	2304	14.6	31.6	46.2

Abbreviations: F = Female; M = Male; T = Total; FGN = Foreign; TB D = TB Deaths.
Sources: Buenos Aires, *Statistical Year-Book 1910 and 1911: 121; Buenos Aires, Anuario Estadístico 1904: 41.*

communities: Italian, Spanish, French, British, German and Uruguayan. The Argentine censuses of 1895 and 1914 listed the foreign population by nationality for the nation.[62] Yet, given the emigrations and the unreliable statistics for foreign population for Buenos Aires, it was very difficult to estimate the exact foreign-born population from particular countries for specific years. If one considers the ratio of Argentine to foreign-born populations there is some evidence that foreign tuberculosis deaths were greater than those of Porteños. Between 1900 and 1911, the foreign-born deaths varied from 46.2 to 48.2 percent of the tuberculosis mortalities. Between 1899 and 1911, tuberculosis deaths of Argentines living in Buenos Aires represented 6.77 to 11.74 percent of total deaths. In contrast, foreign tuberculosis deaths ranged from 11.02 to 14.21 of total deaths. Recent immigrant groups suffered more from tuberculosis than others due to crowded living areas and poor working condition.

Table 3.3 provides the number of pulmonary tuberculosis deaths from 1907 to 1938 in Philadelphia and compares U.S. Caucasian and African-American tuberculosis deaths with the primary countries of immigration. For U.S. Caucasian, the tuberculosis deaths declined steadily and by 1938, there were twenty-four percent fewer deaths compared to 1907. In contrast, the number of deaths of African-Americans actually increased from 381 in 1907 to 461 (121 percent in 1938). Tubercular deaths increased among U.S. Caucasians in 1918 and African Americans from 1914 to 1918. When examining foreign populations, the tubercular deaths of all foreign populations increased between 1914–1918 and 1920–1923 with the exception of German emigrants. Given attitudes of Philadelphians toward Germany during World War I, the statistics on German tubercular deaths are most likely incomplete; German immigrants had reservations on reporting tubercular deaths. From 1920 to 1923, those born in Russia, Italy, Austria-Hungry, and France had another temporary increase in tubercular deaths; these nationals came from countries heavily damaged by the war and affected by the recession of 1920–1921. Immigrants from Sweden/Norway and China/Japan also saw a small increase in tubercular deaths. In contrast, nationals from Ireland, England/Wales and Scotland experienced a continued decrease of tubercular deaths. By 1938, when foreign tubercular deaths were 17.3 percent of total deaths, African-American deaths were two and half times higher.

Tuberculosis Patient Experiences in Buenos Aires and Philadelphia

Foreign and native-born tuberculosis patients had diverse experiences with public health officials in their cities. A comparative analysis of the populations and public health policies of Buenos Aires and Philadelphia demonstrates the similarities of and the differences between their efforts

Table 3.3 Philadelphia Pulmonary TB Deaths by Place of Birth

Year	U.S. Caucas	Af Am	Ire	Ger	Russia	Italy	Eng Wales	CA	AU/HU	PO	Scot	FR	SE/NO	China JP	Misc	Unk	Total FNG	Tot of all Pul Death	FNG% of T Deaths
1907	1868	381	328	143	98	60	76	8	40	34	27	2	12	8	28	44	908	3157	28.76
1909	1710	378	265	110	104	48	73	7	34	26	23	5	14	0	39	27	775	2863	27.07
1910	1793	329	261	110	86	61	57	6	50	26	24	8	12	7	27	16	751	2873	26.14
1914	1600	395	221	91	102	64	58	4	57	19	15	5	7	5	20	21	689	2684	25.67
1915	1619	436	177	91	136	81	47	8	46	23	19	5	6	4	30	26	699	2754	25.38
1918	1844	533	201	81	173	98	56	8	73	32	21	3	15	8	31	80	880	3257	27.02
1920	1270	409	111	40	67	53	38	10	44	40	16	2	5	1	14	10	451	2130	21.17
1923	952	410	101	38	76	58	29	3	53	27	8	4	6	5	25	22	455	1817	25.04
1928	753	454	63	18	39	42	21	3	38	19	7	2	3	2	14	31	302	1509	20.01
1929	658	456	61	20	46	47	22	6	47	31	8	2	6	5	8	28	337	1451	23.23
1930	621	486	43	29	37	43	16	9	40	28	10	1	1	6	9	17	289	1396	20.70
1932	554	444	36	23	39	33	15	4	32	18	7	0	5	5	7	12	236	1234	19.12
1934	600	427	35	16	40	25	20	1	32	18	8	0	3	5	9	24	236	1263	18.69
1936	571	426	24	16	33	18	23	0	39	18	0	0	3	3	8	17	202	1199	16.85
1938	452	461	23	10	44	19	14	1	19	17	0	0	5	3	9	27	191	1104	17.30

Abbreviations: Caucas = Caucasian; Af Am = Africians Americans; Ire = Ireland; Ger = Germany; Eng = England; CA = Canada; AU/HU = Austria/Hungry; PO = Poland; Scot = Scotland; Fr = France; SE/NO = Sweden/Norway; JP = Japan; Misc = Miscellaneous; Unk = Unknown; FNG = Foreign; Tot = Total; Pul = Pulmonary
Source: Philadelphia, *Annual Message of the Mayor 1904, vol. 3: 240; 1912, vol. 3: 109–10; 1939:* 392–3.

to prevent tuberculosis. The diversity in ethnicity of both cities in the 1870–1945 period affected municipal public health campaigns. Both Buenos Aires and Philadelphia attracted many immigrants between 1890 and 1920. However, foreigners comprised forty-five to fifty-two percent of Buenos Aires' population, but less than twenty-six percent of Philadelphia's. More Italian immigrants came to Buenos Aires, and they had a greater influence there. Philadelphians were never as concerned about the tubercular deaths of the foreign-born as were the Porteños. But the foreign population of Philadelphia never exceeded twenty-six percent.[63]

Various ethnicity groups came in different decades to Philadelphia in response to political and religious issues in Europe. The Germans contributed to the growth of Philadelphia in the eighteenth century; by 1880, the Irish represented the largest foreign group in the city. Between 1890 and 1920, the Italians arrived and in 1920, the Russians sought refuge. An examination of foreign deaths in Philadelphia indicated that foreign deaths in 1871 were a high of fifty-three percent of native Philadelphian deaths and a low of twenty-three percent in 1896 with an average from 1870 to 1938 of thirty-eight percent. Thus, foreign-born adult tuberculosis deaths exceeded native Philadelphians.[64] At the same time, Philadelphia expressed concern not about Europeans as carriers of tuberculosis bacteria but about African Americans who were isolated in ghettos due to racism. African Americans comprised 3.29 percent of the Philadelphia population in 1870 and over thirteen percent by 1945. Table 3.1 confirms that the African-American population in Philadelphia increased steadily throughout the first thirty-eight years of the century. Although there were few Afro-Argentines in Buenos Aires, agricultural migrants came from the provinces to Buenos Aires in large numbers during the same time period in which primarily rural African Americans moved to Philadelphia. European discrimination encouraged Jews to emigrate to both Philadelphia and Buenos Aires. Philadelphian sentiment against the Jewish population was never as strong as the prejudice against African Americans.

Often forgetting their own previous status, immigrants who arrived earlier discriminated against those who came later. Immigrants to both Philadelphia and Buenos Aires formed their own community groups to provide aid and support during illnesses and economic difficulties. Philanthropists in both cities supported the building of hospitals and medical institutions. However, the Argentine government funded private charities, whereas those in the U.S. raised their own funds. Because Catholics were immigrating to a primarily Protestant nation, Philadelphia's foreign-born population supported more religious organizations than those in Buenos Aires. In contrast, the percentage of Protestants in Buenos Aires remained relatively small. Unlike the immigrants to Buenos Aires, immigrants to Philadelphia often became citizens and took political action on their own behalf. Elite concerns about working-class immigrants shaped public health and tubercular policies in both Buenos Aires and Philadelphia. However, these concerns failed to recognize the influence of tuberculosis on all ethnicities and classes.

Table 3.4 shows that tuberculosis affected every class and occupation, the unskilled and professionals in both Philadelphia and Buenos Aires. In Buenos Aires, the largest number of tubercular deaths between 1889 and 1897 were in food processing, domestic service, commerce and textiles—occupations that employed the largest number of people. The sizeable number of female tubercular deaths of domestics and textile workers supports anecdotal evidence. In Buenos Aires, from 1912 through 1918, the largest number of tuberculosis deaths was in the public sector; this contrasts with the small number in Philadelphia. In Philadelphia, the largest number of deaths was among domestics. In the cities, workers in skilled professions were vulnerable to tuberculosis. The significant number of deaths of those with unknown occupations in both Buenos Aires and Philadelphia underlines the difficulty of linking tubercular deaths to occupations. The failure of public officials to report the occupation of workers may reflect the stigma attached to pulmonary tuberculosis.

Before 1945, there was no medicine that effectively cured tuberculosis, so initial attempts at treatment centered on prevention. The beginning of the twentieth century witnessed the apex of public health initiatives. The municipal governments of Buenos Aires and Philadelphia expanded health departments in response to public concerns about epidemics and sanitation. Public health workers sought to prevent illness and promote individual health by controlling epidemics and disease and teaching individuals the principles of personal hygiene. The municipal regulations and services of both Philadelphia and Buenos Aires chiefly addressed the poor. The cities' municipal governments faced similar challenges in providing water, sewage removal, housing and health services to the immigrants. Health officials in both cities believed that poor housing, meager diet, long working days, unhealthy working conditions, inadequate urban sanitation and immoral behavior (manifested in alcoholism, prostitution and rowdiness) made individuals susceptible to tuberculosis and a danger to the middle and upper classes.

Philadelphia public health officials were more likely to diagnose African Americans with tuberculosis than Irish immigrants. In contrast to Philadelphia, Buenos Aires public health officials focused on the differences between foreigners and the native-born and failed to recognize that tuberculosis mortality among immigrants to Buenos Aires was only slightly higher than among Argentine nationals. (There was actually no difference. In 1909, forty-six percent of the population was foreign-born and forty-six percent of those dying of tuberculosis were immigrants.) Most immigrants did not actively suffer from tuberculosis when they arrived

Table 3.4 Pulmonary TB Deaths by Occupation of Men and Women Over Ten Years of Age in Buenos Aires and Philadelphia

Industry by year	*1889–1897*		*1912*	*1913*	*1914*	*1915*	*1915*	*1916*	*1917*	*1917*	*1918*	*1918*	*1920*
	BA-M	*BA-F*	*BA*	*BA*	*BA*	*Phila*	*BA*	*BA*	*Phila*	*BA*	*Phila*	*BA*	*Phila*
Agriculture, Fishery, Water	316					33			34		13		9
Building Trades	246		88	83	94	105	76	75	129	67	167	105	94
Clay, Glass, Stone, Minerals	41	9				26			25		6		9
Commerce	517	14	64	103	87	230	97	86	201	72	254	118	163
Domestic	97	709				784			789		893		648
Food Processing	288	137	107	111	80	33	67	58	27	52	21	73	11
Skilled Labor, misc.	630	5				115			131		157		173
Leather	178		8	9	12	37	8	8	32	4	36	6	13
Lumber			40	52	44	29	48	36	17	42	9	39	13
Metal: iron, steel, etc.	197		39	63	61	132	63	55	147	38	152	85	106
Printing	90		14	21	31	31	20	32	35	19	21	34	10
Professionals	52	21	20	20	25	55	23	27	87	23	92	48	46
Public Service			250	250	269	30	242	311	33	226	52	420	47
Soldiers/guards	289												
Textile/clothing	62	267	72	91	109	132	115	101	167	69	166	101	107
Transport	254		92	85	93	167	63	76	144	54	163	93	85
Children and students			284	138	332	143	284	517	204	506	218	383	135
Unskilled	1834	14				337			439	773	519		271
Unknown	947	2680	1553	1964	2037	758	2203	2212	640	1863	411	2727	279
Total	6038	3856	2631	2852	3274	3177	3309	3594	3281	3808	3350	4191	2219

Sources: Lozano, "Estadística," *La Semana Medica*; Philadelphia, *Annual Message of the Mayor*, 1915: 535–7; 1917:442–5; 1918:432–5; 1920:582–6; Gimenez, Consideración, 32.
Abbreviations: BA-M = Buenos Aires Males; BA-F = Buenos Aires Females.

in Argentina; instead they developed the disease a few years after they came to their new country. Social conditions, not ethnicity, defined who was most likely to contract tuberculosis. Cramped living conditions, poor working conditions, meager nutrition, inadequate health care and the stress of relocation contributed to the activation of latent infections. The social diversity within Philadelphia and Buenos Aires neighborhoods and the underreporting of tuberculosis among elites make it difficult to prove that the poor and immigrants were more likely than wealthy natives to contract tuberculosis and die of it.[65]

Both Buenos Aires and Philadelphia implemented disinfection policies and required milk pasteurization. However, Philadelphia was less willing than Buenos Aires to bear the costs of both disinfection regulations and educational programs. That said, it is questionable how effective disinfection programs were in either city. Research in the 1930s demonstrated that in most cases dried sputum did not cause infection, but public health officials continued to hope that tuberculosis could be prevented by removing dust from public places, stopping spitting and disinfecting rooms. Although Buenos Aries required that city merchants sell only pasteurized or sterilized milk five years before Philadelphia, officials in both cities executed pasteurization policies successfully. Milk pasteurization served both the poor and middle classes, reduced tuberculosis among children and substantially contributed to better health in both cities.

Both middle- and working-class sufferers searched for physicians who did not diagnose them as tubercular, and patients often sought to combat their illnesses with folk medicines. Physicians faced difficulty in diagnosing tuberculosis and were generally unwilling to inform the authorities of cases. Initially, many physicians did not believe that tuberculosis was infectious; in any case, they saw no advantage in reporting cases of tuberculosis to the health department when there was no cure for it. Physicians also worried that diagnosing tuberculosis would encourage patients to seek another doctor. Affluent Philadelphians and Porteños who could afford private physicians escaped the supervision of the health department and even the limited mandatory disinfection policies. Landlords rarely reported the death of tubercular patients in their apartments. Thus, both the ill and physicians in Buenos Aires and Philadelphia sought ways to avoid public health mandates.

Both Buenos Aires and Philadelphia established public health clinics to provide basic care for women and children and to detect tuberculosis at the early stages. Health officials visited the homes of the poor and provided detailed instruction on hygiene, food preparation and sleeping arrangements. Ill patients' families often could not afford to take advantage of municipal health services. For instance, when sick people visited dispensaries, they often had to leave work early (and thereby lose pay) and bear the cost of traveling long distances. The emphasis on preventing tuberculosis, focusing as it did on the poor, thus actually made life more difficult for them. Tuberculosis cases were reported only by public clinics serving the poor, a fact that reinforced the belief that the poor were somehow to blame for tuberculosis. Although their living and working conditions made the poor more likely to contract tuberculosis, there is no evidence that the poor caused tuberculosis among the elite. Nor is there evidence that promoting middle-class moral values contributed to a decrease in tuberculosis. However, the common, but faulty belief that the poor spread tuberculosis did lead to the construction of better housing and the creation of green spaces in both cities—developments that improved the quality of living for all groups. Neither Philadelphia nor Buenos Aires was unique in focusing on the poor. Instead both cities were following global accepted policies in their efforts to prevent tuberculosis and reorder urban society.

As services to the tubercular were being redefined, charitable institutions increased their influence in both Buenos Aires and Philadelphia. Charities in both cities supplemented the public health programs that served the neediest. For example, the Henry Phipps Institute's programs and clinics for African Americans served as a model of a successful effort to serve the poor. Buenos Aires charities focused on women and children, because they thought that women and children—more than men—could easily be influenced to change their behavior. The elite expected that women and children who participated in the charities' programs would in turn influence their husbands and fathers. By working with immigrants, especially working-class women and children, the Argentine government hoped to unify and improve the society. But if that goal was achieved, time rather than elite efforts was principally responsible.

Public health professionals in both Philadelphia and Buenos Aires were familiar with the latest scientific discoveries, but they had to institute their policies within an often hostile political environment. Departments of public health in Philadelphia and Buenos Aires both faced political resistance to their programs. For example, Lawrence Flick and Henry Landis could use the Henry Phipps Institute to implement anti-tuberculosis campaigns in Philadelphia before the public health department received state funding to establish prevention programs. Emilio Coni developed an effective anti-tuberculosis campaign in Buenos Aires, but he often aroused political disagreements; he fought with the city council, the mayor and the Sociedad de Beneficencia in trying to implement his health programs. He campaigned to get the government to allocate the resources necessary for fighting tuberculosis but was often frustrated by public officials and private citizens who were unwilling to spend the money that was needed. Coni hoped to enable physicians to analyze sputum at no cost to them—an effective means of tuberculosis diagnosis. But he could not do so. Although hygienists in both cities vocally advocated for social reform and demanded greater government attention to the living conditions of the poor, Coni more effectively shaped his government's commitment to improving Buenos Aires' physical environment than did public health officials in Philadelphia. The latter were constrained by dependence on the private sector. The power brokers of both Philadelphia and Buenos Aires gradually created healthier cities, but they did so by different strategies. Lawrence Flick utilized the Henry Phipps Institute to introduce tuberculosis prevention policies, while Emilio Coni lobbied the Buenos Aires government to finance the municipal's public health efforts.[66]

Philadelphia and Buenos Aires—two major metropolises that developed tuberculosis prevention programs early in the twentieth century—exemplified the focus of health professionals worldwide in combating tuberculosis and the international consensus on how to treat it. The cities' demographic and geographic differences had less impact on the implementation of tuberculosis policies than the personalities of public health officials, the established role of government in promoting public health policies and the traditional power balance between the private and public sectors. However, there was a correlation between tuberculosis deaths and living and working conditions of various ethnic groups in both cities. Decrease in epidemic deaths led to tuberculosis representing a greater percent of mortality rates. At the beginning of the twentieth century, Porteño public health services faced difficulty in meeting the needs of the increasing number of immigrant with the resulting increase in tuberculosis deaths. In contrast, by 1917 when public health policies were still being developed and before the introduction of antibiotics, Philadelphia tuberculosis death rates began to decline sharply. Tuberculosis deaths declined in both Buenos Aires and Philadelphia and within various ethnic groups as the standard of living improved. Although declining tuberculosis death rates correlate with the importance and effectiveness of public health programs, it is the government support of policies which improved the standard of living (rather than any focus on moral improvement or hygiene) that substantially decreased the number of tuberculosis cases.

Notes

1 E. Klappenbach, "Tuberculosis pulmonar: Inyecciones de Gayacol-íodoformado," trans. V. B. Reber. *Anales del Círculo Médico Argentino* 15, no. 5 (May 1892): 231–32.

2 The Catholic University of America, American Catholic History Research Center and University Archives (hereafter CUA); Lawrence F. Flick Papers (hereafter FP); paraphrased from Letters, Vol. 75 July to December 1915, F. M. Kirby, Wilkes Barre, Pa., 27 August 1915 to Flick.

3 Elisa Radovanovic and Alicia Busson, "La Vivienda obrera en Buenos Aires en la decada de 1880, presupuestos teóricos y realizaciones," in *Primeras Jornadas de Historia de la Ciudad de Buenos Aires: Vivienda en Buenos*

Aires (Buenos Aires: Municipalidad de la Ciudad de Buenos Aires, Secretaria de Cultura Instituto Histórico de la Ciudad de Buenos Aires, 1985), 170; David Rock, *Argentina, 1516–1987: From Spanish Colonization to Alfonsín* (Berkeley: University of California Press, 1987), 173–75; José Ceppi, *Guía del emigrante a la República Argentina* (Buenos Aires: Imp. "Roma" de J. Carbone, 1898), 20.

4 See Victoria Mazzeo, *Migración internacional en la ciudad de Buenos Aires 1855–1980* (Buenos Aires: Municipalidad de la Ciudad de Buenos Aires, 1988), 3; and Buenos Aires, Dirección General de Servicio Estadístico Nacional, *Anuario estadístico de la ciudad de Buenos Aires, 1905* (Buenos Aires: Compañía Sud-Americana de Billetes de Banco, 1906), 32; James Scobie, *Buenos Aires, Plaza to Suburb, 1870–1910*, 208–12. Richard J. Walter, *Politics and Urban Growth in Buenos Aires, 1910–1942* (New York: Cambridge University Press, 1993), 10, 235–55 provides an excellent description of Buenos Aires in the 1940s (statistics, 235); Rock, *Argentina, 1516–1987*, 234–35, 283, 312, 331; Carlos Andrés Escudé, "Health in Buenos Aires in the Second Half of the Nineteenth Century," in *Social Welfare, 1850–1950: Australia, Argentina and Canada Compared*, ed. D.C.M. Platt (London: Macmillan Press, 1989), 63; Jose C. Moya, *Cousins and Strangers: Spanish Immigrants in Buenos Aires, 1850–1930* (Berkeley: University of California Press, 1998), 149, 171–72, 182–85, 200, 330.

5 Scobie, *Buenos Aires: Plaza to Suburb*, 135–39, 211–13, 217 and Tables 6 and 7 (265–66); Rock, 7, 159, 186, 196, 239; Samuel L. Baily, *Immigrants in the Lands of Promise: Italians in Buenos Aires and New York City, 1870–1914* (Ithaca: Cornell University Press, 1999), 198.

6 Scobie, *Buenos Aires: Plaza to Suburb*, 231, 235–39; George Reid Andrews, *The Afro-Argentines of Buenos Aires 1800–1900* (Madison: University of Wisconsin Press, 1980), 187–88, 214–15.

7 Baily, 114, 122, 166–67; Fernando J. Devoto, "Programs and Politics of the First Italian Elite of Buenos Aires, 1852–1880," trans. Amy Ferlazzo, in *Italian Workers of the World: Labor Migration and Formulation of Multiethnic States*, ed. Donna R. Gabaccia and Fraser M. Otanelli (Urbana: University of Illinois Press, 2001), 43, 52.

8 Mirta Zaida Lobato, "La Patria degli Italiani and Social Conflict in Early-Twentieth Century Argentina," trans. Amy Ferlazzo, in *Italian Workers of the World*, 75; Baily, 96, 101, 200–1.

9 Devoto, 45, 49–50, 55; Baily, 117, 173, 177, 179,181, 193–95; Congreso Internacional de Medicina e Higiene, *Guía Médica de la República Argentina* (Buenos Ares: Gráfica M. Pastor & Cia., 1910), 231.

10 Baily, 117, 119, 134, 150, 176, 198–99.

11 Moya, 18, 57, 149, 173, 207, 222–23, 247.

12 Moya, 179–81, 183, 284–86, 292; Congreso Internacional de Medicina e Higiene, 119–231.

13 Moya, 288–89, 294–95, 305, 307–8, 313.

14 Eugene F. Sofer, *From Pale to Pampa: A Social History of the Jews of Buenos Aires* (New York: Holmes & Meier, 1882), 4,70, 37, 79–80, 83, 85; Victor Mirelman, *Jewish Buenos Aires 1890–1930: In Search of Identity* (Detroit: Wayne State University Press, 1990), 21–22, 26, 275.

15 Sofer, 36–38, 44, 94–96, 99, 106, 109–10, 118–19, 128; Mirelman, 62–64, 71; Rock, 233; Haim Avni, "Argentine Jewry: Its Socio-Political Status and Organizational Patterns," *Dispersion and Unity* 12 (1971): 144–48.

16 Sofer, 6–7, 72, 134; Mirelman, 76–77, 102–4, 131, 139, 159–60, 162–66, 171–74, 221.

17 Sofer, 130; Mirelman, 82–83, 188–90, 195.
18 Mirelman, 48–49, 52, 55–56, 65, 73; Sofer, 38, 44–45.
19 Hernán Otero, Historia de los franceses en la Argentina (Buenos Aires: Editorial Biblos, 2012), 15, 114–16; J. P. Daughton, "When Argentina Was "French": Rethinking Cultural Politics and European Imperialism in Belle-Époque," *The Journal of Modern History* 80 (December 2008): 843–44.
20 Otero, 204–7, 235, 237, 239–40, 256, 314, 327.
21 Otero, 272–76; Daughton, 838–40. 847–48.
22 Benjamin Bryce, *To Belong in Buenos Aires: Germans, Argentines, and the Rise of a Pluralist Society* (Stanford: Stanford University Press, 2018), 22–23.
23 Eduardo O. Ciafardo, "Las damas de beneficencia y la participación social de la mujer en la ciudad de Buenos Aires 1889–1920," *Anuario IEHS-Tandil* 5 (1990): 161–63; B. Bryce, 30–40.
24 Argentina, Comisión directiva del censo nacional, *Segundo censo de la República Argentina, mayo 10 de 1895* (Buenos Aires: J. Peuser, 1896), 1, 643–44.
25 Vera Blinn Reber, *British Mercantile Houses in Buenos Aires, 1810–1880* (Cambridge: Harvard University Press, 1979), 41, 44, 48, 50, 120–21, 127; Rock, 169.
26 Andrews, 66, 183–86, 209, 217.
27 Andrews, 190–91, 196–98, 200, 204.
28 Andrews, 209–10.
29 The concept of "degenerate space" is discussed in Diego Armus, "Salud y anarquía: la tuberculosis en el discurso libertario argentino, 1870–1940," in *Salud, cultura y sociedad en América Latina* ed. Marcos Cueto (Lima: Instituto de Estudios Peruanos, 1996), 93–97, 106–7, 111–15, and in Diego Armus, "La idea del verde en la ciudad moderna: Buenos Aires, 1870–1940," *Entrepasados* (Buenos Aires) 5, no. 10 (1996): 9–18. Kristin Ruggiero, *Modernity in the Flesh: Medicine, Law and Society in Turn-of-the-Century Argentina* (Stanford: Stanford University Press, 2004), discusses moral contagion, 84–114, as does Andrew R. Aisenberg, *Contagion: Disease, Government and the "Social Question" in Nineteenth-Century France* (Stanford: Stanford University Press, 1999), 10–12, 29–30, 66–112, 128–32, 147–48. "Moral contagion" and "degenerate space" are analytical concept of historians; Porteños did not use those phrases.
30 Emil R. Coni, "La campaña contra la tuberculosis en la República Argentina," *La Semana Médica* 16, no. 40 (7 October 1909): 1398–99; "Casas par obreros en el barrio de los Patricios," *Alianza de Higiene Social* 9, nos. 3–4 (August/September, 1909): 112–16; Donna J. Guy, "Emilio and Gabriela Coni: Reformers, Public Health, and Working Women," in *The Human Tradition in Latin America: The Nineteenth Century*, eds. Judy Ewell and W. H. Beezley (Wilmington, DE: Scholarly Resources, 1989), 236–40; Ernest Allen Crider, "Modernization and Human Welfare: The Asistencia Pública and Buenos Aires, 1883–1910" (PhD diss., Ohio State University, 1976), 229–39.
31 Emilio R. Coni, "Hospitalización y aislamiento de los tuberculosos pulmonares en Buenos Aires," *La Semana Médica* 9, no. 43 (27 October 1904): 1139–40; "La Desinfección pública en la tuberculosis," *Revista de la Tuberculosis* 1 (1902): 283–84; Emilio R. Coni, *Código de higiene y medicina legal de la Republica Argentina para uso de los médicos, abogados, farmacéuticos, etc.* (Buenos Aires: Etchepareborda, 1891), II: 50–51; Emilio

R. Coni, "Higiene y Salubridad en la República Argentina," in *Primer Congreso Médico Latino-Americano, Santiago de Chile 1 al 9 de enero de 1901* (Santiago: Congreso Médico Latino-Americano, 1901), 76; Coni, "La campaña contra la tuberculosis en la República Argentina," (7 October 1909): 1412; José Penna and Horacio Madero, *La Administración sanitaria y asistencia pública en la ciudad de Buenos Aires* (Buenos Aires: Guillermo Kraft, 1910), 2, 145–49.

32 Liga Argentina contra la tuberculosis, *Revista de la Tuberculosis*, I (November 1901): 217; Samuel Gache, "Profilaxis antituberculosa en Buenos Aires," *La Semana Médica* 10, no. 42 (15 October 1903): 977–84; Emilio R. Coni, "La Lucha antituberculosa en la América Latina," *Alianza de Higiene Social* 9 (August/September 1909): 143–54.

33 "Liga Argentina contra la tuberculosis: Informe, anual de su presidente correspondiente al año 1907," *Alianza de Higiene Social* 7 (1907–1908): 333; Enrique Foster, "Dispensario de Lactantes: la Gota de Leche," *Archivos Latinoamericanos de Pediatría* 1, no. 1 (March 1905): 342–51; Emilio R. Coni, "La Lucha antituberculosa en la América Latina," *Alianza de Higiene Social*, 75–77; Ricardo Schatz, "Higiene pública y policía sanitaria: Profilaxis de la tuberculosis en los tambos de Buenos Aires," *Anales del Círculo Médico Argentino* 18, no. 1 (January 1895): 55–62; Emilio R. Coni, "The Campaign against Tuberculosis in Argentina," in *Transactions of the Sixth International Congress on Tuberculosis, Washington, September 28 to October 5, 1908* (Philadelphia: William F. Fell Company, 1908), 4, 51, 60–61.

34 Eduardo Ciafardo, "La práctica benéfica y el control de los sectores populares de la ciudad de Buenos Aries, 1890–1910," *Revista de Indias* 54, no. 201 (May/August, 1994): 388–96, 399, 408; Cynthia Jeffress Little, "The Society of Beneficence in Buenos Aires, 1823–1900" (PhD diss., Temple University, 1980), 47–48, 249–50, 269–74; Sociedad de beneficencia de la capital, *República Argentina: álbum histórico de la Sociedad de Beneficencia de la capital, 1823–1910* (Buenos Aires: Lit. A Bianche, 1910); Sociedad de Beneficencia de la Capital, *Memoria del Año 1905* (Buenos Aires: Imprenta, Litografía y Encuadernación G. Kraft, 1906), 48.

35 Ciafardo, "La práctica benéfica y el control," 399–400; Karen Mead, "Gender, Welfare and the Catholic Church in Argentina: Conferencias de Señoras de San Vicente de Paul, 1890–1916," *The Americas* 58, no. 1 (July 2001): 93–96, 99, 104–9, 112–14.

36 Eduardo O. Ciafardo, "Las damas de beneficencia y la participación social de la mujer en la ciudad de Buenos Aires 1880–1920," *Anuario IEHS*-Tandil 5 (1990): 165, 169; Ciafardo, "La práctica benéfica," 391–92, 393–94, 404; Donna J. Guy, "Mothers Alive and Dead: Multiple Concepts of Mothering in Buenos Aires," in *Sex and Sexuality in Latin America*, eds. Daniel Balderston and Donna J. Guy (New York: New York University Press, 1997), 155–58.

37 Ciafardo, "Las damas de beneficiencia," 161–63, 166–70; Ciafardo, "La práctica benéfica," 387.

38 For statistics for Philadelphia see Nathaniel Burt and Wallace E. Davies, "The Iron Age 1876–1905," in *Philadelphia: A 300-Year History*, ed. Russell Weigley (New York: W.W. Norton & Company, 1982), 488, and Caroline Golab, "The Immigrant and the City," 203–4; for Buenos Aires, see Scobie, *Buenos Aires: Plaza to Suburb*, 263.

39 Hepp, *The Middle Class City*, focuses on the middle class, but see particularly 144–45, 180–81; Simon, *Philadelphia: A Brief History*, 43; Sutherland, "Housing the Poor in the City of Homes," 180–81.

40 Caroline Golab, "The Immigrant and the City: Poles, Italians and Jews in Philadelphia, 1870–1920," in *Peoples of Philadelphia: A History of Ethnic Groups and Lower-Class Life, 1790–1940*, eds. Allen F. Davis and Mark H. Haller (Philadelphia: Temple University Press, 1973), 204–7.

41 Mark H. Haller, "Recurring Themes," in *Peoples of Philadelphia: A History of Ethnic Groups and Lower-Class Life 1790–1940*, eds. Allen F. Davis and Mark H. Haller (Philadelphia: Temple University Press, 1973), 277–81; Golab, 211; Thomas Wirth, "Urban Neglect: The Environment, Public Health and Influenza in Philadelphia, 1915–1919," *Journal of Pennsylvania History* 73 (2006): 326.

42 La Vern J. Rippley, *The German-Americans* (Boston: Twayne Publishers, 1976), 130–34; Herbert A. Strauss, "Transplanted and Transformed: German-Jewish Immigrants since 1933," in *America and the Germans: An Assessment of a Three Hundred Year History*, Volume 2, *The Relationship in the Twentieth Century*, eds. Frank Trommler and Joseph McVeigh (Philadelphia: University of Pennsylvania Press, 1985), 245, 250; Henry F. Page, "The German Hospital of the City of Philadelphia," *Founders' Week Memorial Volume: Containing an Account of the Two Hundred and Twenty-Fifth Anniversary of the Founding of the City of Philadelphia, and Histories of Its Principal Scientific Institutions, Medical Colleges, Hospitals, etc.*, ed. Frederick P. Henry (Philadelphia: City of Philadelphia, 1909), 652–59; Gail Farr Casterline, "St. Joseph's and St. Mary's: The Origins of Catholic Hospitals in Philadelphia," *The Pennsylvania Magazine of History and Biography* 108, no. 3 (July 1984): 305–11; Barbara Bates, *Bargaining for Life: A Social History of Tuberculosis, 1876–1938* (Philadelphia: University of Pennsylvania Press, 1992), 66, 149.

43 Maxwell Whiteman, "Philadelphia's Jewish Neighborhoods," in *The Peoples of Philadelphia: A History of Ethnic Groups and Lower Class Life 1790–1940*, eds. Allen F. Davis and Mark H. Haller (Philadelphia: Temple University Press, 1973), 235, 237, 239, 246; Lloyd M. Abernethy, "Progressivism, 1905–1919," *Philadelphia A 300 year History*, ed. Russell F. Weigley (New York: W.W. Norton & Company, 1982), 529; Arthur P. Dudden, "The City Embraces 'Normalcy' in 1919–1929," in *Philadelphia: A 300-Year History*, ed. Russell F. Weigley (New York: W.W. Norton & Company, 1982), 588; Henry N. Wessel, "The Jewish Hospital Association of Philadelphia," in *Founders' Week Memorial Volume: Containing an Account of the Two Hundred and Twenty-Fifth Anniversary of the Founding of the City of Philadelphia, and Histories of Its Principal Scientific Institutions, Medical Colleges, Hospitals, etc.*, ed. Frederick P. Henry (Philadelphia: City of Philadelphia, 1909), 664, 668, 677; E. Digby Baltzell, Allen Glicksman and Jacquelyn Litt, "The Jewish Communities of Philadelphia and Boston: A Tale of Two Cities," in *Jewish Life in Philadelphia, 1830–1940*, ed. Murray Friedman (Philadelphia: Institute for the Study of Human Issues, 1983), 304.

44 Dennis J. Clark, "The Philadelphia Irish: Persistent Presence," in *The Peoples of Philadelphia: A History of Ethnic Groups and Lower Class Life 1790–1940*, eds. Allen F. Davis and Mark H. Haller (Philadelphia: Temple University Press, 1973),138–39, 141–42; Burt and Davies, 488; Joseph M. Spellissy, "The St. Joseph's Hospital," in *Founders' Week Memorial Volume: Containing an Account of the Two Hundred and Twenty-Fifth Anniversary of the Founding of the City of Philadelphia, and Histories of Its Principal Scientific Institutions, Medical Colleges, Hospitals, etc.*, ed. Frederick P. Henry (Philadelphia: City of Philadelphia, 1909), 614, 618–19, 627–29; Casterline, 290–91, 295, 299, 303–4.

45 Joan Younger Dickinson, "Aspects of Italian Immigration to Philadelphia," *The Pennsylvania Magazine of History and Biography* 90, no. 4 (October 1966): 445–56; Richard A. Varbero, "Philadelphia's South Italians in the 1920s," in *Peoples of Philadelphia: A History of Ethnic Groups and Lower Class Life 1790–1940,* eds. Allen F. Davis and Mark H. Haller (Philadelphia: Temple University Press, 1973), 255–60; John F. Sutherland, "Housing the Poor in the City of Homes: Philadelphia at the Turn of the Century," in *The Peoples of Philadelphia: A History of Ethnic Groups and Lower-Class Life, 1790–1940*, eds. Allen F. Davis and Mark H. Haller (Philadelphia: Temple University Press, 1973), 186; Whiteman, 243–44; Franklin Stahl, "St Agnes' Hospital," in *Founders' Week Memorial Volume: Containing an Account of the Two Hundred and Twenty-Fifth Anniversary of the Founding of the City of Philadelphia, and Histories of Its Principal Scientific Institutions, Medical Colleges, Hospitals, etc.*, ed. Frederick P. Henry (Philadelphia: City of Philadelphia, 1909), 706–8; John St. George Joyce, *Story of Philadelphia* (Philadelphia: Rex Printing House, 1919), 452; Bates, *Bargaining for Life*, 56, 65.

46 Wirth, "Urban Neglect," 328; Henry R. M. Landis, "The Tuberculosis Problem and the Negro," *Virginia Medical Monthly* (January 1923), rpt. in Sixteenth Report of the Henry Phipps Institute (Philadelphia, 1924): 2; David McBride, *Integrating the City of Medicine: Blacks in Philadelphia Health Care, 1910–1965* (Philadelphia: Temple University Press, 1988), 57–58.

47 Golab, 208; Carolyn Adams et al., *Philadelphia: Neighborhoods, Divisions, and Conflict in a Postindustrial City* (Philadelphia: Temple University Press, 1991), 11; Abernethy, 532; Jerome P. Bjelopera, *City of Clerks: Office and Sales Workers in Philadelphia 1870–1920* (Chicago: University of Illinois Press, 2005), 31; McBride, *Integrating the City*, 70.

48 McBride, *Integrating the City*, 63–64; 78–80; Bates, *292;* Emily K. Abel, *Tuberculosis and the Politics of Exclusion: A History of Public Health and Migration to Los Angeles* (New Brunswick: Rutgers University Press, 2007), 126.

49 Vanessa Northington Gamble, *Making a Place for Ourselves: The Black Hospital Movement, 1920–1945* (New York: Oxford University Press, 1995), 21–28, 33; Bates, 290, 298, 303–9, 338; McBride, *Integrating the City*, 73–77; 128–29.

50 Paul Starr, *The Social Transformation of American Medicine* (New York: Basic Books, 1982), 180–82; James H. Cassedy, *Charles V. Chapin and the Public Health Movement* (Cambridge: Harvard University Press, 1962), 68, 126–28; Philadelphia City Archives, Philadelphia Information Locator Services, "Guardians of the Poor," 8 November 2000; David McBride, *Integrating the City*, 236; Charities, Bureau of City of Philadelphia www.phila.gov/phils/docs/inventor/graphics/agencies/A065.htm (18 December 2014).

51 Wirth, 318–19, 324; Abel, *Tuberculosis and the Politics of Exclusion*, 32; Guy Hinsdale, "Tuberculosis in Pennsylvania," *Journal of the American Medical Association* 35, no. 16 (20 October 1900): 996–99; Elizabeth Fee and Evelynn M. Hammonds, "Science, Politics, and the Art of Persuasion: Promoting the New Scientific Medicine in New York City," in *Hives of Sickness: Public Health and Epidemics in New York City*, ed. David Rosner (New Brunswick: Rutgers University Press, 1995), 160–63, 172, 182.

52 Wirth, 328–29; Pennsylvania Society for the Prevention of Tuberculosis, "How Hotel Keepers Can Aid in Preventing the Spread of Tuberculosis" (Philadelphia: The Historical Society of Pennsylvania, 1910); Georgina

D. Feldberg, *Disease and Class: Tuberculosis and the Shaping of Modern North American Society* (New Brunswick: Rutgers University Press, 1955), 50, 83–90; Katherine Ott, *Fevered Lives: Tuberculosis in American Culture since 1870* (Cambridge: Harvard University Press, 1996), 116–20.

53 Theodore B. Sachs, "The Official Responsibility of the City in the Tuberculosis Problem," in The National Association for the Study and Prevention of Tuberculosis, *Transactions of the Eleventh Annual Meeting, Seattle, Washington, June 14–16* (Baltimore: Wiliams & Wilkins Company 1915), 278–83; Hermann M. Biggs, *Brief History of the Campaign against Tuberculosis in New York City* (New York: New York City Department of Health, 1908), 4–5, 12, 14; John S. Billings, Jr., *The Registration and Sanitary Supervision of Pulmonary Tuberculosis in New York City* (New York: New York City Department of Health, 1912), 8–9, 11, 23–24.

54 Cynthia A. Connolly, "Nurses: The Early Twentieth Century Tuberculosis Preventorium's 'Connecting Link,'" *Nursing History Review* 10 (2002): 133–37, 141.

55 Whiteman, 245; Wirth, 317, 320–21; Lawrence Francis Flick, "Report of the Committee on Tuberculosis," *Annual Report of the American Public Health Association* (1897), 1–2.

56 Wirth, 321–23, 326–29.

57 David McBride, "Henry Phipps Institute, 1903–1937: Pioneering Tuberculosis Work with an Urban Minority," *Bulletin of the History of Medicine* 61, no. 1 (Spring 1987): 83–88, 95; Frank Craig, *Early Days at Phipps* (Philadelphia: University of Pennsylvania Press, 1952).

58 McBride, "Henry Phipps Institute," 78, 83–84, 87–88, 90; Bates, 296–300; Table 3.1: Comparison of White and Black TB Pulmonary Deaths in Philadelphia.

59 "Work Among the Negroes of Philadelphia," 12; Wirth, "Urban Neglect," 327; McBride, "Henry Phipps Institute, 1903–1937," 96–97; Table 3.1.

60 Pennsylvania Society for the Prevention of Tuberculosis, *Annual Report 1898* (Philadelphia: Society for the Prevention of Tuberculosis, 1898), 7; Pennsylvania Society for the Prevention of Tuberculosis, *Annual Report 1911* (Philadelphia: Society for the Prevention of Tuberculosis, 1911), 4; Pennsylvania Society for the Prevention of Tuberculosis, *Annual Report 1920* (Philadelphia: Society for the Prevention of Tuberculosis, 1920), 4–8; Samuel Kelton Roberts, *Infectious Fear: Politics, Disease and the Health Effects of Segregation* (Chapel Hill: University of North Carolina, 2009), 42–62, provides an excellent analysis of the racial interpretation of disease in the U.S.

61 Vera Blinn Reber, "Blood Coughs, and Fever: Tuberculosis and the Working Class of Buenos Aires," *Social History of Medicine* 12, no. 1 (April 1999): 82–85 has a detailed discussion of living conditions in various districts.

62 B. Bryce, Table 1, 2 "Foreign Nationals," 16, 17.

63 Mazzeo, *Migración internacional*, 3; Daniel M. Fox, "Social Policy and City Politics: Tuberculosis Reporting in New York, 1889–1990," *Bulletin of the History of Medicine* 49, no. 2 (1975): 175; Godias J. Drolet and Anthony M. Lowell, *A Half Century's Progress against Tuberculosis in New York City, 1900–1950* (New York: New York Tuberculosis and Health Association, 1952), VII, LXII, LXIV–LVI, 4; Golab, 205; Buenos Aires, *Anuario estadístico de la ciudad de Buenos Aires* (Buenos Aires: Compañía Sud-Americana de Billetes de Banco, 1910): 119–23.

64 See Table 4.2: Pulmonary Tuberculosis Deaths of Adults.

65 Buenos Aires, *Anuario estadístico de la ciudad de Buenos Aires* (Buenos Aires: Compañía Sud-Americana de Billetes de Banco, 1900), 32.

Calculations for 1909 were based on data provided by Buenos Aires, *Statistical Year-Book of the City of Buenos Aires* (Buenos Aires: Compañía Sud-Americana de Billetes de Banco, 1910), 121–24; Pennsylvania Society for the Prevention of Tuberculosis, *Annual Report of the Commissioner of Health of the Commonwealth of Pennsylvania* (Harrisburg: Government Printing Press, 1920); Table I; Nicholas B. King, "Immigration, Race and Geographies of Differences in the Tuberculosis Pandemic," in *The Return of the White Plague: Global Poverty and the New Tuberculosis,* eds. Matthew Gandy and Alimuddin Zumla (London: Verso, 2003), 49.

66 Emily K. Abel, "Taking the Cure to the Poor: Patients' Responses to New York City's Tuberculosis Program 1894 to 1918," *American Journal of Public Health* 87, no. 11 (November 1997): 1809, 1811–13; Reber, "Blood, Coughs and Fever," 89–91; Guy, "Emilio and Gabriela Coni," 239–40; Barron H. Lerner, "New York City's Tuberculosis Control Efforts: The Historical Limitations of the 'War on Consumption,'" *American Journal of Public Health* 83, no. 5 (May 1993): 759–61.

4 Tuberculosis Treatment in Buenos Aires and Philadelphia

Patient and Physician Experiences

> George E. Macklin, 21 June 1904: I did as I was told, as I usually do and put on a fly-blister: as a result I am now minus over the top of my right lung, four by five inches of skin, and the surface very much resembles porterhouse steak, and it is not necessary for me to say to you that it is sore...left the plaster on about an hour and a half... You want this done once a week... I would be glad to know where you want to take the next piece of skin off; or if you can kindly tell me where I erred...I will promise you, if it makes me sore as this one you will have to change your prescription. Otherwise, I am feeling tiptop.[1]

> Maria E. Lombardo, aged seventeen years, an Argentine student, entered the hospital on 23 November 1918; initiated treatment of tuberculin starting with a l/10 solution and increasing until injection 1 cc; three administrations daily resulted in the cure taking nine months and patient put on weight of ten pounds.[2]

The previous statements provide insight into patient treatment from two different perspectives. The first case was that of George Macklin, a wealthy general manager of the Pressed Steel Car Company in Pittsburgh who consulted Dr. Lawrence Flick in the spring of 1903. He could afford to take time off from work, confer with one of the best-known tuberculosis experts and follow whatever treatment was recommended. In contrast, Maria Lombardo came from a working-class family. Rather than protesting any treatment, she was subject to physical experimentation in 1917 in Hospital Municipal Doctor Tornú. These cases illustrate the frustration of patients, the trial-and-error proceedings of physicians who could not promise a cure and the greater options available to the wealthy. Because there was no cure for tuberculosis, patients sought to shape their own treatments.[3]

The late nineteenth century witnessed a transition between humoral and biomedical procedures. The experiences of George and Maria reflected that transition. The theory of humorism contended that the human body contained four basic substances (black bile, phlegm, yellow bile and blood), which are in balance when an individual is healthy. In contrast, biomedical theory applied new understandings of infection to clinical medicine, as is seen in Maria's tuberculin treatment. Between 1870 and 1945, Porteño and Philadelphia physicians increasingly employed biomedical treatments on their patients.

Although physicians disagreed among themselves about specific remedies for tuberculosis, they shared a common discourse. By the end of the nineteenth century, western-trained physicians emphasized clinical medicine—in particular, the use of patent and laboratory-produced medications, surgery and disease-prevention procedures. Tuberculosis treatments fell into two broad categories: medications/surgical procedures and fresh air/diet regimens. Both approaches reflected increased understanding of how tuberculosis affects the human body and were utilized worldwide. One set of treatments utilized medications; the other assumed that a strong body could resist the disease. Neither of the treatments was particularly effective, but patients could choose between them. The tubercular ill in Buenos Aires and Philadelphia adapted strategies that best fit their economic and social needs. The working class utilized clinics in order to stay at home, entered sanatoriums if there was a hope of cure, avoided hospitals until there was no hope, and ignored efforts that aimed to improve their morals. Those patients like Macklin, who could afford the best care, complained about treatment and ignored directives that they disliked or found ineffective. In both Philadelphia and Buenos Aires, middle-class and elite patients had access to the latest therapies but were often aware that different physicians favored different treatments.

Gender, class and age modified and influenced diagnosis, choice of treatment and patient response. Age, gender, health and vocation determined if and when the tubercle bacilli entered the body and if it became active or not. In Philadelphia and Buenos Aires, the diagnosis was particularly difficult before Koch's discovery of the tubercle bacillus in 1882. Although tuberculosis could be found in any organ, physicians focused on pulmonary tuberculosis—the most common variety. They could base their analysis only on symptoms. Beginning in the 1870s, physicians used the stethoscope with some success to detect tuberculosis. Family histories provided additional medical information.[4]

Since extended rest and a nutritious diet were the most effective treatments, early diagnosis was extremely important. Too often physicians could do little when the spitting of blood finally led them to diagnose tuberculosis. Between 1870 and 1945, physicians in Buenos Aires and Philadelphia generally discerned three stages of tuberculosis, which differed in terms of the symptoms that were observed and the perceived potential for cure. In the first stage—rarely treated and difficult to distinguish from other diseases—patients suffered from a dry persistent cough, pain in the shoulders and chest, a small increase in the pulse rate, an abnormal daily temperature range, indigestion and weight loss. In the second stage—which was often confused with bronchitis—patients coughed harder leading to hoarseness, a fluctuating fever and the spitting up of mucus material. In the third stage—physicians could finally diagnose pulmonary tuberculosis: the patient was now spitting up blood and had a distinct cough, hollow-sounding lungs, a rapid pulse, diarrhea and constant pain in the joints.[5] Both patient and physician viewed the third stage as most serious. However, patients suffered and bore the anguish of pain and the worry about the seriousness of the disease through all three stages.

Beginning in the 1890s—when saliva could be tested for the bacillus and tuberculin could be used to diagnose the presence of *Mycobacterium tuberculosis*—physicians had more useful diagnostic tools. In 1907, Clemens von Pirquet introduced an improved tuberculin skin test which allowed physicians to identify the presence of tuberculosis at an early stage; however, the test did not distinguish between those who had latent tuberculosis and those who had the disease. The availability of the X-ray, invented in 1895, further refined diagnostic techniques. Unfortunately, X-ray plates provided only blurred images until the 1920s. Interpreting the blurry images was a challenge: at times, physicians mistook the stomach for the lungs. Even in the 1930s, general practitioners might not use X-radiation and would diagnose tuberculosis simply because a patient's temperature increased in the afternoon. In some instances, inadequately trained physicians did not even check sputum or examine the lungs. Diagnosing tuberculosis did, however, become progressively easier and more accurate and thus encourage prevention efforts.[6]

While new procedures made the identification of tuberculosis more accurate, they did not solve the problems of treatment. The treatment was based on the physician's evaluation of the stage of a patient's tuberculosis. Early diagnosis meant that the patient could be treated at home with regular visits to a clinic. If the physician felt that the disease could be cured, he often recommended a sanatorium. Medical personnel sought to persuade patients with advanced tuberculosis (and without families to care for them) to go to a hospital; if the individual insisted on staying at home, he was taught how to disinfect his room and told that no one else should sleep in his room. By 1898—when Buenos Aires' physicians viewed tuberculosis as contagious rather than hereditary—tubercular husbands and wives with children were told to go to a hospital, so as not to infect their children; Public Assistance then took responsibility for the children.[7]

Tuberculosis Treatment for Women, Manual Workers and the Aged

From 1870 to 1945, tuberculosis diagnosis and treatment posed special challenges for three particular groups: women, low-paid foreign workers and the aged. Table 4.1 shows that adult tubercular deaths as a percent

Table 4.1 Pulmonary Tuberculosis Deaths of Adults, Age 20–100, in Buenos Aires from 1900 to 1911

Year	Age 20–29						Age 30–39						Age 40–49						Age 50–59						Over 60						Total Death 20–100			Total Deaths	%TB Deaths
	Arg		Fng		Total		Arg		Fng		Total		Arg		Fng		Total		Arg		Fng		Total		Arg		Fng		Total						20–100
	F	M	F	M	F	M	F	M	F	M	F	M	F	M	F	M	F	M	F	M	F	M	F	M	F	M	F	M	F	M	F	M	T		
1900	166	112	72	130	238	242	58	84	49	123	107	207	22	45	34	116	56	161	10	16	16	55	26	71	5	5	4	21	9	26	436	707	1143	16504	6.93
1901	159	156	90	108	249	264	71	78	68	135	139	213	28	41	47	138	75	179	6	12	18	84	24	96	9	6	5	32	14	38	501	790	1291	15807	8.17
1902	178	110	88	138	266	248	69	118	81	81	159	229	24	131	35	31	59	162	12	81	17	14	29	95	7	30	13	13	20	43	533	777	1310	14097	9.29
1903	212	126	110	130	322	256	61	132	59	77	120	209	32	135	47	36	79	131	15	66	18	18	33	84	7	32	8	10	15	42	569	722	1291	13996	9.22
1904	201	116	82	135	283	251	75	148	76	97	151	245	30	148	46	49	76	197	17	74	14	18	31	92	4	41	9	12	13	53	554	838	1392	14313	9.73
1905	235	130	103	155	338	285	96	147	72	101	168	248	36	131	48	54	84	185	18	70	22	25	40	95	6	45	13	11	19	56	649	869	1518	15916	9.54
1906	245	153	65	160	310	313	85	153	74	107	159	260	32	152	57	52	89	204	17	92	33	22	50	114	6	42	16	11	22	53	630	944	1574	17916	8.79
1907	227	163	111	161	338	324	82	164	82	112	162	276	36	154	55	65	91	219	16	104	13	27	29	131	16	51	15	9	31	60	651	1010	1661	18616	8.92
1908	209	158	110	176	319	334	101	167	79	107	180	274	34	151	48	62	82	213	24	100	18	23	42	123	10	44	13	14	23	58	646	1002	1648	18139	9.09
1909	177	177	105	163	282	340	90	156	68	98	158	254	30	150	48	64	78	214	5	85	25	32	30	117	5	34	13	6	18	40	566	965	1531	18959	8.08
1910	236	188	97	189	333	377	70	204	67	115	137	319	37	187	36	80	73	267	16	94	8	27	24	121	7	41	8	10	15	51	582	1135	1717	20968	8.19
1911	267	220	138	218	405	438	84	173	85	108	169	281	39	156	38	68	77	224	9	103	26	27	35	130	1	26	16	11	20	37	706	1110	1816	22869	7.94

Source: Buenos Aires, *Year-Book, 19101911*, 119–20.
Abbreviations: Arg = Argentine; Fng = Foreign; F = Female; M = Male; T = Total.

of all deaths varied between 6.93 and 9.73 percent. Argentine and foreign women (considering 1 to 2 ratios between foreign men and women) died in the largest number due to pulmonary tuberculosis between the ages twenty and twenty-nine. From 1900 to 1911, the pulmonary deaths of Argentine women increased by sixty-one percent, while population growth was approximately forty percent; more women than men between the ages of fifteen and twenty-nine died of tuberculosis, while more men died between the ages of thirty and forty-nine. Foreign men died of pulmonary tuberculosis in the largest numbers between ages twenty and thirty-nine; Argentine men died in the largest numbers from ages thirty to forty-nine. In Buenos Aires, gender was a significant factor in determining the likely age at which one died of tuberculosis.

Table 4.2 does not provide a gender breakdown by specific ages. However, the table does provide a total of pulmonary female adult deaths. From 1870 to 1883, the deaths of women exceed those of men in six years. The largest number of female pulmonary tubercular deaths occurred during the child-bearing years. During youth and early adulthood, the mortality rates from tuberculosis were usually greater for women than for men in both Buenos Aires and Philadelphia.[8] From 1900 to 1914, adult tubercular deaths as a percent of all deaths varied from 9.42 to 10.68 percent. Before World War I, adult pulmonary tuberculosis deaths in Philadelphia began to decrease. After a small increase during the war years, Philadelphia adult pulmonary deaths decreased rapidly from 9.20 percent of all deaths in 1915 to 5.91 in 1923. However, the number of deaths of African Americans remains high through 1938. Between 1870 and 1945, physician attitudes toward women and their health varied considerably.

In the nineteenth century, women's bodies were viewed as threatening; female sexuality was considered dangerous. Emotional and respiratory diseases—including whooping cough and tuberculosis of the lungs—were thought to affect females more than males. By 1922, Doctor César Sánchez Aizcorbe of Argentina argued that physical education was more necessary for women than men to prepare them for childbirth. The primary task assigned to women was to bear and nurture children. As a result, women's bodies were thought to be better suited to the domestic spheres and ill-suited for public careers.[9] In the late nineteenth century, it was thought that pregnancy might cure tuberculosis in women. In 1920, Lawrence Flick argued that tuberculosis did not shorten a mother's life, but that her condition should nevertheless be carefully monitored. Tuberculosis was to be treated during pregnancy; and if the disease was active, the woman should have complete bed rest. But by the late 1920s, medical science concluded that pregnancy needed to be interrupted in order to cure tuberculosis. Because of lowered resistance, childbirth was believed to aggravate the disease.[10] (Currently, physicians treat tuberculosis in pregnant women because the infection is dangerous

Table 4.2 Pulmonary Tuberculosis Deaths of Adults, Age 20–100, in Philadelphia for Various Years from 1870 to 1938

Year	Age						TB Deaths 20–100			Af/Am	Place of Birth			Tot PulTB	Adult %	Total Death	AdTB % Tot
	20–29	30–39	40–49	50–59	60–69	70+	F	M	Total		U.S.	Fng	Ukn	TBDeath	TB D		Death
1870	681	548	366	231	116	63	1020	985	2005	153	1406	732	170	2308	86.87	15317	13.09
1873	715	547	328	217	128	59	1018	976	1994	187	1391	729	171	2291	87.04	15224	13.10
1877	754	585	364	203	111	53	1036	1034	2070	152	1508	689	152	2349	88.12	16004	12.93
1878	735	647	361	236	142	62	1143	1040	2183	201	1604	766	121	2491	87.64	15743	13.87
1880	877	634	424	241	151	66	1192	1201	2393	205	1816	767	109	2692	88.89	17711	13.51
1882	900	688	445	264	150	80	1268	1259	2527	108	1877	797	135	2809	89.96	20059	12.60
1883	896	682	424	276	153	71	1267	1235	2502	199	1890	786	122	2798	89.4%	20076	12.50
1885	928	671	411	250	155	90	1215	1290	2505	219	1915	769	137	2821	88.80	21392	11.71
1889	765	656	383	230	146	58	1059	1179	2238	181	1685	689	158	2532	88.39	20536	10.90
1890	815	675	493	241	146	83	1128	1325	2453	201	1926	719	119	2764	88.75	21732	11.29
1892	824	695	356	269	158	71	1095	1278	2373	185	1957	672	80	2709	87.60	24305	9.76
1896	745	632	398	238	131	65	997	1212	2209	194	1981	465	68	2514	87.87	23982	9.21
1899	829	725	466	240	152	72	1083	1401	2484	238	2083	621	114	2818	88.15	23796	10.44
1900	696	728	453	272	156	57	1053	1309	2362	287	2035	643	39	2717	86.93	25078	9.42
1901	750	808	522	269	153	77	1135	1444	2579	299	2302	621	23	2946	87.54	24137	10.68
1902	731	784	487	251	135	75	1059	1404	2463	339	2199	613	13	2845	86.57	23847	10.33
1903	828	766	530	294	171	63	1112	1540	2652	293	2143	865	45	3053	86.87	25510	10.40
1904	830	774	524	334	160	58	1123	1557	2680	340	2265	827	25	3117	85.98	25976	10.32
1905	714	747	497	284	158	60	1060	1400	2460	312	2043	762	33	2838	86.68	24807	9.92
1907	750	847	570	327	164	42	1079	1621	2700	381	2249	864	44	3157	85.52	27750	9.73
1914	653	660	577	348	154	51			2443	395	1995	668	21	2684	91.02	26918	9.08
1915	635	672	546	325	168	72			2418	436	2055	673	26	2754	87.8%	26287	9.20
1917	692	725	622	350	172	56			2617	510	2234	748	37	3019	86.68	29681	8.82
1918	848	782	655	381	212	64			2942	533	2377	800	80	3257	90.33	42643	6.90
1920	576	516	398	261	124	50			1925	409	1679	441	10	2130	90.38	26516	7.26
1923	406	404	333	258	123	44			1568	410	1362	455	22	1817	86.30	26513	5.91
1936	290	239	221	113	129	46			1038	426	571			1199	86.57		
1938	242	231	174	171	91	56			965	461	452	164	27	1104	87.41		

Sources: *Philadelphia, Annual Message of the Mayor*, for various years incl. 1904 v. 3: 240; 1912, v.3: 109–10

Abbreviations: F = Female; M = Male; Af/Am = African Americans; Fng = Foreign; Ukn = Unknown; D = Deaths; Tot = Total; Pul = Pulmonary; Ad = Adults.

to both the mother and the developing fetus.)[11] In the first half of the twentieth century, wealthy women were seen as fragile and unsuited to physical activity, yet working-class women toiled long hours in crowded workshops and factories.[12] Since the society generally valued men more highly than women, men received more to eat than women when there was a food shortage. When food was widely available, women improved their diet, which helped reduce mortality from infectious diseases. The immune systems of well-rested women more easily warded off diseases. As basic services, such as running water, sewerage, electricity, and domestic appliances became commonly available, working-class women did less physical labor. The improved housing also benefited women's health.[13] In the twentieth century, social attitudes gradually changed: although women's child-bearing responsibilities were still emphasized, it came to be understood that women needed good health and education to raise their children successfully.

Class and ethnicity also shaped society's understanding and treatment of women. In Philadelphia, ethnicity often defined which women sought employment. Italians had the smallest proportion of women working outside the home because Italian men thought that daughters and wives should remain under their protection. In Buenos Aires, Italian women were garment workers but did the work in their homes. Although Polish women in Philadelphia also often remained at home, Polish families took in boarders to supplement the family income. African-American women were more inclined than women in any other group to work outside the home. In Buenos Aires and Philadelphia, single women had always worked in factories and as clerks, teachers and servants.[14]

Immigrant women in Buenos Aires, like those in Philadelphia, sought paid labor in factories and workshops to contribute to the family income. Even though immigrant women comprised only nineteen percent of women in Argentina in 1895, they outnumbered native-born women in employment by two to one. Women were active in cigar wrapping, shoemaking and the food industry and also worked as domestic servants and laundresses. Before the 1930s, factories remained small, and immigrant women often sewed items piecemeal in their homes or toiled in sweatshops. In the 1940s, female migrants to Buenos Aires from elsewhere in Argentina—like immigrants at the beginning of the century—found work as domestic servants and predominated in the clothing and textile industries. Women tended to work longer hours than men and had difficulty finding time to care for their families. When women had little time to prepare proper meals, families purchased food from street vendors. Women earned sixty percent less than men for skilled and semi-skilled work, and at least ten percent less for unskilled work. The death or illness of a male often left a family destitute. Status, the financial situation of the family, the children's ages and the type of childcare available influenced the decisions of women to obtain paid labor.[15]

In Argentina, political reformers sought to protect poor women through legislation that limited working hours and improved factory conditions. Poorly enforced legislation, however, left women unprotected. Lengthy work days, lack of rest, circulatory problems during pregnancy and work in (match, burlap, and tobacco) factories with poor air circulation contributed to the spread of pulmonary tuberculosis in women.[16] But legislation also discriminated against working-class mothers. In the 1920s, a law required that a tubercular Argentine woman give up her baby or at the least place it temporarily in a non-tubercular home. Class was clearly an issue in seven cases discussed in a 1926 medical journal. A baby girl was given immediately to one mother, the wife of a doctor, while working-class mothers had their babies taken from them by Public Assistance. Those who were considered cured could take their babies home. However, most mothers with tuberculosis gave birth at home and subsequently cared for their babies.[17] Working women faced many special challenges in supporting themselves and caring for the ill. In 1911, Buenos Aires, a widow with several daughters who earned her living by sewing at home had to decide how to care for a daughter who contracted tuberculosis and was diagnosed in the late stage. The mother asked the doctor to let the daughter die at home, but the physician convinced the mother to place her in a hospital so that the other children would not be exposed to the disease. Because the hospital was far from their home, family members could not visit often. When the mother visited the following week, the daughter had died and already been buried, because the family did not arrive in time to take charge of the cadaver.[18] Although this may have been a particularly egregious case, working-class men and women often had difficulty finding the time and transportation fare to travel across the city to visit relatives in the hospital.

Loss of life adversely influenced both working-class families and the Argentine economy more broadly. In Buenos Aires from 1899 to 1911, sixty-one to sixty-seven percent of all tubercular deaths fell among those aged between twenty and fifty. Extended illnesses and deaths occurred among those who were most skilled, who were then replaced by less experienced workers. New immigrants sometimes benefited, finding positions vacated by tuberculosis victims. At the same time the tubercular, who worked as long as they were able, were less productive than the healthy.[19] Tuberculosis contributed to a decline in the standard of living: on average an adult with tuberculosis lost three to four months of work per year, which led to a twenty to thirty percent decrease in annual household income. Tuberculosis affected all classes, but it was particularly debilitating for the working class, because workers needed to continue to work while being treated.[20]

Age also influenced the diagnosis and treatment of tuberculosis. In Buenos Aires, in the 1940s, physicians found that latent cases tended to become active when individuals reached old-age. The aged had decreasing immunity and increasing physical problems, which reduced their resistance to tuberculosis. Diagnosis was more difficult because of the presence of other diseases, and older people were sometimes less willing to accept new treatments. If there was a history of tuberculosis within family, the long exposure eventually ensured the infection of its members. In families where children developed tuberculosis, the disease often came from an older family member. Age affected treatment, as physicians were less inclined to perform surgery on older patients; doctors instead advised better hygiene, diet and sanatorium treatment.[21] Women posed a challenge for male physicians. In the nineteenth century, doctors in Buenos Aires and Philadelphia initially believed that the different physiologies of men and women required them to be treated differently. Physicians incorrectly thought that female organs (the uterus and the ovaries) were responsible for most women's illnesses including headaches, sore throats, indigestion and tuberculosis. They also too often believed that the digestive organs were responsible for men's diseases. Environmental factors were thought to cause tuberculosis in men, but tuberculosis in women was thought to relate to menstruation. (It is true that menstruation causes women to need more protein; and when women's diet was lacking in protein their resistance to disease declined.)[22] In fact, working and living conditions contributed to tuberculosis susceptibility in both men and women. Although physicians commonly exaggerated the differences between the sexes, tuberculosis treatments were rarely gender-specific. Physicians saw no contradiction in believing that lower-class women should do manual labor, whereas elite women should rest. Male public officials treated immigrant and the poor paternalistically. Although the medical profession sought to treat all groups, it was class rather than gender that most influenced the differences in the treatment of the tuberculosis patients.

George E. Macklin: Treatment Options of the Wealthy

During the twentieth century, wealthy patients could afford to try various cures. They traveled to different locations seeking a healthier climate, lived at sanatoriums, hired nurses and servants for personal assistance, questioned their treatments and changed physicians. The poor, in contrast, accepted the treatments offered with fewer complaints. The two-year correspondence between Lawrence Flick and George Macklin illustrates the type of tuberculosis treatments used by both Argentine and United State physicians. In spite of physicians using the most promising and recent remedies, a patient's health often declined rapidly.[23]

Macklin wrote regularly to Flick and described his weight, temperature, pulse, the nature of his sputum and various colds that he contracted. He requested prescriptions and set up appointments to see Flick. (Appointments were often canceled, because of business commitments or because Macklin did not feel well enough to travel.) He complained about various medications and sought to direct his own treatment. On 30 December 1903, he wrote that he was almost out of the tonic, the "dark brown sticky stuff," and requested an alternative treatment to replace sleeping outdoors. He questioned whether sleeping out in the cold and walking to his house through the snow in bare feet was a "humane treatment?"[24]

On 1 June 1904, Macklin wrote that he was having oil rubbed on his whole body, not just his arms and legs. He noted that "I have slept in the hot summer nights with better things than a skin full of grease, but they tell me that is what a fellow with a 'busted' lung is up against."[25] On 19 August, Macklin wrote Flick

> I want to notify you that a stick of dynamite, taken internally will probably have better results on me.... All my friends in the West, I am quite sure, feel that I am dying in slow stages in the Eastern country. They all think I ought to be back in the dry country. I tell them one might as well be dead as to lie out in that country, so it doesn't make much difference whether you die a slow death here or live a long time out there. The only thing I kick about is that your rules are so rigid that while I am doing this dying I cannot have a good time. I wish you would hurry up and fix that dose that will kill or cure so that I can once more get out and look around with the boys.[26]

As his condition worsened, Macklin thought he might go to Italy to be treated by a new serum. After consultation, Flick decided that Maragliano's serum, still in an experimental stage, should instead be given in the U.S. A new sanatorium had opened at Glenside, outside of Philadelphia. If Macklin went to the sanatorium, another physician would give the injection, but Flick would still supervise Macklin's care. Furthermore, Flick thought that three months rest would do Macklin good. Macklin reported that he would try to get his business in order, so he could go to a sanatorium.[27] By November Macklin was in a sanatorium, and he wrote, "this place is ok, as long as one has to be away from home; milk, eggs and meals are as good as could be and beautifully cooked and served in a way that makes one want to eat." But as Christmas neared, he asked Flick for permission to have a quiet Christmas with his family. He planned to leave Friday at noon on the Penn Limited, so as to arrive in Pittsburgh in the morning. After spending Saturday and Sunday at home, he would leave early Monday morning to return to Glenside. He promised not to go to his office.[28]

When his stay at Glenside failed to improve his health, Macklin traveled in February 1905 to Camden, South Carolina. His nurse, Charles Bacher, and his wife, Elizabeth, cared for him at the Kirkwood Hotel under the direction of Flick. Macklin's health continued to deteriorate and in mid-February, he hemorrhaged extensively. When Macklin had a major coughing spell (he discharged four ounces of thick red bloody mucus), Bacher injected him with 1/100 grain of nitroglycerine, gave him ice chips to suck and required him to remain flat on his back with a bag of cold water on his chest. The following morning when Macklin was feeling better, he received his usual treatment: fifty creosote drops in hot water followed by a cold sponge bath, and then his milk/egg diet. He sat on the porch on the morning and did a little walking; after lunch, he went to bed. When he awoke, he had a massage for thirty minutes, followed by a hypodermic injection of Maragliano's serum and his afternoon meal. At eight P.M. Macklin felt good with a pulse of 108, but at 8:30 he had another hemorrhage, spitting up six ounces of bloody mucus. His nurse gave him table salt in a glass of water and sent for a local doctor who ordered 1/100 grain of nitroglycerin and 1/100 grain of ergot to be given every four hours as long as the patient was awake. To calm the patient, the nurse was to give him a quarter grain of morphine and l/150 grain of atropine. Flick disagreed with the local doctor and telegraphed that the atropine, morphine and ergot be stopped immediately, as they endangered tuberculosis patients. Flick wanted the drugs to be replaced with Epsom salts and recommended that a half dram of sulfate of magnesium be given hourly to help Macklin purge his bowels. He further recommended that Macklin consult a local tuberculosis expert.[29]

By early March, Macklin wrote that he felt better. In spite of a persistent cough, he spent time sitting on the porch. However, his condition continued to worsen, and Mrs. Macklin and Charles Bacher clashed over his care. Bacher complained that Mrs. Macklin insisted on his leaving the room. When he returned, she was either in Macklin's bed or expressing affection and pity for him. Bacher wrote that Elizabeth and George Macklin spent several hours every morning looking at advertisements and letters, which did not contribute to Macklin's improvement. Macklin wrote Flick that he would come north around the first of April and give up his business. Macklin wanted to buy a farm in Ebensburg, Pennsylvania, at an elevation of 1400 feet. After another major hemorrhage, Elizabeth decided to move her husband to the north with Bacher's help. On 17 April 1905, Macklin arrived by sea and was met by an ambulance. Macklin was now directly under Flick's care, so the correspondence between them ceases. In spite of the best care available, Macklin died on 26 June 1905 in St. Joseph's Hospital, Philadelphia.[30]

Although George Macklin was an affluent patient who could afford the best care, his treatments failed to cure him. Wealth permitted Macklin to try any treatment that might be effective and to enjoy any climate that might improve his health. At the same time, his responses to treatment resemble those of many other tubercular patients. He continued to work in spite of Flick's recommendation to the contrary, and he resisted going to a sanatorium. He protested when treatments were uncomfortable and ineffective, but willingly utilized all experimental treatments.

Medication Options for Tuberculosis

Physicians in both Buenos Aires and Philadelphia used drugs such as heroin, morphine and opium to combat pain. To decrease nighttime coughing, 1/24 to 1/8 of a gram of heroin might be given two to three times a night. To reduce night sweats, atropine, zinc oxide and camphor acid might be given; atropine was used to stop hemorrhaging; iodoform, ichthyol and tannalbin were used to prevent diarrhea. Mostly administered orally, drugs could also be inhaled, rubbed on the body or injected into the lungs. By the 1880s, there were more than thirty types of vaporizers, and patients used inhalers regularly. Medical journals and manuals in Buenos Aires provided physicians with the newest treatments for tuberculosis, including a variety of both local and European formulas. Mixed in large batches, the substances were often combined with wine, alcohol and water to make them taste better. Patients frequently ingested the formulas before eating, subsequently complaining about their taste and ineffectiveness.[31]

Although physicians and public health officials generally agreed as to causes and general treatment of tuberculosis, there was disagreement, as to specific medications. Physicians developed their own approaches to tuberculosis. Flick recommended many of his preferred treatments in the Macklin case. He placed great faith in rubbing oil. Rubbing a patient nightly was a demanding task for a nurse. Flick also used creosote, calomel, potassium iodide, quinine, iodoform, lead water and laudanum from opium. He believed that drugs should be used in moderation and that opiates, stimulants and depressants should be used cautiously. To build up the body, Flick might prescribe strychnine, arsenic, phosphorus, digitalis and iron. Most importantly, Flick emphasized diet; he saw a clear relationship between the lungs and the stomach. He believed that if the stomach failed, so did the lungs. Although drugs might be helpful, he thought that nutrition was most important. Rest, moderate exercise and fresh air were also significant.

Once a consumptive was "cured," a continuing nutritious diet was important to prevent recurrence.[32]

Physicians wanted tubercular patients to eat three large meals a day. Milk was easily digested and viewed as the perfect food. It helped build up weight and was often provided free to poor patients. Eggs were considered to be the next best food. Early twentieth-century physicians recommended that patients each day drink three to six quarts of sterilized milk and eat six to twelve fresh eggs, as well as vegetables and fruits. Some patients could not tolerate the quantity of milk and eggs; furthermore, even with support from charity organizations, the poor could not afford such a diet. Although there is some evidence that individuals on high protein diets were less likely to contract tuberculosis, there is no proof that a diet of eggs and milk cured tuberculosis.[33]

Physicians were continually evaluating the effectiveness of medications and experimenting with new ones. They debated the value of heavily advertised creosote, which patients took orally or inhaled to reduce coughing during all stages of pulmonary tuberculosis. It was initially thought to destroy the tubercle bacilli; creosote was also reputed to improve a patient's appetite and to diminish spitting. Although Flick prescribed creosote for Macklin, most physicians decreased its usage after 1900 as it destroyed the pancreas and was ineffective against the tubercle bacilli.[34] Maragliano's serum, made from the blood of horses or cattle, which contained tuberculosis antibodies, also failed to destroy the tuberculosis bacteria in humans; it was yet another of many experimental medications thought to cure tuberculosis that physicians used both with and without patients' permission.[35]

In addition to medications created by physicians, patients also bought patent medicines. Patent medicines seemed to patients to be as effective as those prescribed by doctors; in addition, they were usually less painful and certainly more affordable. By the late 1930s some of the patent medicines resembled those prescribed by physicians for pulmonary tuberculosis early in the century. Commercials made the medicines sound like miracle drugs; they were said to cure tuberculosis, convulsions, rheumatism, constipation and other widespread ailments. Advertisements for tuberculosis patent medicines promised to cure coughs and all illnesses of the chest and throat; it was claimed that the medicines had been used in hospitals in Brussels, Paris, Vienna and Lisbon. Testimonials extolled the success of these over-the-counter medications. Within three months bleeding and coughs would end; a former patient would then be fat, healthy and fully recovered. Chemical analysis suggests that the over-the-counter medicines often contained vitamins and patients believed that they reduced fatigue and strengthened the body. Patent medicines included a small amount of poison to destroy the tuberculosis bacteria and all utilized various substances, including gold, calcium, copper and silver, which were suspended in oil. Various herbs, including seaweed, were also popular ingredients. Patent medicines could be rubbed on the skin, swallowed or injected. Non-traditional medicines and over-the-counter drugs did little harm to patients; to the extent that they made the patient more comfortable, they were even useful.[36]

In rurals area with few physicians, patients with chronic illnesses often turned to healers and inexpensive non-traditional medicine. Healers who combined folk traditions with biomedicine provided hope. Many patients could not distinguish between healers and physicians since one group did not cure disease more successfully than the other. Among the healers were students who had abandoned their studies at the Buenos Aires Faculty of Medicine and foreigners who had not confirmed their degrees. The urban poor also turned to healers, since few patients survived hospitals stays early in the twentieth century. In addition, the urban poor had difficulty accessing doctors; doctors were also thought to stigmatize the poor.[37] The rural ill consulted healers more than did urban patients.[38] The tubercular often simultaneously consulted physicians, pharmacists and healers.

Vaccines and Surgery

From the first recognition that germs cause tuberculosis, physicians sought a cure for it. In the late nineteenth century, the hope was for an inoculation. The August 1890 rumors that Robert Koch had developed an anti-tuberculosis vaccine generated worldwide excitement. Physicians went to Germany to obtain tuberculin, a sterile liquid that contains the products of substances extracted from the tubercle bacillus. Physicians injected it into their patients to generate antibodies to fight the tuberculosis bacteria and thereby provide a cure. After reading descriptions of Koch's method, Buenos Aires' physicians obtained the serum from Berlin. As early as February 1891, they began experiments with tuberculin and were among the first in South America to use the new treatment. The Board of Trustees of the German Hospital in Philadelphia sent its chief resident to Berlin to study Koch's method; Koch gave him several vials with which to begin treatment.[39]

The case studies published in medical journals illustrate physician experiments with vaccines. In 1897, a Buenos Aires physician, Dr. Antonio Chiocconi, gave thirty-three injections of tuberculin to Juan A., a twenty-year-old, working-class immigrant from Uruguay, who entered the Casa de Aislamiento (Hospital Muñiz) in Buenos Aires. Juan had had measles at ten, and later minor colds; there were, however, no indications of health problems until six months before he entered the hospital, when he came down with a bad cold, cough and fever. His first doctor diagnosed influenza, and Juan remained in bed for fifteen days, coughing bloody mucus and sweating at night. His weight loss and fever led him to enter the hospital. Dr. Chiocconi contended that his tuberculin treatment enabled patients, like Juan, to improve their appetites and to gain weight within a few weeks. Patients' coughs and expectorations diminished, bacteria disappeared from saliva and some former patients were able to return to work. Although his patients were not completely cured, Chiocconi thought that additional time would ensure a cure. Unfortunately, that proved to be a false hope for Juan.[40]

As late as 1911, Dr. Federico Marugo used tuberculin on José F., a thirty-four-year-old Spanish immigrant laborer, who went to the Hospital Rawson for out-patient services. José lived in miserable, unsanitary conditions and appeared to suffer from malnutrition. His daughter had died of pulmonary tuberculosis at the age of two years. For two years, he coughed greenish-yellow, blood-streaked mucus. He got tired easily, was weak and needed help to get up and down tram steps. His nighttime sweating was so profuse that he had to change bed clothes every night. The tuberculin injections appeared initially to improve his condition and to make him more comfortable. But he could not be cured since his lungs were too damaged.[41] Although physicians could not duplicate Koch's findings, tuberculin remained a widely used remedy between 1890 and 1925. Initially, Argentine physicians argued that Koch's serum helped tubercular patients. Nevertheless, extensive testing and a variety of experiments by Argentine physicians proved Koch's serum to be a disappointment. By 1911, most physicians had concluded that the injections were dangerous for patients and hastened deaths.[42]

With increasing medical agreement that Koch's tuberculin did not cure, Argentine physicians sought to identify other injectable chemicals that might restore health to patients. Thus, Dr. César Rollino treated Manuela R., aged thirty years, an ironer, who entered a hospital in 1902, with Richet's serum, cacodylate of soda, overfeeding and then creosote in an enema. Manuela R.'s mother had died in childbirth, and there was no information on the health history of her father. As a child, she twice had measles as well as smallpox. Manuela had married at the age of twenty and delivered a son by normal birth, but he had died of pneumonia at three months. Two months after giving birth, she began to bleed from the uterus, suggesting some type of malignancy in the genital tract; one year later she had an operation for an abdominal tumor. Her tuberculosis had begun six months earlier with pain on the right side, a dry cough, fatigue, and fever in the afternoon, nighttime sweating, expectoration and hemorrhaging of the lungs. Within five months of starting Rollino's treatments, her health had improved.[43]

Dr. Federico Marugo injected Pilar F. (a sixteen-year-old Argentine) daily for twenty days with five grams of calcium chloride followed by another fifteen injections to replenish her calcium loss. She entered Hospital Rawson in 1910. Her father had died of tuberculosis in September and a brother in October, which provided strong epidemiological evidence that she also had tuberculosis. She had always lived in poor and unsanitary housing. She had first sought outpatient treatment, after three months of losing weight, coughing, sweating, pain in her shoulders and weakness. Dr. Marugo followed the injections by using tuberculin for eight more days and supplemented medications with food and rest. Although Pilar F. appeared to be cured, later indications were that she continued to carry tuberculosis bacilli and that the treatment had failed.

Philadelphia and Buenos Aires physicians also promoted surgery as a way to cure tuberculosis. Surgeons most commonly utilized artificial pneumothorax, a procedure which involved putting air in the pleural cavity to collapse the diseased lung, so it could rest. The procedure remained dangerous; many things could go wrong, including the puncturing of a vein, a lung, the stomach, the heart or the liver. By 1910, many of the technical problems had been solved, but patients were frightened and fatigued by the procedure. When Edward Trudeau, one of the best-known tubercular physicians, underwent the treatment in 1912, its popularity increased. By the 1920s, pneumothorax machines were portable and efficient, and Philadelphia physicians often used the procedure. Physicians thought that the treatment reduced a patient's fever, cough and expectoration, and improved the patient's appetite.[44]

Whether to use the pneumothorax treatment generated much discussion. Argentine doctors noted that pregnant patients posed an additional challenge. In the 1920s, physicians at Hospital Municipal Doctor Tornú recommended the immediate use of pneumothorax after the birth of a baby, when the mother had lung lesions and clearly diagnosed tuberculosis. They also used the procedure early in pregnancies. For example, C.C., a nineteen-year-old domestic who was married, in the fourth month of her pregnancy had a pneumothorax treatment, which led to a normal temperature and ended the hemorrhaging of her lungs. M.M., a twenty-six-year-old unmarried house servant, had had respiratory infections for at least six years. Beginning in her eighth month of pregnancy, she had increased temperature, nighttime sweating, coughing and bloody saliva. Immediately after she gave birth, she underwent an artificial pneumothorax procedure. Both women immediately improved.[45]

From 1910 to 1945, no more than ten percent of the U.S. sanatorium patients, and even fewer in Argentina, endured artificial pneumothorax procedures, because most physicians preferred to use other approaches.[46] Those most likely to undergo the surgery were patients who had not responded to other therapies or for whom a rest cure was too expensive. Only anecdotal evidence suggests that the pneumothorax treatment actually cured any patients, and the pain associated with the remedy made it unpopular with patients. Although the treatment did not permanently cure, it probably extended the lives of those who underwent it. The treatment was based on the same philosophy as the sanatorium regimen: it was thought that resting the lungs enabled the body to combat the disease.

BCG: An Effective Tuberculosis Vaccine

Without a cure, physicians hoped for a vaccine that would prevent tuberculosis. The efficacy of the smallpox vaccination certainly contributed to patient and physician optimism. Leon C.A. Calmette and Camille Guérin developed the Bacille Calmette Guérin (BCG) in 1908. By the early 1920s, this weakened form of a live bovine tuberculosis bacillus proved successful in stimulating the body's immune system to combat tuberculosis without causing the disease. Initially, BCG was given by mouth, but eventually, it was injected. In contrast to the acceptance of tuberculin, public health officials in Argentina and the U.S. generally rejected BCG. However, Argentine physicians utilized BCG in Buenos Aires more often than in Philadelphia. For example, between 1925 and 1938, Buenos Aires' health agencies injected 57,000 children from families with tuberculosis with BCG, and the maternity service of the Hospital Tornú also injected the newborns of tubercular mothers.[47]

A shocking disaster in 1930 in Lubeck, Germany—in which seventy-three out of 249 infants died after being vaccinated with a contaminated BCG strain—greatly reduced interest in BCG. The usage of this vaccine decreased until the 1940s for three reasons: safety concerns, the fact that BCG invalidated the tuberculosis skin test by creating tuberculosis antibodies, and concerns about the cost of efforts to immunize the population. But after World War II, the vaccine was used worldwide; an effective clinical trial—conducted by the Institut Pasteur which vaccinated the Muslim population in Algiers in the 1930s—did much to legitimize the use of BCG, although it did not conclusively prove its efficacy.[48]

Although some physicians in Argentina and the U.S. argued for using BCG where tuberculosis was particularly prevalent or to protect children, both countries resisted vaccination campaigns. U.S. public health officials challenged BCG's safety and efficacy; they also noted that—even if BCG protected against tuberculosis—it was unclear how long the protection lasted. The U.S. government was still evaluating BCG in the 1940s when new anti-tuberculosis drugs proved far more effective. By the 1950s, the U.S. Public Health Service promoted antibiotics rather than BCG. By the 1960s, clinical trials suggested that BCG was sixty to eighty percent effective in preventing tuberculosis for a five-to-fifteen year span; it reduced mortality in infants born into tubercular families and decreased cases of tuberculosis meningitis and miliary tuberculosis. Because the vaccine is inexpensive, easy to administer and somewhat effective, the World Health

Organization currently supports BCG vaccination for children who live in countries in which tuberculosis is highly endemic.[49]

Jesús Pueyo was among the researchers who failed to develop a therapeutic vaccine in the 1930s. Pueyo—who worked in the laboratory of the Facultad of Medicina of the University of Buenos Aires—thought that he had developed an injectable medicine that would cure tuberculosis. After animal trials in 1936, Pueyo offered his vaccine on an experimental basis free of charge to physicians. Although most of the medical establishment rejected the vaccine as ineffective, many patients argued that the remedy offered some benefits and posed no danger. The controversy grew so heated that in the winter of 1941 patients and their families marched on Argentina's National Congress shouting, "We want the vaccine Pueyo." But the vaccine ultimately proved ineffective. The 1941 demonstrations nevertheless illustrate the desperation of families who were seeking a cure for tuberculosis.[50]

Working-Class Tuberculosis Treatment: Home and Clinic

The finances of working-class patients limited their treatment options. Poor patients in Buenos Aires and Philadelphia first sought treatment at public clinics near their homes. Although women generally went to clinics earlier than men, many working-class patients in Buenos Aires did not visit dispensaries until the disease was at an advanced stage. Patients tended to go to hospitals only when their health deteriorated; on the other hand, they were more willing to enter affordable public sanatoriums. Both poor and wealthy patients preferred to be treated at home. Physicians thought that patients who carefully followed prescribed routines for three to five years could be treated successfully if treatment began when the disease was at an early stage.[51]

Home treatment consisted of rest outdoors, proper nutrition and the use of sputum cups. Both the wealthy and poor were encouraged to live outdoors in tents (on their roofs or in their yards) and to turn porches into sleeping areas. With a focus on cleanliness, public health workers taught patients to take cold douches, to cover their mouths and noses when coughing and to place tissues in paper bags, to burn sputum cups and to clean cup holders in boiling water. One problem with home treatment was that patients were likely to catch colds, influenza and pneumonia from other members of their households. Such additional infections complicated the treatment of tuberculosis. On the other hand, home treatment decreased the cost to the patient and family. Among Flick's home treatment cases in a six-year period, eighteen percent appeared to be cured, thirty-six percent were much improved, nineteen percent were temporarily improved, and only twenty-seven percent were unimproved.[52] These statistics support anecdotal evidence that home treatments did extend the lives of some patients.

Tuberculosis clinics in both Buenos Aires and Philadelphia sought to diagnose and treat tubercular patients who lived at home. Charities and governments increased the number of tuberculosis clinics because they provided the most economical and practical health care for the working poor. The Porteño dispensaries—one-story buildings with a laboratory and waiting and consulting room—are representatives. They provided a variety of services to poor tubercular patients and their families. The clinics were patronized by Argentine and foreign nationals, women and men, and workers in all professions; however, clinic patients most commonly worked as day laborers, seamstresses and domestics. Working with the public health authorities, the Argentine Anti-Tuberculosis League opened four clinics in primarily working-class districts of Buenos Aires between 1902 and 1908. The number of patient office visits at the three largest clinics grew from 1,381 in 1902 when there were 1,619 pulmonary tuberculosis deaths in the city to 2,812 in 1908 when there were 2,081 deaths. In 1920, the city of Buenos Aires had six clinics, five operated by the league and one by the national. Although the number of tuberculosis patients served by the clinics was impressive, Buenos Aires needed more clinics.[53]

Philadelphia and Buenos Aires clinics tried to prevent tuberculosis by identifying and diagnosing it, and by educating and treating the working poor. The clinics proceeded as follows. Once a patient had provided medical and family histories, a physician gave the patient a physical exam and received from the patient a sputum sample for examination. After patients were taught about the infectious nature of tuberculosis, the means of disinfecting living quarters and the dangers of tobacco and alcohol, they were sent home with some medicine, sputum cups and a reminder to visit the clinic on a regular basis. In Buenos Aires, patients who were mobile were required to go to the clinic every two weeks to be weighed; but invalids were treated by clinic personnel in their homes. When necessary, Buenos Aires' clinics gave patients bedding and clothing, helped pay their rent, and dispensed pasteurized milk, beef, bread, medicine, soap, and disinfectants. Although the clinics treated patients at all stages of tuberculosis, individuals at earlier stages of tuberculosis tended to go to clinics; those at later stages went to hospitals. Porteño inspectors and Philadelphia home nurses made follow-up visits to patients' residences to ensure that preventive measures were being followed, to prevent the further spread of disease. Those in Buenos Aires who failed to follow the regulations were ineligible for further clinical services after the second offense.[54]

Philadelphia slowly expanded the number of charity and state clinics. In 1873, the Board of Trustees of the area's Episcopal Church opened the first tuberculosis dispensary; in 1882, it established another dispensary.

Also, in 1873, a Philadelphia church in connection with its dispensary inaugurated a kitchen which provided nutritious meals for the sick. Philadelphia charities provided tuberculosis patients with food, clothing and blankets, and also helped with other expenditures. The Kensington Dispensary, supported by the Lutheran Church and staffed by volunteer physicians, opened in 1906 to treat the tubercular. The Kensington Dispensary provided outpatient care to recent immigrants. Staffed by visiting nurses, the clinic emphasized the importance of fumigation and provided patients with a variety of articles, including sputum cups, milk, false teeth, spectacles, cots and blankets. Kensington also donated clothing to patients going to sanatoriums, secured employment, and referred to the city's Children's Bureau families who needed financial assistance. In 1915, the Kensington Dispensary treated 4,829 patients with pulmonary tuberculosis.[55]

The work of the Kensington Dispensary is illustrated by the case of Mrs. H., who was diagnosed with tuberculosis in 1911. She was able to work because her child was being cared for in the clinic's nursery. When she came down with a bad cold, Mrs. H. was hospitalized, and her child was left in the care of a friend. When a visiting nurse arrived to check on the child, she was distressed to find that the caregiver was in a drunken stupor, and the child was near the edge of the bed. The nurse then placed the baby with the mother in the hospital. When she recovered, Mrs. H. returned to work, leaving the baby in the hospital's nursery. When Mrs. H. became sicker, her mother (who lived on a farm in Belleville, Arkansas) agreed to care for her daughter and child but provided no money to transport them. The dispensary raised the money and sent them to Arkansas on New Year's Day 1913. Mrs. H. arrived safely, and her health improved.[56]

Pennsylvania did not open its first state-run dispensary in Philadelphia until 1905. Within two days after a patient's first visit to a dispensary, a nurse went to the home to demonstrate proper prevention procedures to the infected patient and the other family members. Each dispensary had its own physician and nurses to treat patients. By 1917, there were 116 state tuberculosis dispensaries with an enrollment of 12,000 patients located throughout Pennsylvania. Between 1907—when the official Pennsylvania campaign against tuberculosis began—and 1917, 97,655 patients were admitted to dispensaries. Of those 22,348 were transferred to sanatoriums, and 7,802 were discharged with the disease "arrested" or "cured." State dispensaries provided information on prevention and diet and made referrals to welfare organizations, fresh air schools, the Mount Alto Sanatorium and the Philadelphia General Hospital.[57] By 1919, Philadelphia had four dispensaries with sixteen nurses. Five years later, the Philadelphia Department of Health had ten tuberculosis clinics. The number of clinics—located throughout the city—made it possible to require patients discharged from state sanatoriums to visit a dispensary at least once every six months. By the 1930s—as the number of tubercular patients declined and exposure lessened—clinics evolved into social service bureaus that employed workers to provide home care for consumptives, free milk, preventive measures and education. By 1941, the city's twenty-seven clinics primarily served immigrants, African Americans and the poor.[58]

Philadelphia dispensaries also performed experimental treatments, which were more typically done in Buenos Aires' hospitals. For example, in 1910, a Philadelphia dispensary utilized tuberculin with limited success. Beginning in 1910, a fifty-year-old foreman received twenty-nine injections in eight months. Three months after the first treatment, he felt better and was able to work as a watchman. On completion of his injections, he returned to work as a foreman. But by the end of 1912, he developed a slight cough and had lost two-and-a-half pounds. In contrast, after spending three months at the Mont Alto Sanatorium a twenty-one-year-old single woman returned to Philadelphia still feeling weak and unable to work. After thirty-six tuberculin injections in nine months, she returned to work as a bookbinder. One year after the last injection, the patient felt fine and was a full-time employee. She had not missed a day of work in a year.[59]

Physicians found it challenging to get patients to follow instructions. Invalids often failed to spend time outdoors; some worked when they should have been resting because their families depended on them; others failed to follow dietary regimes.[60] Philadelphia tuberculosis clinics utilized visiting nurses to teach patients preventive methods and make certain that they followed instructions. Visiting nurses also taught the tubercular how to avoid infecting others, instructed families in cooking and nutrition and if necessary solicited help from charities. Nurses visited impoverished patients without charge. By contrast, middle-class patients were expected to pay streetcar fare and an hourly wage for nurses. From 1893 to 1897, more than ninety percent of the visiting nurses' patients were maternity cases, but the number of tuberculosis patients steadily increased. By 1907, nurses were conducting classes for twenty-five to thirty patients at churches and dispensaries to teach tuberculosis prevention. Between March 1908 and February 1909, a nurse responsible for 238 tubercular patients recorded the following outcomes: forty-three patients were treated at home; thirty-six were referred to hospitals or sanatoriums; fourteen were sent to the country; eleven were examined and found not to be to tubercular, eleven were transferred to other agencies; sixty died; and sixty-three remained under the nurse's care. In 1917, visiting nurses saw 298 patients in the advanced stage of pulmonary tuberculosis, but by 1923, that number decreased to fourteen—indicating that few of the most serious patients were remaining in their homes.[61]

Treatment for tuberculosis was similar in Buenos Aires and Philadelphia, but the organizations providing it differed. In Buenos Aires, clinics were created by the private secular Anti-Tuberculosis League; the nation and city government were slow to support the creation of public dispensaries. In Philadelphia, the first dispensaries were all administered by private religious charities, with the exception of the Phipps Institute. Eventually, Pennsylvania supported public clinics in Philadelphia. Nevertheless, the function, purposes and services of the two cities' clinics were similar. Patients in both cities complained about the cost of transportation to visit clinics and the need to leave work early, which led to lost wages. Some immigrants also had difficulty communicating with physicians. In spite of the challenges in Buenos Aires and Philadelphia, the number of medical consultations, office visits, home visits, prescriptions and food supplements increased steadily in the early part of the twentieth century. Because of early diagnosis at the clinics, some patients were able to improve enough to resume work.[62]

Hospital Care in Buenos Aires

Until 1891, pulmonary patients were admitted to all Buenos Aires hospitals. However, Porteño physicians recommended the Hospital Muñiz for seriously ill tuberculosis patients who needed public assistance. Acknowledging the contagiousness of tuberculosis, in April 1902, the Buenos Aires municipal government passed an ordinance requiring that—as of January 1904—pulmonary tubercular patients be admitted only to hospitals that could isolate patients.[63] Initially, most hospitals did not have facilities to segregate tubercular patients. Tuberculosis patients had to go to Hospital Muñiz, Hospital Rivadavia or the newly established Hospital Municipal Doctor Tornú, which together had only 700 beds for an urban population of 1,306,680 in 1910.[64] The military hospital had to send its patients to the Hospital Muñiz. All other hospitals were encouraged to send tubercular patients in the disease's early stages to the Hospital Tornú, and patients with advanced cases to the Hospital Muñiz. Because of the increasing number of tuberculosis patients, Hospital Muñiz had difficulty providing separate spaces for patients with other contagious diseases. In 1900, almost half of the 235 patients in the Hospital Muñiz were tubercular; patients with other contagious diseases continued to be admitted. There were not enough beds in the city to isolate tubercular patients, so all hospitals continued to accept them. From 1906 to 1917, 9.5 percent of the patients in municipal hospitals were diagnosed with tuberculosis.[65]

In 1904, the Hospital Muñiz inaugurated a new pavilion for 100 tubercular patients. This facility provided patients with their own wards, sitting areas, dining rooms, laboratories and surgery as well as special facilities for mothers and children. Between 1901 and 1905, when 8,686 individuals died of pulmonary tuberculosis in Buenos Aires, 3,125 tubercular patients of both sexes entered Hospital Muñiz. Of these fifty-two percent were Argentines, eighteen percent Italians, seventeen percent Spanish and thirteen percent of other nationalities. Because of expanding need in 1910, the national government began constructing a 220-bed tuberculosis hospital in the Province of Buenos Aires. The Hospital Vicente López y Planes, serving tubercular women and children, was inaugurated in 1916 to supplement the Hospital Muñiz in caring for the very ill.[66]

As hospital facilities improved, the number of tubercular patients who entered hospitals increased—in spite of the high mortality from tuberculosis. From 1892 through 1918, fifty-seven percent of the tubercular patients who entered a hospital died; forty-three percent died at home. More patients died in November through January (the hot summer months), because heat placed stress on the body. Although during the sixteen-year period, hospital deaths varied by month and decreased, in some years, hospital deaths remained high. The most deaths (twenty-six percent in 1918) occurred in the Hospital Muñiz—suggesting that the medical profession was successfully encouraging the most serious cases to go to the contagious disease hospital of Buenos Aires. Public health officials believed that the increased number of deaths in hospitals (as opposed to deaths at home) pointed to the success of their prevention efforts; in effect, those dying in hospitals were less likely to infect others.[67]

Hospital Care in Philadelphia

Buenos Aires and Philadelphia faced similar challenges of providing hospital care for the tubercular. However, Philadelphia hospitals were initially less willing to accept tuberculosis patients, and religious organizations played a more important role in providing treatment. As of 1870, the Philadelphia General Hospital— which primarily cared for poor consumptives—mingled tubercular patients with others (just like hospitals in Buenos Aires). But by the 1890s, many Philadelphia hospitals rejected the tubercular: it was hard to care for them, and they posed a risk to other patients.[68] The first private Pennsylvania institution to treat tuberculosis was the House of Mercy for consumptive men, founded in 1876 by the Philadelphia Protestant Episcopal City Mission. The Chestnut Hill Home for consumptive women opened in 1886 and began to accept men in 1907. Originally, these homes offered basic care for both chronic and incurable patients, emphasizing the provision of fresh air and nourishing food. Eventually, physicians also offered medications, baths, ointments, and gas and air inhalation. Between 1894 and 1904, a little less than a third of the admittees were discharged as cured or improved.[69]

In order to get more hospitals to accept an increased number of tubercular patients, in 1895, Lawrence Flick organized the Free Hospital for Poor Consumptives, which paid for the care of patients in hospitals that would segregate them from other patients. In 1901, the Free Hospital for Poor Consumptives was paying five dollars a week to provide care for forty patients in various Philadelphia hospitals. Flick was a Catholic, and he secured the co-operation of the three Catholic Hospitals of Philadelphia: St. Joseph, St. Mary and St. Agnes, as well as the Rush Hospital for Consumption and Allied Diseases. The Jewish hospital opened special wards in 1890, in which it housed thirty-five tubercular patients; and by 1897 it cared for 104 consumptives.[70]

In 1903, The Philadelphia General Hospital began to offer expanded treatment for consumptives who were housed in six glass pavilions. Soon the General Hospital was accepting tubercular patients from other hospitals. In 1908, it accommodated two hundred male patients and seventy female patients at a time. Although the hospital doubled its capacity between 1904 and 1916, there was still a shortage of beds. By 1933, during the Great Depression, all Philadelphia's hospitals admitted tubercular patients, including those who could not pay. Patients did not remain long, as they came primarily for diagnosis and surgical procedures. About a fourth of these tubercular patients had pneumothorax therapy. When lung collapse therapy could not be used, physicians during the 1930s used other forms of surgery including removing scar tissue, so pneumothorax could be performed or removing ribs to sink a chest wall to decrease the lung's mobility. Philadelphia General had a waiting list for tubercular patients until 1954; at that time new drugs had eliminated the need for hospital beds.[71]

Although Philadelphia's hospitals cared for the acutely ill with the latest medications and technology, they still faced patients' complaints. For example, in 1901, the University Hospital recommended that a patient, Mr. Hopkins—whose care was paid for by the Free Hospital for Consumptives—be transferred to the surgical ward for an operation for his arthritic and tubercular joints. When he resisted surgery, he was informed that he would be discharged if he did not accept the transfer. Francis Fisher reported in 1900 that at Rush Hospital he received medicine only twice a day (not five times a day, as he should have) and that his temperature was often not taken. He requested an egg instead of stew meat, which he could not eat, but he was told to eat what he was given. At about the same time another patient complained that he could not get enough to eat and had to buy food to supplement his meals. As these stories indicate, patients sought to shape the quality of their hospital care by resisting surgery, evaluating medications, questioning procedures, determining the length of hospital stay, and seeking to improve the quality and quantity of food.[72]

Philadelphia and Buenos Aires tubercular and their families preferred home treatment to hospital care. The availability of public nurses, local clinics and charity institutions in both cities allowed poor and working-class patients to continue to live at home until they became too sick for family care. Wealthy patients had greater choices and could afford nursing care at home for a longer period. Hospitals in both cities originally served the very ill poor who went there to die. Gradually, however, hospital treatments improved. As hospitals offered new technologies unavailable in clinics or homes, they became more acceptable to patients of all classes. The availability of private hospitals for particular religious or ethnic groups gave patients increased choices. Although class continued to define the quality and type of health care available for the tubercular between 1870 and 1945, increasingly the wealthy—like Macklin, chose to die in hospitals.

Physician and Patient Attitudes toward Tuberculosis Treatment

In 1911, Lawrence Flick summarized the understanding of tuberculosis treatment that was common before the discovery of streptomycin. He thought that physicians should understand the general principles of tuberculosis, the available treatments and the stages of disease experienced by patients. Physicians were expected to ensure that the bowels were active so that microorganisms infecting a patient's system could be excreted. Diet and exercise should be appropriate to the individual. Drugs should be used only when advantageous, and experimental vaccinations should be used with caution; depressants, stimulants and opiates were to be avoided. Rest and fresh air were always important. Patients in a poor home environment should be moved to a sanatorium. Treatment should not be stopped when health improved.[73]

Because no medication or vaccination existed to cure tuberculosis, physicians found it difficult to counsel patients and their families. Nevertheless, medical professionals wanted to give clear instructions to their patients; they emphasized that patients should follow their orders to seek a cure. In spite of the efforts of physicians to help their patients, the main way of curing tuberculosis was to prevent an individual from contracting tuberculosis in the first place. Physicians, public health officials, hospitals, clinics and various private entities including labor organizations and life insurance companies provided the public with brochures. The Metropolitan Life Insurance Company, for example, in 1912 published a pamphlet entitled *A War on Consumption: Its Cure and Prevention.*

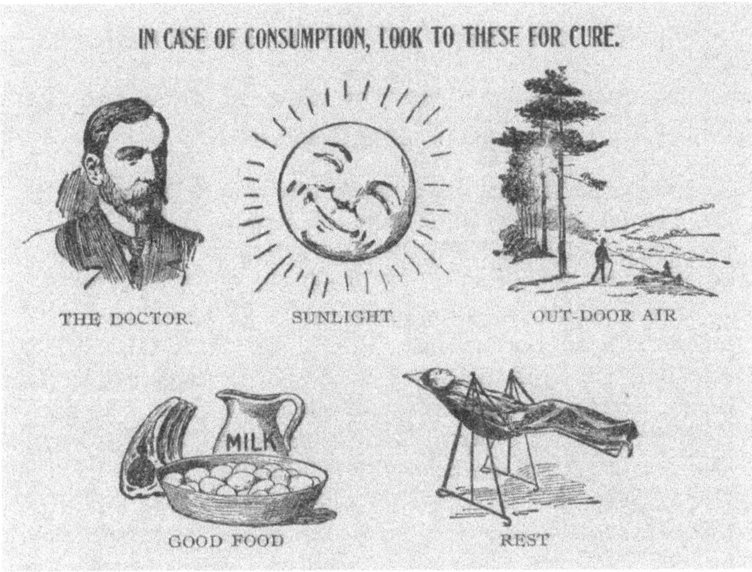

Figure 4.1 "In Case of Consumption, Look to These for Cure," Metropolitan Life Insurance Company, A *War on Consumption: Its Cure and Prevention* (New York 1912):12. This image is used by the kind permission of The College of Physicians of Philadelphia.

This fifteen-page pamphlet, prepared for policyholders, used pictures and diagrams to explain the nature of tuberculosis, its threat to lives, its spread, prevention, and cure. The pamphlet reveals the state of understanding of the disease in the early twentieth century (tuberculosis was a germ; it was not hereditary), called on individuals to take the necessary steps for both prevention and cure, and advised tuberculosis patients to follow the advice of their physician. Figure 4.1 illustrates the explanations and advice provided tuberculosis patients seeking a cure for tuberculosis. The pictures emphasized five factors for a successful cure: the physician, sunlight, out-door air, good food and rest.

Figure 4.2: "A Careful Consumptive—Not Dangerous to Live With," spoke directly to the concerns of family members who lived with and cared for a patient. The pamphlet advised taking five specific actions: cover coughs, spit and sneeze into paper or cloth; burn, boil or disinfect contaminated items; wash hands before and after eating; provide the patient with the same dishes and boil them in water before washing them with other dishes; and have the patient sleep alone. An examination of both illustrations, suggests that they were prepared for middle-class patients. The individuals are Caucasian; the table setting with two plates, cup and knife, fork and spoon is of middle class, as is the stove and bed.

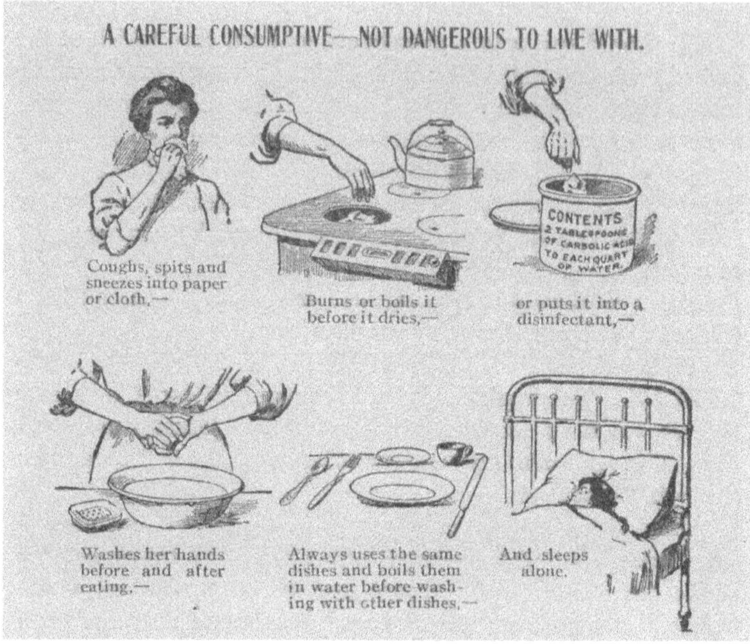

Figure 4.2 "A Careful Consumptive—Not Dangerous to Live With," (New York 1912):13. This image is used by the kind permission of The College of Physicians of Philadelphia.

The Metropolitan Life Insurance pamphlet provided the standard information that general practitioners gave their patients.

From 1870 to 1945, patients and their families in both Buenos Aires and Philadelphia would have seen and heard a variety of information about tuberculosis and all patients shared some similar experiences with the disease. At the same time, individual treatment experiences differed. In part, this was because of patients' different classes and genders, and the different stages of the disease; but it was also because of physician preferences and the changing evaluations of the efficacy of various medicines. Treatments actually differed as much within Buenos Aires and Philadelphia as they did between them. Neither Argentina nor the U.S. chose to implement a national vaccination program for BCG: in both countries, the elites and middle classes blamed the poor and immigrants for tuberculosis, and public health officials did not want to pay for a national vaccination program or subject everyone to it.

Buenos Aires and Philadelphia physicians and patients hoped for a cure for tuberculosis and were willing to take risks with experimental drugs. Treatment was intended both to heal and to relieve pain.

However, cures remained elusive. In Buenos Aires and Philadelphia, tuberculosis killed the young at the prime of their social and economic lives. In both cities women of child-bearing age, twenty to twenty-nine, were more likely to die of tuberculosis than at any other age. Men were more likely to die between the ages of thirty and thirty-nine. From 1870 to 1923, pulmonary tuberculosis deaths as a percent of all deaths increased in Buenos Aires from 4.66 percent in 1870 to 11.86 percent in 1923. In Philadelphia, adult deaths decreased from 13.09 percent in 1870 to 5.91 percent in 1923.[74] Although tubercular deaths decreased much more rapidly in Philadelphia than in Buenos Aires, it was the decrease in the contagious spread of tuberculosis rather than treatment that led to fewer deaths. Medications might lessen pain, but dying from tuberculosis was painful: patients experienced sweating, diarrhea, hemorrhaging and feelings of suffocation. Philadelphia and Buenos Aires' medical journals debated the effectiveness of new medications, but there was little evidence that they were useful. Although life expectancy for the seriously ill tubercular patient was longer in the twentieth century than the nineteenth, it was usually less than five years.[75] The placebo effect may have operated, some patients improved, others did not. Scientists continued to search for vaccines that would prevent tuberculosis and for medicines that would cure.

Porteño and Philadelphia physicians and patients hoped that lives could be extended by medication and surgical procedures and by fresh air and diet regimens. The ill and their families began to follow physician instructions and to expect doctors to diagnose their illness and to cure. During the late nineteenth century, both wealthy and poor tuberculosis patients in Buenos Aires and Philadelphia often ignored their doctors' recommendations and many physicians had difficulty earning a living. Only gradually did families visit clinics or send their tubercular members to hospitals. Physicians had less influence over their patients between 1870 and 1945 than they would have later on, when the authority of physicians increased as medical care became more effective.[76]

Diagnosing patients with tuberculosis increased their families' anguish. In the 1870–1945 era, patients and their families viewed tuberculosis as both shameful and deadly. In both Buenos Aires and Philadelphia, it was common to prefer a diagnosis of pneumonia rather than tuberculosis. Patients might choose to ignore medical advice and treatment became it damaged family relationships, affected job opportunities or was unaffordable. Patients were particularly prone to ignore medical advice when they had been diagnosed with a chronic disease such as tuberculosis, which could not be treated successfully. Patients tried to affect their treatments by leaving a facility in which they received care and even filing formal complaints. Most families understood that there was no remedy for tuberculosis, and that a cure was unlikely. All this began to change in

1943 when researchers discovered a treatment for tuberculosis. The utilization of streptomycin with PAS (introduced in 1946), and isoniazid (first used in 1951) overcame the tubercle bacilli and avoided toxic reactions.[77] The treatments of the sick and their actions illustrate the shared experiences of tuberculosis patients in both Buenos Aires and Philadelphia.

Notes

1 The Catholic University of America, American Catholic History Research Center and University Archives, (hereafter cited as CUA), Lawrence F. Flick Papers (FP), Second Series, Vol. 14 (June–September, 1904), 21 June 1904, George E. Macklin to Lawrence F. Flick.

2 Oscar P. Aguilar, "La tuberculina como diagnostico pronostico y tratamiento de la tuberculosis pulmonar," trans. Vera Blinn Reber (MD diss., Facultad de Medicina, Universidad de Buenos Aires, 1918).

3 CUA, FP, 30 April 1903, Macklin to Flick; Aguilar, 102–3.

4 CPP, FCR, Lawrence Francis Flick, "Early Recognition of Tuberculosis," *University Medical Magazine* (November 1893), 4; CPP, FCR, Lawrence Francis Flick, "Differential Diagnosis between Tuberculosis of the Lungs and Diseases Which Resemble It," *International Clinics* 4, no. 12 (1903). Antonio Cetrángolo, *Treinta años curando tuberculosos* (Buenos Aires: Librería Hachette, 1944), 140–41, 147.

5 Sheila M. Rothman, *Living in the Shadow of Death: Tuberculosis and the Social Experience of Illness in American History* (Baltimore: John Hopkins Press, 1995), 16–17; Katherine Ott, *Fevered Lives: Tuberculosis in American Culture since 1870* (Cambridge: Harvard University Press, 1996), 25–26, 142; Domingo Salvarezza, *Tisis Pulmonar*, MD diss., Facultad de Medicina, Universidad de Buenos Aires, 1866 (Buenos Aires: Imprenta de Buenos Aires, 1866), 23–29; CPP, FCR, Lawrence Francis Flick, "Home Treatment of Tuberculosis," *Procedures of the Philadelphia County Medical Society* (February 1901): 3.

6 Ott, 93–94; Helen Bynum, *Spitting Blood: The History of Tuberculosis* (London: Oxford University Press, 2012), 203; Jorge Plaza, *Tratamiento higiénico de la tuberculosis pulmonar*, MD diss., Facultad de Medicina, Universidad de Buenos Aires (Buenos Aires: La Semana Médica, 1912), 29–31; Abram H. Persky, "The Diagnosis and Treatment of Pulmonary Tuberculosis," *Transactions of the College of Physicians*, Third Series, 47 (1925): 568–70.

7 Buenos Aires, Dirección General de la Asistencia Pública, *Instrucciones para los inspectores sanitarios* (Buenos Aires: El Correo Español, 1898), 4–6.

8 Nicole L. Smith, "The Problem of Excess Female Mortality: Tuberculosis in Western Massachusetts, 1850–1910" MA thesis, University of Massachusetts-Amherst concluded that tuberculosis was the prime cause of greater female mortality between ages 10–19 and 30–39.

9 Deborah Lupton, *Medicine as Culture: Illness, Disease and the Body in Western Society* (London: Sage Publications, 1994), 132–33; César Sánchez Aizcorbe, "La cultural fiscal de la mujer en la profilaxis de la tuberculosis," in *Primer Congreso Pan-Americano de la Tuberculosis Córdoba 10–16 Octubre, 1922*, Vol. 3 (Córdoba: Imprenta de la Universidad, 1922), 259–62; Sandra McGee Deutsch, "The Catholic Church, Work and Womanhood in Argentina, 1890–1930," *Gender and History* 3, no. 3 (Autumn 1991):

306; Richard J. Walter, *Politics and Urban Growth in Buenos Aires, 1910–1942* (New York: Cambridge University Press), 13–14, 248.

10 CPP, FCR, vol. 1 (1920), 3–4, Lawrence Francis Flick, "Pregnancy in Tuberculosis," *Hospital Progress*; *La Semana Médica* 20, no. 1 (2 January 1913): 57.

11 "Tuberculosis Treatment during Pregnancy," (28 December 2014), www.webmd.com/baby/tc/treating-tuberculosis-in-pregnant-women-topic-overview.

12 Ludmilla Jordanova, *Sexual Visions: Images of Gender in Science and Medicine between the Eighteenth and Twentieth Centuries* (Madison: University of Wisconsin Press, 1989), 78–79, 83; Justino Ramos Mexia, "Higiene y educación fisica de la mujer" (MD diss., Facultad de Medicina, Universidad de Buenos Aires, 1898), 21, 26.

13 William D. Johnston, "Tuberculosis," in *The Cambridge World History of Human Disease*, ed. Kenneth F. Kiple (New York: Cambridge University Press, 1993), 1060; Lesley Doyal, *What Makes Women Sick: Gender and the Political Economy of Health* (New Brunswick: Rutgers University Press, 1995), 1–2, 19, 31–35; Jordanova, 25; Lupton, 137.

14 Mark H. Haller, "Recurring Themes," in *The Peoples of Philadelphia: A History of Ethnic Groups and Lower-Class Life, 1790–1940,* eds. Allen F. Davis and Mark H Haller (Philadelphia: Temple University Press, 1973), 289; Caroline Golab, "The Immigrant and the City: Poles, Italians and Jews in Philadelphia, 1870–1920," in *The Peoples of Philadelphia: A History of Ethnic Groups and Lower-Class Life, 1790–1940,* eds. Allen F. Davis and Mark H. Haller (Philadelphia: Temple University Press, 1973), 215; Arthur P. Dudden, "The City Embraces 'Normalcy' in 1919–1929," in *Philadelphia: A 300-Year History*, ed. Russell F. Weigley (New York: W.W. Norton & Company, 1982), 567, 591–92.

15 Donna J. Guy, "Women, Peonage and Industrialization: Argentina, 1810–1914," *Latin American Research Review* 16, no. 3 (1981): 77, 80; "Trabajo de la mujer a domicilio," *Boletín del Departamento Nacional del Trabajo* 19 (31 December 1911): 788–91; Augusto Bunge, "El trabajo industrial en Buenos Aires: Informe presentado al Departamento Nacional de Higiene," *Anales del Departamento Nacional de Higiene* 11, no. 9 (September 1904): 399–403.

16 Guy, "Women, Peonage and Industrialization, 77, 81; Donna J. Guy, "Emilio and Gabriela Coni: Reformers, Public Health, and Working Women," in *The Human Tradition in Latin America: The Nineteenth Century*, eds. Judy Ewell and W. H. Beezley (Wilmington: Scholarly Resources, 1989), 234; Hèctor Recalde, *Las condiciones de trabajo*, vol. 2 of *Mujer condiciones de vida de trabajo y salud* (Buenos Aires: Centro Editión de America Latina, 1988–89), 214–15, 224–29.

17 Alejandro A. Raimondi and Tristán González, "Tuberculosis y embarazo. El nuemotórax en el embarazo y en el parto," *Revista de la Sociedad Argentina de Tisiología* 1 (August 1925): 31–43.

18 "Trabajo de la mujer a domicilio, 790.

19 Buenos Aires, *Statistical Year-Book of the City of Buenos Aires* (Buenos Aires: Compañía Sud-Americana de Billetes de Banco, 1919), 110–23; Victoria Mazzeo, *Migración internacional en la ciudad de Buenos Aires 1855–1980* (Buenos Aires: Municipalidad de la Ciudad de Buenos Aires, 1988), 19; Samuel Gache, *La tuberculose dan la République Argentine* (Buenos Aires: Augustin Etcheparebarda, 1899), 147–150, 156–60.

20 Léopold Blanc and Mukund Uplekar, "The Present Global Burden of Tuberculosis," in *The Return of the White Plague: Global Poverty and the "New"*

Tuberculosis, eds. Matthew Gandy and Alimuddin Zumla (London: Verso, 2003), 95.

21 Luis L. Boffi, *Tuberculosis de los viejos* (Buenos Aires: Lotito Hermanos y Cia., 1942), 13–16, 20–28.

22 Arturo Balbastro, *La Mujer Argentina (Estudio Médico-Social)*, MD diss., Facultad de Medicina, Universidad de Buenos Aires (Buenos Aires: Imprenta Sud-Americana, 1891), 11–12; Johnston, "Tuberculosis," 1060; Barbara Ehrenreich and Deirdre English, *For Her Own Good: 150 Years of Expert Advice to Women* (New York: Doubleday, 1978), 112, 122; Flick, "Pregnancy in Tuberculosis," 1–4.

23 For the correspondence between Macklin and Flick, see CUA, FP Second Series, Vols. 12–16; essentially the same story in more detail is told by Bates, *Bargaining for Life*, 214–30.

24 CUA, FP, 30 December 1903, G. E. Macklin to Lawrence F. Flick.

25 CUA, FP, vol. 14, Pittsburgh, PA, 1 June 1904, G.E. Macklin to Flick.

26 CUA, FP, 19 August 1904, G.E. Macklin to Flick, Pittsburgh, PA.

27 CUA, FP, 27 August 1904; 3, 26, 28 September 1904, Macklin to Flick.

28 CUA, FP, 3 October 1904, 17 October 1904, 5 November 1904, 14 December 1904, Macklin to Flick.

29 CUA, FP, Camden S.C., 16, 19 February 1905 Charles Bacher to Flick; Also see Bates, 223–24, 387, note 31.

30 CUA, FP, 14 February 1905, 12, 15, 18 March 1905, Macklin to Flick; CUA, FP, Elizabeth Macklin to Flick, 2 February 1905, 26 February 1905, 30 March 1905, 6 April 1905, 17 April 1905, Charles Bacher to Flick, 16 February 1905, 18 March 1905, CUA; date of death is provided by Bates, 230.

31 University of Pennsylvania (hereafter UP) University Archives and Record Center (hereafter GA), Archives General, 1909, Phipps Institute (hereafter AGPI), Beverley Robinson, "Creosote Treatment of Pulmonary Tuberculosis," reprinted from the 1909 *Medical Record*, 1–2; Ott, 45–50; "Tuberculosis," *Anales del Círculo Médico Argentino* 15, no. 9 (September 1892): 667; "Formulario," *Anales del Círculo Médico Argentino* 15, no. 8 (August 1892): 575; *Guía Médica de la Repúblic Argentina, 1890–1891* (Buenos Aires: Casa Editora, 1890), 93; Sebastián Esoin, "Tratamiento de la tuberculosis pulmonar" (MD diss., Universidad de Buenos Aires, 1914), 41–43; Federico Marugo, *Tratamiento de la Tuberculosis Pulmonar por la recalcificación*, MD diss., Facultad de Medicina, Universidad de Buenos Aires, 1911 (Buenos Aires: Establecimiento Gráfico de Alberto Monkes, 1911), 47–52. Among the best sources on the treatment of tuberculosis in Buenos Aires are the dissertations for the degree of Doctor in Medicine. Although they appear to have been published, the editions were small and are now rare. The most complete collection of Argentine medical dissertations is to be found at the Central Library of the Facultad de Medicina of the Universidad de Buenos Aires.

32 Frank Craig, *Early Days at Phipps* (Philadelphia: University of Pennsylvania Press, 1952), 18–19; CPP, FCR, Lawrence Francis Flick, "Hygiene of Phthisis," *Transactions of the Philadelphia County Medical Society* (11 January 1886), 10–14; CPP, FCR, Lawrence F. Flick, "The Treatment of Tuberculosis," *Medical News* (2 September 1899): 2; CPP, FCR, Lawrence F. Flick, "Some New Points in the Treatment of Tuberculosis," *Transactions of the Philadelphia County Medical Society*, 2; CPP, FCR, Lawrence Francis Flick, "Home Treatment," 7.

33 CPP, Joseph Walsh Papers (hereafter JWP) 1925–1936, 6 (25 September 1934), "The Advantage of Milk," 25 September 1934; CPP, FCR, Lawrence Francis Flick, "Home Treatment," 1–2, 5; Persky, 572–73.

34 For contemporary discussions of creosote, see Alfred Careño Croftan, *Clinical Therapeutics; a Handbook on the Special Treatment of Internal Disease* (Chicago: Cleveland Press, 1907), 322–23; Maurice Fishberg, *Pulmonary Tuberculosis*, 2nd ed. (Philadelphia: Lea & Febiger, 1919), 621–27. CPP, pamphlet collection, E. M. R. Gavott, "Where Creosote Succeeds;" suggested positive results in fifty-four out of ninety-three cases with samples being sent to registered physicians on request; CPP, pamphlet collection, "Creosotide" (Nelson, Baker & Co., Detroit, Mich.) was a "chemical compound of Creosote and Iodine...an amorphous brownish powder, practically insoluble in water and almost free from odor and taste."

35 For further discussion of the serum see M. F. Ravenel, "Maragliano's Method of Producing a Specific Serum for the Treatment of Tuberculosis and of Vaccinating against Tuberculosis; with Observations upon the Treatment Carried Out with Serum in Professor's Maragliano's Clinic," in *Second Annual Report of the Henry Phipps Institute for the Study, Treatment, and Prevention of Tuberculosis* (Philadelphia: Henry Phipps Institute, 1905). It was Flick's association with Maragliano that allowed for the treatment to be done in Philadelphia; he sent Ravenel to Genoa to observe his methods.

36 For discussion of medications, see *La Tribuna*, 25 January 1875, 16 February 1875, 31 May 1875, 4 June 1875 and 22 June 1875; *Actualidades Médicas* 4, no. 38 (December 1934); 7, no. 80 (September 1938); Diego Armus, *Ailing City: Health Tuberculosis and Culture in Buenos Aires, 1870–1950* (Durham: Duke University, 2011), 29–38; *Schenck's Almanac* (Philadelphia: J. H. Schenck & Sons, 1870), various advertisements; Thomas Dormandy, *The White Death: A History of Tuberculosis* (Washington Square: New York University Press, 2000), 273–83.

37 Ricardo González Leandri, *Curar, persuadir, gobernar: La construcción histórica de la profesión médica en Buenos Aires, 1852–1886* (Madrid: Consejo Superior de Investigaciones Científicas Centro de Estudios Históricos, 1999), 48–53; Armus, *Ailing City*, 47–48.

38 González Leandri, 48 indicated that the Argentine census of 1869 reported 1047 male and female healers and 453 physicians in the whole country, but only 9 healers and 154 physicians in the city of Buenos Aires, while the province of Buenos Aires had 118 healers and 89 physicians.

39 "Comunicación detalles sobre un medicamento contra la tuberculosis, por el profesor R. Koch, de Berlin," *Anales del Circulo Medico Argentino* 14, no. 1 (January 1891): 16–27; Diógenes Decoud, "El método de Koch en la clinica del Profesor Pirovano," *Anales del Círculo médico Argentino* 14, no. 2 (February 1891): 43–59; Eliseo Cantón, *Historia de la medicina en el Río de la Plata desde su descubrimiento hasta nuestros días*, vol. 4 (Madrid: Imp. G. Hernández y Galo Saéz, 1928), 242–43; Albert G. Miller, *History of the German Hospital in Philadelphia and its Ex-Resident Physicians* (Philadelphia: Press of J.B. Lippincott Company), 52.

40 Antonio R. Chiocconi, "La tuberculina residual en el tratamiento de la tuberculosis" (MD diss., Universidad de Buenos Aires, 1898), 44–45, 48–49.

41 Marugo, 115–17.

42 Marino R. Castex, "Nuevos casos de oftalmo-reacción a la tuberculina de Koch," *Departamento Nacional de Higiene* 14, no. 8 (August 1907): 277–78; Esoin, 85–89; Ott, 62; Georgina D. Feldberg, *Disease and Class: Tuberculosis and the Shaping of Modern North American Society* (New Brunswick: Rutgers University Press, 1955), 56–58.

43 César Rollino, "Pronóstico de la tuberculosis pulmonar" (MD diss., Facultad de Medicina, Universidad de Buenos Aires, 1902), 40–42.

44 Ott, 94–99; Dormandy, 255–62; J. Woodrow Savacool, "Philadelphia and the White Plague," *Transactions and Studies of the College of Physicians*, ser. 5, 8, no. 3 (1986): 174–75.

45 Raimondi and González, "Tuberculosis y embarazo," El Neumotórax artificial en el embarazo y el parto 33–39.

46 Ott, 99; Raimondi y González, "Tuberculosis y embarazo," 39.

47 Daniel Priano, "La bacteriología de la tuberculosis vacunación preventiva y curativa," *La Semana Médica* 48, no. 23 (5 June 1941): 1315–24; Armus, *Ailing City*, 59, 64; Bynum, *Spitting Blood*, 175.

48 David S. Barnes, *Making of a Social Disease: Tuberculosis in Nineteenth-Century France* (Berkeley: University of California Press, 1995), 4, 101, 119–20, 174, 208–12, 248; Clifford Rosenberg, "The International Politics of Vaccine Testing in Interwar Algiers," *The American Historical Review* 117 (June 2012): 689, 695.

49 "Estado actual de los tuberculosis pesquisados en el dispensario," *La Semana Médica* 44, no. 41 (14 October 1937): 908; Feldberg, 154–55, 160–61, 175–76, 186, 193, 202, 211, 214; Frank Macfarlane Burnet and David O. White, *Natural History of Infectious Disease* (Cambridge: Cambridge University Press, 1972), 222; Graham A. Colditz, Timothy F. Brewer, Catherine S. Berkey, et al., "Efficacy of BCG Vaccine in the Prevention of Tuberculosis," *Journal of American Medical Association* 271 (1994): 698–702; Laura C. Rodrigues, Vinod K. Diwan and Jeremy G. Wheeler, "Protective Effect of BCG against Tuberculous Meningitis and Miliary Tuberculosis: A Meta-Analysis," *International Journal of Epidemiology* 22 (1993): 1154–58.

50 Diego Armus, "Historias de enfermos tuberculosos que protestan Argentina, 1920–1940," in *Avatares de la medicalización en América Latina 1870–1970*, ed. Diego Armus (Buenos Aires: Lugar Editorial, 2005), 84–90; Armus, *Ailing City*, 101–11.

51 "La asistencia de tuberculosos pobres," *Alianza de Higiene Social* 7 (1907–1908): 193–95; Emilio R. Coni, "La campaña contra la tuberculosis en la República Argentina," *La Semana Médica* 16, no. 41 (14 October 1909): 1437–52; CPP, FCR Lawrence Francis Flick, "Hospital for Advanced Cases of Tuberculosis," *International Clinics* 19, S.V. I: 3. The terms dispensary and clinic are used as synonyms.

52 S. Adolphus Knopf, *Tuberculosis: A Preventable and Curable Disease* (New York: Moffat, Yard and Company, 1909), 56–57; Craig, *Early Days at Phipps*, 16–17, 22; CPP, FCR, Lawrence F. Flick, *Diagnosis and Treatment of Early Cases of Tuberculosis* (Philadelphia, 1907), 638; CPP, FCR, Lawrence Francis Flick, "Home Treatment," 1–2, 9–10.

53 "Liga argentina contra la tuberculosis: Informe anual de su presidente correspondiente al año 1907," *Alianza de Higiene Social* 7 (1907–1908): 333; the number of office visits is greater than the number of individuals visiting clinics. "Liga Argentina contra la tuberculosis" *Alianza de Higiene Social* 9 (January/February 1910): 232–33; Héctor Recalde, *Vida popular y salud en Buenos Aires 1900–1930* (Buenos Aires: Centro Editor de América Latina, 1994), 74. Emilio R. Coni, *Higiene Social: Asistencia y previsión social Buenos Aires caritativo y previsor* (Buenos Aires: Imprenta de Emilio Spinella, Ed., 1918), 432–34, discusses the founding of clinics.

54 "Dispensario Dr. Enrique Tornú," *La Lucha Antituberculosa* 2, no. 1 (June 1902): 12–14; "La Liga Argentina contra la tuberculosis," *La Lucha Antituberculosa* 2, no. 4 (September 1902): 148–49; Emilio R. Coni, "La Lucha antituberculosa en la República Argentina," *La Lucha Antituberculosa* 5,

nos. 4–8 (1905): 160–62; Karl Schaffle, "The State Tuberculosis Dispensary an Asset to the Municipality," *Spunk* 9, no. 7 (October 1917): 8–9; Gibson Smith, "The Ideal Tuberculosis Clinic," *The Listening Post* 4, no. 35 (February 1926): 16.

55 Kensington Dispensary for the Treatment of Tuberculosis (Philadelphia), Board of Managers, *Ninth Annual Report of the Kensington Dispensary for the Treatment of Tuberculosis* (Philadelphia: Press of P.C. Stockhausen, 1915): 8, 12–13, 16, 35; Savacool, 150, 170.

56 Kensington Dispensary for the Treatment of Tuberculosis, 19–20.

57 B. Franklin Royer, "The Work of the State Department of Health in the Tuberculosis Campaign," *Spunk* 5, no. 12 (March 1914): 9; "Information for the Public," *Spunk* 9, no. 1 (April 1917): 1; Schaffle, "The State Tuberculosis Dispensary," 11–13; Savacool, 164.

58 Savacool, 171; Lawrence F. Flick, "The Crusade against Tuberculosis in Philadelphia," presented to the Philadelphia County Medical Society on 23 November 1932, privately printed; "Tuberculosis Work in Philadelphia," *Monthly Bulletin of the Department of Public Health and Charities of the City of Philadelphia* 4, no. 6 (June 1919): 86; David McBride, *Integrating the City of Medicine: Blacks in Philadelphia Health Care, 1910–1965* (Philadelphia: Temple University Press, 1988), 129.

59 Albert P. Francine and H. J. Hartz, "Results with Tuberculin (Dixon's) in Advanced Chronic Ambulatory Tuberculosis," read before the College of Physicians of Philadelphia 4 December 1912, 8.

60 Lawrence F. Flick, "The Work of the Year," *Second Annual Report of the Henry Phipps Institute for the Study, Treatment, and Prevention of Tuberculosis* (Philadelphia: Henry Phipps Institute, 1905), 47.

61 Visiting Nurse Society of Philadelphia Records, Center for the Study of the History of Nursing (hereafter VNS), UP, Series, IX, Box 39, News Clippings and Publications, folder 7; *Eleventh Annual Report of the Visiting Nurse Society of Philadelphia*, MC 5/I, folder 18; UP, VNS, *Twenty-Third Annual Report of the Visiting Nurse Society of Philadelphia for Year Ending February 28, 1909*, MC5, Box 4; UP, VNS, MC5 Box 3, "Report of Special Nurse on Tuberculosis, March 1, 1908 to February 28, 1909"; Anna Drake, "Nursing in Tuberculosis," *Listening Post* 5, no. 4 (July–August 1927): 3–8.

62 "La asistencia de tuberculosos pobres," *Alianza de Higiene Social* 7 (1907–1908): 194–95; Coni, "La Lucha antituberculosa en la República Argentina," 162; Alice M. O'Hallaron, "The Work of the Dispensary Nurse," *Spunk* 6, no. 1 (April 1914): 10–11; Schaffle, 8–9; CP, manuscript William H. Hutt, "First work in America for the Relief of Tuberculosis," 1905. "Liga argentina contra la tuberculosis," *Alianza* (1910): 229–32, provides specific data on the medical consultations, office visits, prescriptions, food distributions, and sputum analysis of the tuberculosis clinics between 1902 and 1909.

63 Emilio R. Coni, "Hospitalización y aislamiento de los tuberculosos pulmonares en Buenos Aires," *La Semana Médica* 9, no. 43 (27 October 1904): 1139–40.

64 "La Tuberculosis en los Hospitales de la Capital," *Revista de Ciencias Médicas* IX, no. 101 (September 1926): 191–92.

65 "La asistencia pública de los tuberculosos en Buenos Aires," *Revista de la Tuberculosis* 1, no. 4 (September 1901): 118–19; Alberto B. Martínez, *Censo general de población edificaciones, comercio e industrias de la ciudad Buenos Aires, levantado en los días 11 y 18 septiembre de 1904* (Buenos Aires:

Cía. Sudamericana de Billetes de Banco, 1906), 317–38; Coni, "La lucha antituberculosis en la República Argentina," 156–58; "La Tuberculosis en los Hospitales de la Capital," *Revista de Ciencias Médicas* 9, no. 101 (September 1926): 191–92.

66 Samuel Gache and J. A. Muñiz, "Sanatorio para mujeres y niños," *La Lucha Antituberculosa* 6, nos. 4&5 (September/October 1906): 149–50; Coni, La campaña contra la tuberculosis" (14 October 1909): 1444. Table 2.1: Comparative Demographics, Buenos Aires and Philadelphia 1870–1938. Archivo General de la Nación Argentina (hereafter AGN), Hospital Vicente López y Planes (hereafter HVLP), Buenos Aires, Sociedad de Beneficencia, legajo 150–52, provides detailed information on the construction and operation of this hospital.

67 For 1895, "Mortalidad por enfermedades infecciosas en la ciudad de Buenos Aires durante los años 1895 y 1896," *Anales al Departamento Nacional de Higiene* 6, no. 25 (1 July 1896): 403–9, 424–28; 6, no. 27 (16 July 1896): 495–96; 6, no. 30 (8 August 1896): 522–24; 6, no. 34 (8 September 1896): 610–12; 6, no. 37, 38, 39 (1, 8, 16 October 1896): 721–23; 6, no. 42 (8 November 1896): 800–802, 862–64; 7, no. 1, 2 (1, 8 January 1897): 20–23; 7, no. 5, 6 (1, 8 February 1897): 87–89. For 1904, Coni, "La lucha antituberculosa" (1905), 156–58; for 1908, Coni, "La campaña contra la tuberculosis," (14 October 1909), 1438; for 1913–1919, Domingo Cabred, *La tuberculosis en la República Argentina, Informe presentado al Ministerio de Relaciones Exteriores y Culto, el 31 de mayo de 1918* (Buenos Aires: Imprenta y Encuadernación del Hospicio de la Mercedes, 1919), cuadro I.

68 CUA, FP, Tuberculosis Letters, vol. 14, 1901, pt. 3 Philadelphia 18 November 1901, Lawrence F. Flick to John T. Morris, 724; Guy Hinsdale, "Tuberculosis in Pennsylvania," *Journal of the American Medical Association* (20 October 1900): 996–99.

69 CPP, FCR, Lawrence F. Flick, "The Crusade against Tuberculosis in Pennsylvania," annual address of the President of the Free Hospital for Poor Consumptives, delivered on 9 March 1908; "Summary of the Consumptive Department for the Year Ending April 15, 1904," *1904: 34th Annual Report: The Philadelphia Protestant Episcopal City Mission*, 25; Savacool, 151–52; Craig, *Early Days at Phipps*, 7.

70 Bates, 43, 56, 61, 65–66, 253; "Twenty-first Annual Report of the Rush Hospital for Consumption and Allied Diseases from 1 June 1912 to 1 June 1913 and the Women's Board of the Rush Hospital of Philadelphia," 2; CPP, LFP, Tuberculosis Letters, vol. 10 1900, pt. 1; President of the Jewish Hospital Association to Flick, 3 February 1900; UP, GA,AGPI "Minutes of Board of Directors of the Phipps Institute," 6 July 1911; Charles K. Mills, "The Philadelphia Almshouse and the Philadelphia General Hospital from 1854–1908," in *Founders' Week Memorial Volume* (Philadelphia: City of Philadelphia, 1909): 506–7.

71 Bates, 286–87; Savacool, 168.

72 CUA, FP, *Tuberculosis Letters*, vol. 10, 1900, pt. 2 Francis Fisher to Flick, 30 June 1900; CUA, FP, Tuberculosis Letters, vol. 12 1901, pt. 1, Philadelphia 18 April 1901 James Tyson to Flick, 251.

73 CPP, FCR Lawrence Francis Flick, "Tuberculosis as It Concerns the Physicians," *Interstate Medical Journal* 18, no. 2 (1911): 7–10.

74 Table 2.1: Comparative Demographics.

75 There is scientific literature on life expectancy of those with tuberculosis related to the current epidemic, but little for the early twentieth century. See Marc Arnold, *Disease, Class and Social Change: Tuberculosis in Folkestone*

and Sandgate, 1880–1930 (Newcastle upon Tyne: Cambridge Scholars Publishing, 2012), 119; Albert P. Francine, "Results on January 1, 1913 in Philadelphia Patients Discharged from Mont Alto in 1909," in *Transactions of the National Association for the Study and Prevention of Tuberculosis, Ninth Annual Meeting, Washington D.C., May 8–9, 1913* (Philadelphia; William F. Fell, 1913), 285.

76 Paul Starr, *The Social Transformation of American Medicine* (New York: Basic Books, 1982), 30, 60, 137.

77 Juan Alsina, "La Santa Cristina en casos avanzados de tuberculosis pulmonar," *La Semana Médica* (4 November 1926): 1241–42; William Feldman, "Studies in Chemotherapy of Tuberculosis including Use of Streptomycin," *Transactions and Studies of the College of Physicians of Philadelphia*, Fourth Series, 14, no. 3 (December 1946): 81–97; Bynum, 190–216.

5 The Sanatorium Age
Argentina and Pennsylvania

> I was surprised in the middle of my work by a violent vomiting of blood...that confirmed a suspected illness.... Gathering together in whatever manner a few pesos, reducing the expenses of the family that I left.... I arrived at Cosquín for the first time in the month of May of 1897.... The imponderable climate of these hills began to produce a miracle! After two months I found myself feeling better every moment and all the symptoms began to disappear and my weight increased by eight kilos.[1]

> There stands an institution
> In the Pennsylvania hills
> That has made so many happy
> By curing of their ills
>
> It has stood for many years now
> It has often times been tested
> Many cases have been cured
> And a number too arrested
>
> These mortals now made happy
> Mont Alto's praise have sung
> It has built up many a system
> And patched up many a lung[2]

The quotations reflect how tubercular individuals experienced their illnesses and recoveries. The first passage is a translation of a letter written by the Porteño director of the Post and Telegraph office who in 1897 traveled to the province of Córdoba and stayed in a hotel. He could afford only a three-month stay, so he returned to work in Buenos Aires, knowing that his sojourn had been too short. By 1899, he was again very ill, and his doctor arranged for him to return to Córdoba. From 1900 to 1905, he was healthy and comfortably established in Córdoba; and having benefitted by rest and the climate, he decided to marry. The poem, published at the Mont Alto State Sanatorium in a monthly magazine produced by patients gave hope to those living in Pennsylvania's public sanatoriums. Philadelphians traveled to the hills of Pennsylvania, expecting that fresh air and a sanatorium's protein diet would restore them to health. Both accounts imply that climate and a sanatorium stay would cure tuberculosis; such positive outcomes were, unfortunately unusual.[3]

Public health officials and physicians advocated constructing sanatoriums to cure the tubercular. Medical and popular beliefs initially encouraged building sanatoriums in cold or dry climates. In Pennsylvania, entrepreneurs and public officials supported the building of sanatoriums in mountainous regions. By the early nineteenth century, the hot, dry climate of the interior Argentine provinces of Córdoba and Mendoza became the location of choice for many tubercular Porteños. Travelers even suggested that the hills of Córdoba, some 4,000 feet above sea level with a moderate winter climate, were as beneficial for tuberculosis patients as mountain retreats in Europe. By 1869, a British traveler reported that European consumptives could benefit from Córdoba by traveling by steamer from a European port to Argentina. Although the ocean trip to Buenos Aires took thirty-four days, the vacationer needed only a day to travel to Córdoba. The relaxed pace of life in resort areas and their moderate temperatures might extend the lives of the tubercular, but the climate did not contribute to a cure. The death rate from tuberculosis in Córdoba was actually higher than that in Buenos Aires—but that was in part the result of the many tubercular patients who came from other cities.[4]

Sanatoriums total institutions[5] in which individuals of similar circumstances lived together, subject to the institution's rules, separated from the outside world—came to be viewed as a means of preventing and curing tuberculosis. They drew their inspiration from infectious disease hospitals that isolated individuals, asylums that aimed to be therapeutic and resorts that created a comfortable living environment. Like hospitals, they provided specialized short-term care for the seriously ill and inexpensive care for the moderately ill. Sanatoriums did not quarantine patients, who were free to leave when they chose. Thus, both private and public sanatoriums needed to make themselves attractive to patients. Privately run sanatoriums created a resort atmosphere, and even public sanatoriums offered entertainment, educational opportunities and employment training. Between 1860 and 1945, public health officials and physicians in the Western world believed that sanatorium care was providing the best option for curing tuberculosis.

History of Sanatorium Development

Germany provided the prototype for public and private sanatoriums in the U.S. and Argentina. Hermann Brehmer, a German physician, began treating tuberculosis in 1854; by 1856, he had established the first sanatorium for treating tuberculosis in the village of Göbersdorf in the Prussian province of Silesia. Brehmer developed the basic treatment that sanatoriums employed worldwide, basing it on how he treated his own illness. His program of daily walks in the clear mountain air coupled with periods of rest and a nutritious diet sought to create strong bodies that would resist tuberculosis.[6] Although many of the tubercular chose to live in hotels or rent apartments and homes in hot dry climates, physicians advised their patients to live in a sanatorium that enforced rest periods and regulated their diet.

When the Commonwealth of Pennsylvania concluded that it should finance the building and operation of sanatoriums, it constructed the buildings at Mont Alto and several smaller institutions. Argentina financed the building of several sanatoriums, including Sanatorio Nacional de Tuberculosos Santa María, Hospital Sanatorio de Llanura Vicente López y Planes and Hospital Dr. Enrique Tornú. Patients in Philadelphia and Buenos Aires could choose to go to either government-run sanatoriums or private ones. They could decide on a sanatorium in their home city or travel elsewhere. Patients were treated similarly in public and private sanatoriums and in rural and urban institutions, although wealthy patients might receive more luxurious care in private resorts.

Because physicians had difficulty diagnosing tuberculosis and the poor did not seek to enter sanatoriums on their own, the initial system—in which "incipient" cases were assigned to sanatoriums and "advanced" ones were assigned to hospitals—failed. Public health officials accordingly favored sending both types of patients to sanatoriums, since they could treat a wide variety of tubercular cases.[7] Sanatoriums filled a need: hospitals were too expensive for most patients, and the number of tuberculosis patients requiring inexpensive care was increasing. Furthermore, the poor lacked space in their own homes to separate tuberculosis patients from the rest of the family. Sanatoriums were useful, because they isolated the contagious, cared for poor patients and taught the patients' families how to prevent tuberculosis. They also offered opportunities to investors, who could profit by investing in expanded treatment in sanatoriums. Sanatoriums, therefore, appealed to the government, the medical community, and both the wealthy and the poor.[8]

There were two types of sanatoriums. Privately operated sanatoriums resembled resorts such as the German health spas; they appealed to the middle and upper classes. By contrast, the government-run sanatoriums served the poor and the terminally ill. Joseph Walsh (physician, tuberculosis specialist and medical director of White Haven Sanatorium) investigated sanatoriums in Europe when he attended the International Tuberculosis Congress in Paris in 1905. He compared European and U.S. sanatoriums and reported that Europe had many more sanatoriums than the U.S. For example, in 1905 Germany had seventy-two government sanatoriums with six thousand beds and twenty-five private sanatoriums with 1500 beds. In comparison, in 1900, the U.S. had only thirty-four private and state sanatoriums with 4,485 beds. (By 1925, the U.S. had 536 sanatoriums with 673,338 beds.) Walsh also noted that cut the Britain, Germany, and France spent much more government money on sanatoriums than the U.S. did. U.S. tuberculosis patients faced three problems: the shortage of beds in sanatoriums, the uneven quality of care and the limited facilities available for African Americans. In 1934, there were 21,099 African American tuberculosis deaths in the U.S. (427 in Philadelphia), but only 3,334 beds in sanatoriums.[9]

U.S. state governments recognized that many patients could not afford private sanatoriums and, therefore, began building sanatoriums to treat impoverished patients. The Channing Home, the first public sanatorium focusing exclusively on treating the tubercular poor, began treating patients in Boston in 1857; a year after, Brehmer opened his sanatorium. In 1898, Massachusetts opened the first state sanatorium at Rutland. This facility had a capacity of 400; each patient was charged $4.00 per week. Other states soon followed suit; Pennsylvania opened Mont Alto in 1908.[10] The first private U.S. sanatorium began operations in Asheville, North Carolina, in 1857. But it was Edward Livingston Trudeau's sanatorium that became a model for later efforts. In 1873, Trudeau moved to a summer hotel in the Adirondacks where he rested in the winter and treated patients in the summer. Concluding that the Adirondack climate and opportunity to rest improved his health, in 1884, he established the Adirondack Cottage Sanitarium at Saranac Lake, New York. By 1894, the sanatorium offered nine cottages with their own bathrooms, an open-air pavilion for patient recreation, an infirmary that could treat ten people and a house for a resident physician. Soon a library, a workshop, a bacteriology laboratory, an X-ray facility and a nursing school were added.[11]

Trudeau's sanatorium looked like an upscale summer hotel. By the 1920s, it catered to social and financial elites. Nevertheless, Trudeau's customers were not altogether satisfied. Patients had little to do except look out the window and eat the trays of food that arrived five times a day. Even reading was forbidden; boredom led some patients to leave prematurely. Although most patients paid their own expenses, the reasonable cost and the subsidies offered to a few enabled some people of moderate means to stay at the sanatorium. Trudeau's experiences showed that people could recover temporarily from tuberculosis. He emphasized a holistic approach. Patients needed to leave the environment that produced tuberculosis and work on building their bodies by resting and eating healthy food. Physicians prescribed specific drugs to address the symptoms of coughing, night sweats, spitting blood, and weight loss. Because Trudeau probably contracted tuberculosis in 1865 (when he cared for his tubercular brother and shared his bed), the sanatorium's physicians regularly asked patients if they slept alone.[12]

States followed one of two plans. They either placed the burden of managing sanatoriums on local agents (as in Massachusetts) or built and financially supported sanatoriums and dispensaries (as in Pennsylvania). Increasingly, the U.S. treated the poor in state-financed sanatoriums, as opposed to treating them in hospitals funded by private charities and local governments. State and federal sanatoriums grew rapidly. Privately run sanatoriums faced competition from public institutions, other private facilities and residential hotels. To support private sanatoriums in 1901, Pennsylvania's government paid a weekly fee to private sanatoriums that cared for lower- and middle-class patients. Although sanatorium regimens successfully cured some individuals in the beginning stages of tuberculosis and isolated infected individuals from the community, public institutions were available for only a small fraction of tuberculosis patients; 3-month waiting periods for admission were not unusual.[13]

Day Camps

Those who were awaiting space at a sanatorium and those who wanted to supplement home treatment were encouraged to attend day camps that followed the fresh air, diet and rest regimen. In 1905, Boston opened the first day camp for tuberculosis patients. Patients at the camp rested or did light exercise in the outdoors and ate nutritious meals. Nurses cared for them and physicians regularly examined them. Many patients were reluctant to go to day camps; they found them inconvenient and resented the enforced routine. Nevertheless by 1911, thirty-seven-day camps operated in the northeast as well as a night camp in Pittsburgh, Pennsylvania.[14]

Philadelphia opened its first out-door treatment center in 1911 under the direction of the Philadelphia Central Dispensary. In April, a large tent was erected and furnished with camp chairs. Located on a pier near the river, it operated until December 1, when it became too cold for patients to stay outdoors. Thirty patients attended the camp each day in the summer, although ninety registered to attend; this discrepancy suggests that many patients came irregularly or for only a short time. The convalescents arrived at 9 A.M. and stayed until 5 P.M. The program, funded by private contributions, provided patients with trolley fares, adjustable steamer chairs, blankets and drinking glasses. The tubercular received milk during the day and a meal at noon. A trained nurse supervised care and took each patient's pulse and temperature twice a day.[15]

Pennsylvania patients desiring public sanatorium treatment were required to go to the dispensary nearest to their home to obtain a smallpox vaccination and to fill out an application. In one to three months, the state notified an individual of his acceptance in a directive that placed his name on a waiting list. In contrast to private sanatoriums, only residents of Pennsylvania (with preference given to U.S. citizens) were accepted. The state provided the tubercular with the sanatorium rules and a list of necessary winter and summer clothing. Since food and shelter were free, the only expenses for patients were for transportation, clothing, laundry and incidentals.[16]

A Private Sanatorium: White Haven

Lawrence F. Flick founded the White Haven Sanatorium as a semi-private sanatorium in 1901 to treat poor and middle-class patients, regardless of race, ethnicity or religion. After spending six years of caring for the dying in hospitals and facing difficulty getting hospitals to accept tuberculosis patients, Flick wanted to found an institution that focused on treating Philadelphians in the early stages of tuberculosis. A philanthropist gave Flick a large farm 116 miles north of Philadelphia, near the Lehigh River in the Green Mountains, 2,335 feet above the sea level. Flick was expected to raise the money to build the sanatorium.[17]

Initially, the buildings at White Haven were primitive, consisting only of a dilapidated barn and a small farmhouse. Then the Pennsylvania legislature funded the construction of three brick cottages, each of which could accommodate sixteen patients. The legislature also gave financial support for the needy Pennsylvania tubercular patients. Private gifts paid for a sewage plant, the remodeling of the barn (which then housed a large dining room and a kitchen) and additional patient rooms (increasing the sanatorium's capacity to ninety-eight beds). Because Pennsylvania provided only thirty percent of the care costs for poor patients, Flick raised additional funds. When Pennsylvania shifted its funding to state sanatoriums, it decreased its support for White Haven. As a result, the facility increasingly went into debt. By 1908, the sanatorium accepted only paying patients. Patients could, however, pay less for their care by working at the sanatorium. Convalescents who worked eight hours per day actually paid nothing, but patients were usually too weak to work so many hours when they first arrived. The work done by patients enabled the institution to hire twenty-eight fewer employees. Physicians viewed one to two hours of work per day for patients as healthy. Flick also opened a school for nurses at White Haven in 1907, to help address White Haven's need for more workers.[18]

At first, White Haven accepted patients from Pennsylvania, Ohio and New York. Patients ranged between nine and sixty years of age; most were between twenty and fifty. The admission policy favored poor patients and those in the early stages of tuberculosis. White Haven did not accept children and transferred pregnant women to hospitals, because it did not have appropriate medical facilities for such patients. To attract more patients, White Haven eventually accepted both moderate and advanced cases. According to Flick, most patients who remained at the sanatorium over three months improved their health and could often return to their jobs. Some patients, however, stayed for less than a week, because they did not like the discipline or found the weather too cold or the conditions too primitive. Some patients were discharged because they failed to follow the instructions or argued with nurses and other patients.[19]

Sanatorium treatment began by obtaining accurate medical histories from patients. Patients supplied information about their families, their childhood diseases, their vaccinations for smallpox and typhoid, their health complaints and the condition of their respiratory system. Patients were asked whether they liked outdoor activity and were also asked to provide the information about the age at which they began working, their occupation, the age at which they married, and the number of their children and their children's ages.[20] Physicians classified the stage of the patient's tuberculosis, so as to more effectively treat the disease. To restore a person to a healthy state and establish greater resistance to the disease, patients followed a strict routine. They were required to eat large amounts of nutritious food, to spend most of their waking hours in fresh air and to balance their time between rest and exercise. Staff took patients' pulses and their temperatures both morning and night and weighed patients weekly. Patients with rising temperatures were prohibited from exercising. Incipient cases, who could recover in a short time, were separated from advanced cases. Nurses gave medications after meals. All convalescents were required to use spittoons and paper napkins; spitting on the sanatorium grounds was cause for expulsion. To relieve patients of boredom and prepare them for returning home, they also received some education and job training.[21]

White Haven is, perhaps, the best known of Pennsylvania's private sanatoriums for Philadelphia patients. But there were others. In 1884, the Philadelphia Episcopal City Mission opened a convalescent retreat for the tubercular at Glen Mills, Pennsylvania. Lawrence Flick sent some of his patients to Gabriels, a Catholic sanatorium opened by the Sisters of Mercy in 1897 in the Adirondacks. By 1919, Hill Crest, Fern Cliff and Sunnyrest (private sanatoriums that charged between $15 and $40 a week), also served Philadelphia patients.[22]

Flick opposed the construction and expansion of state sanatoriums. He argued that the private sector should build and operate them. He contended that state sanatoriums were too large to be run efficiently, were operated by people who knew little about tuberculosis, were administered on a political basis and failed to provide patients with information on preventive methods. (Needless to say, he was not an impartial observer.) State funding for White Haven decreased because the legislature chose to support state sanatoriums. As a result, Flick had to compete with other private sanatoriums by appealing to middle- and upper-class invalids. Flick's opposition to state-run sanatoriums led him to clash with Dr. Samuel Gibson Dixon (1851–1918), who in 1905 became the first Commissioner of Health of Pennsylvania and subsequently presided over the expansion of state sanatoriums. Dixon had been one of Flick's earliest supporters, but by 1909, their differing approaches to tuberculosis treatment drove a wedge between the two.[23]

Mont Alto: State Sanatorium of Pennsylvania

Mont Alto Sanatorium had a humble beginning. In late 1901, Dr. J. T. Rothrock opened at South Mountain a small private camp for patients in the early stages of tuberculosis. The camp was located near Waynesboro in the heart of a 55,000 acres forestry reserve, 160 miles west of Philadelphia. In its first year, patients with no medical supervision lived in tents and provided their own furnishings and food. In the following year, with the financial support from the state legislature and women's organizations, Rothrock built ten-foot-square cabins. Tuberculosis patients often came with family members, who lived in tents and cared for those residing in the cabins. The Pennsylvania legislature continued to invest money in the private camp by funding construction of a kitchen, a dining room, a spring house (one room building constructed over a spring which provides refrigeration) and an office. However, by 1905, the Commonwealth decided to build its own facilities and purchased Mont Alto. In June 1907, the state legislature transferred 500 acres of forest land (including the location of the original camp) to the Department of Health. In May of the same year, the legislature also provided funds to create and support a sanatorium to provide free care for Pennsylvanians with tuberculosis.[24]

During the early part of the twentieth century, the Pennsylvania legislature supported a number of private sanatoriums, including both White Haven and South Mountain. Once the state purchased the South Mountain Sanatorium at Mont Alto, it expanded rapidly: it accommodated twenty-six patients in 1907, 140 in 1908, 753 in 1910 and 960 in 1912. Beginning in 1912, Mont Alto provided free care to the state's tuberculosis patients. By 1913, it had become the largest public tuberculosis sanatorium in the U.S., with 1,055 beds. By 1916, there were 1,130 patients and almost 200 staff members. In January 1916, sixty-five percent of the patients were male and thirty-five percent female. The construction of a children's preventorium and an adult hospital building brought the total capacity to 1,700 beds in 1946. Mont Alto received patients at all stages of tuberculosis, but the number of patients in the late stages of tuberculosis continued to increase.

By 1924, Pennsylvania was operating three tuberculosis sanatoriums, including Cresson in the Allegheny Mountains (with a capacity of 475 adults and 225 children) and Hamburg in Berks County (with space for 450 adults). By 1926 Pennsylvania—which offered over 2,000 free beds to tuberculosis patients—had more public funded beds than any other state. Nevertheless, because there were only 4,300 beds in public and private sanatoriums, a significant shortage remained. Over fifty counties and most cities with fewer than 100,000 residents had no public or private sanatoriums.[25] African American patients came primarily from Philadelphia and comprised only 7.4 percent of Mont Alto's population in 1920. Between 1907 and 1914, Mont Alto treated 445 African Americans, fairly evenly divided between men and women. Although no minority patients in the early stages of tuberculosis died at Mont Alto, the eighty-eight percent of minority patients who were considered to have moderate or advanced cases died at twice the rate of Caucasian patients. People from all walks of life—ranging from laborers to doctors—shared a common experience at Mont Alto. A patient reported, "... they all associated together and enjoyed the same privileges without anyone considering himself more than the other or trying to domineer the place in any way or form."[26]

Built on 600 acres, Mont Alto at its height included a dining room that served 600 patients daily, an infirmary with 200 beds that handled advanced cases of tuberculosis, a general hospital, an administration building, a children's preventorium, seventy cottages, sixteen pavilions, fifteen tents, four bath houses, a chapel, a laundry, an electric power house, nurses' and doctors' accommodations and a medical director's house. The cottages represented an innovation in patient care. Erected to allow as much air as possible to circulate and the sun to shine at some time during the day in each of the four square rooms, each cottage housed eight people, who were among the healthier sanatorium residents. Although patients complained about the extreme cold in the winter (they placed newspapers between the mattresses and springs to keep warm), the cottages were popular with residents because of the homelike conditions.[27]

Patients arriving at Mont Alto received a physical examination to ensure that they were assigned to the proper cottage or ward. The healthiest could go to the dining room for their meals; the moderately ill could go only for breakfast; and the seriously ill were required to stay in bed and to receive all meals in their rooms. In 1915, physicians judged that 126 (12.8 percent) of the patients were incipiently ill and that 458 (46.4 percent) were moderately ill; 402 (40.8 percent) were thought to be advanced cases. Physicians classified the patients according to the answers to the following questions: "How long have you been ill? Did you ever spit blood? Have you lost weight? Are you able to do light work? Do you cough or expectorate much? Are you feverish and how often?"[28]

The rules and regimen for patients were extensive. Patients were to spit only in the appropriate receptacles and were not to remove furnishings from cottages or to wash clothes or take baths in the cottages. But they were to take a bath twice weekly, and those confined to bed were to be sponged daily with a cleansing bath once a week. All were to wash their hands and faces before each meal; hair was to be washed frequently, nails cleaned, and clothes changed regularly; and teeth were to be brushed on rising and after each meal. Convalescents were to use their own cups to gargle with antiseptics before eating in the morning and before retiring in the evening. Drinking alcohol, using obscene language, gambling or possessing firearms were grounds for dismissal. In between meals and snacks and prescribed treatments and activities, men and women rested in separate camps on steamer chairs in the open air. Physicians experimented with treatments in a search for a cure and initially favored heliotherapy treatment—at first to treat surgical patients and then to treat all patients. They were supposed to enjoy direct natural sunlight outdoors for as long a time as possible.[29]

Women patients might crochet when resting, and men might read. Healthier patients played sports or joined groups to present musicals and plays. Residents also participated in light work, such as caring for poultry, painting or gardening. Patients raised chickens, pigeons, pheasants and guinea pigs for those who could not eat a regular diet. While some patients enjoyed working outdoors, others preferred photography or took short walks in the mountains. Convalescents also attended weekly motion pictures and participated in the resident orchestra. Patients took classes in shorthand, typewriting, spelling, English and penmanship to develop skills to use when they left the sanatorium. Patients could attend religious services in the chapel which was built in 1911; Episcopal services were held twice monthly, Catholic Mass was held every Sunday and there were prayer meetings for Protestants on Wednesdays. In addition to formal religious services, Sunday school was held on alternate Sundays in the dining room. The Mont Alto administration believed that rituals and group activities contributed to a sense of community and therefore promoted holiday celebrations, including Washington's Birthday, St. Patrick's Day, Fourth of July, Thanksgiving, and of course, Christmas and New Year's.[30]

Mont Alto was unique in that its patients published a monthly magazine, *Spunk*, which existed from 1909 until 1963. Residents provided news about their experiences through short stories, essays, poems and cartoons. J. H. Wilcox in the first verse of his poem "The Spunk Cure," described the residents of Mont Alto as follows: "Upon a spunky mountain, In a spunky commonwealth, There's a camp of spunky people, Who are spunking up their health." Reporters described general happenings, offered advice, and commissioned educational articles by specialists on subjects such as proper diets, contagiousness of tuberculosis and the dangers of spitting. *Spunk* included biographical sketches of some patients who died, noted marriages and shared general community gossip. There was a children's page, as well as black-and-white photos of the sanatorium and its activities. Resident poets saw their work in print.

Special holiday celebrations were reported in detail. For example, an article on Fourth of July celebrations spoke of picnicking, games, cottages decorated with flags and a performance by the American Legion band of Harrisburg. Another article reported that Thanksgiving was celebrated with a special service in the chapel, followed by a dinner of "stewed chicken, mashed potatoes, cranberries, lima beans, celery, bread, butter, tea cake and ice cream." *Spunk's* Christmas issue noted that there was a special performance, caroling, greetings and messages and gifts from surrounding communities.[31] *Spunk* articles and poetry emphasized the importance of keeping one's spirits up in order to facilitate a cure. In the final verse of his poem, "The Spunk Cure," Wilcox wrote: "There's spunk for every sickness, A cure for every ill, And spunk flies to the rescue; the Way comes with the will."[32]

At the end of 1921, *Spunk* added "The Question Box" to its format, a feature that allowed patients to ask questions that were answered by physicians in the following month. Patients were less anxious and resentful about their time at Mont Alto when doctors answered their questions about artificial pneumothorax, arrested cases, pulse rates and the drainage of lungs.[33] *Spunk* also enabled patients to critique their treatment, but grievances were generally reflected in satire rather than informal complaints. Leroy Sutcliffe in "Mont Alto Jingles" wrote "And then we have the nurses: A grand and jolly staff, They chase us out to cure and then stand and laugh," ending with "And now I think I'd better stop Before someone gets vexed. If you want to hear the rest of this, It's continued in our next." Nurses were indeed very important in sanatoriums. They ensured that patients followed the regime and cared for them after surgery. Nurses saw themselves as both controlling patients and working with them to combat the disease.[34]

Patients were required to stay at Mont Alto at least four months and encouraged to stay until their disease was "arrested." Public health officials considered a patient's disease arrested when tubercular bacilli were absent from sputum for three months. An individual who remained free of the tubercular bacilli for two years was considered cured. In 1909, the average stay of incipient patients from Philadelphia was six and one-half months; moderately advanced patients stayed for eight months, and advanced patients stayed for seven and one-half months. Once patients left the sanatorium, they were required to report to a clinic near their home so that their progress could be tracked. Patients returning home were encouraged to work outdoors, to get fresh air, to stay away from crowds and dusty places, to work in sunny and airy places, to keep regular hours, to rest after eating and not to get too tired. Often patients were discharged without being cured. Of the 399 patients, in 1909, who returned home to Philadelphia from Mont Alto, only twenty-eight percent were classified as cured or arrested. Forty-four percent of the returnees died within five years. Advanced-case patients often returned home to die.[35]

Sanatorium staff emphasized that when patients left prematurely they imposed a high cost on both families and taxpayers. Patients who departed before they were cured could spread infection and see their own health deteriorate. By the 1940s, articles in medical journals expressed rising concern about patients leaving sanatoriums against medical advice. In December 1960, *Spunk* reported that one-third of all tuberculosis patients left sanatoriums against medical advice due to failure to adjust to institutional rules or dislike of the regimen; individuals would state "I just can't take it any longer; I must get out of the hospital or explode." Others would leave because: "(m)y family needs me."[36]

One of the challenges for patients whose tuberculosis was "arrested" was to find suitable employment, particularly, light outdoor work with time for rest. At the same time, many patients who returned home were still too weak to work at regular jobs. Mont Alto and other sanatoriums established a two-year course of study in nursing care for former patients. In 1926, five students graduated from the Mont Alto Training School: three were former patients at Hamburg and two at Mont Alto. The school celebrated a ten-year reunion in October 1929. The school was not accredited and did not prepare students for general hospital work, but it did provide training for jobs in sanatoriums. Some recovered patients took jobs at Mont Alto rather than return to Philadelphia.[37]

Routines and amusements changed little at Mont Alto in the first half of the twentieth century. Although one could sleep later in the 1940s (when breakfast was at 8:30 A.M.), strict regulations remained. Men were not to have beards or mustaches. Patients had to take daily baths, brush their teeth twice a day and "sleep between the sheets." Various denominational services were held on Sundays, and Bible study sessions were offered during the week. Patients continued to write articles for *Spunk* on sanatorium activities and to inform patients about tuberculosis. Patients were attracted to Mont Alto from all parts of the state (only about forty percent came from Philadelphia) because it offered excellent care. In 1948, Mont Alto—renamed the Samuel G. Dixon Sanatorium—offered state-of-the-art medical treatment and attracted patients with amenities such as bowling alleys and a golf course.[38]

Between 1870 and 1945, public and private sanatoriums in the U.S. competed for the same middle-class patients who were only moderately ill. Although its smaller size enabled White Haven to provide more individual attention to patients than Mont Alto, it could not compete with the public sanatoriums in terms of the prices it charged and the benefits it offered. Mont Alto provided more educational programs, entertainment and activities than White Haven. Treatment gradually changed as new medications were tried and surgery was thought to be more useful. The medical staff developed specific criteria to decide when to operate. Factors included the age of patients, the stage of the disease, the effectiveness of drugs combating the illness, patients' breathing capacity and complications from other diseases. The clinical laboratory provided important information relating to diagnosis and successful surgery. The use of X-rays became more common over time and aided the decision as to whether to operate. With the discovery of the effectiveness of isoniazid, the need for patients to take their medications regularly became increasingly important. Although medications to fight tuberculosis were being developed, Mont Alto continued to emphasize educating patients about tuberculosis as the means to eradicate it. By the 1960s, physicians thought that the public better understood the nature of tuberculosis; early detection with X-rays and tuberculin tests allowed individuals to seek help sooner, thus making patients more willing to confront the disease.[39]

Sanatorio Nacional de Tuberculosos Santa María

The first public sanatorium in Latin America (the Hospital Municipal Doctor Tornú, which was located on the outskirts of Buenos Aires) opened in 1904. In 1910, the Argentine national government purchased the Santa María sanatorium from an entrepreneur and began expanding the institution to provide more space for tuberculosis patients traveling to Córdoba. In 1916, the national government also established the Hospital de Llanura Vicente López y Planes in the province of Buenos Aires. Argentine physicians like their counterparts in the U.S. had come to believe that regimen, not climate, contributed to a cure and that the government ought to build sanatoriums.[40]

In the 1860s, tuberculosis patients in Buenos Aires with modest financial resources made the 24-hour train trip to the hills of Córdoba hoping that good food and fresh air would improve their health. They resided in hotels, boarding houses, private homes and small houses. Residents of small towns (like Cosquín, Cruz de Eje, Capilla de Monte and Santa María Punilla) soon made money boarding the ill. At times, more patients visited towns in the province of Córdoba than could be accommodated, which posed dangers to public health. Thus, the provincial government appointed a medical director and sought to regulate the establishments that were feeding and caring for the sick. Eventually, the government concluded that proper precautions were being taken, and that tuberculosis patients were not spreading the disease. However, visitors feared that hotels, which accommodated both tubercular patients and healthy visitors, were not taking the necessary steps to prevent the spread of tuberculosis. By the early twentieth century, the Argentine national government and the Buenos Aires municipality recognized that Córdoba's provincial hotels could not adequately care for the ill. The national government, therefore, helped to finance the Sanatorio Nacional de Tuberculosos Santa María, which opened in June 1900. This private sanatorium, located near the town of Cosquin, could accommodate 200 patients.[41]

School teachers, members of the military and public employees who sought admission to Santa María were given priority. Santa María accommodated 440 patients by 1915 and 1000 by 1917. Although the sanatorium sought primarily to serve patients in the early stages of tuberculosis, many patients arrived in poor health and soon died. In 1916, twenty-five percent of the patients died within thirty days of admission; an additional fifteen percent within ninety days. From 1912 until 1917, thirty-three percent of the patients died before they had been at the sanatorium for three months. Clearly, many patients with advanced cases were not healed by coming to Córdoba.[42]

Santa María's pavilions accommodated patients, the facility's staff, a laboratory, workshops, a dairy, a kitchen, a laundry and a garage. Patient pavilions of several floors each were divided into six bedrooms. All the rooms had wide galleries for sunning; shared bathrooms were at the end of each floor with a dining room on the first floor. Some patients paid all their expenses, while the government subsidized others. Santa María offered beds to members of groups that supported it. For example, the Liga Israelita Argentina Contra Tuberculosis paid a fee to Santa María; in return, the sanatorium agreed to accept annually thirty Jewish patients. Although additional sanatoriums opened in Argentina, they had too few beds to accommodate all who sought entry.[43]

Medical staff at Santa María imposed a strict regimen. Patients were to wash, brush their teeth, make their beds and dress before breakfast. Leisure activities available to patients included reading, writing, playing dominos or cards, embroidering and listening to music. Music was, however, prohibited if it bothered other patients, and discussion of politics and religion was forbidden. Although dining tables were segregated by sexes, residents ate in a common dining room. Patients were not to smoke, drink alcoholic beverages or spit on the ground. Doors and windows were to remain open unless a doctor ordered otherwise. No one was to leave the sanatorium without permission. Patients who violated the rules faced various penalties, including dismissal from the facility.[44]

As was true of Mont Alto, tuberculosis was uppermost in the minds of Santa María patients. The ill might not completely understand how tuberculosis spread, but they took care to cover their mouths when coughing and to refrain from physical contact with visitors. Information gathered from other tuberculosis patients led some individuals to reject treatments that seemed ineffective and instead to request others that seemed more promising. Patient involvement in treatment is illustrated by the case of a young man who first rejected the pneumothorax treatment but subsequently came to accept it. He was eventually cured. Surgery, including the pneumothorax treatment, was performed at Santa María. Nevertheless, remedies were on the whole simpler and more economical; patients ingested various medicines and were encouraged to sit in the sun and to consume large quantities of milk and eggs.[45]

Patients were also taught new skills, to enable them to earn a living when they were cured. Thus, the sanatorium taught patients to become printers, bookbinders and basket weavers. The institute also published a short-lived monthly literary magazine, *Reflexiones*, which focused on art, science and literature, issues related to tuberculosis and life within the sanatoriums. The magazine included short stories and poems written by patients, as well as educational articles about personal hygiene and treatment options.[46]

Sanatorium Protests

In contrast to Pennsylvania sanatoriums residents (who complained verbally or through *Spunk*), patients in Argentine public sanatoriums demonstrated and utilized political pressure to affect the quality of food and care. Nevertheless, most protests at Santa María and Hospital Tornú were individual complaints about regimen, food and medical treatment. Santa María patients first expressed dissatisfactions to physicians in the pavilions in which they resided. If that effort failed to produce change, complaints went to the hospital director. When all else proved unsuccessful, patients and their families demonstrated publicly and lobbied government officials and the national congress.[47]

La Vanguardia—the most influential socialist publication in Argentina—investigated conditions at public sanatoriums. As early as 1912, *La Vanguardia* pointed out that the state paid 8,000 pesos per month per patient at Santa María, but that the best meal available was boiled meat stew. The newspaper also noted that patients were not receiving proper food and that they had to pay for eggs or milk. Only the most seriously ill were receiving rations of one liter of milk and two eggs per day. In that year, the sanatorium's medical staff was limited to the medical director, one intern and several nurses. According to the newspaper, Santa María's problems stemmed from the fact that the government bought the sanatorium from an entrepreneur. The sanatorium's failings—lack of compassion for tuberculosis victims and poor medical care given them—were blamed on the government, which was thought to have focused primarily on aiding the entrepreneur who sold it.[48] *La Vanguardia's* concluded that Santa María was poorly designed and too large to be run efficiently—a view that was shared by many Argentine tuberculosis experts.[49]

Despite the controversy over Santa María, the first major collective patient protests occurred in Buenos Aires's Hospital Tornú. In 1914, the hospital expelled a patient for complaining to the ward physician about the poor quality and scarcity of food. Four years later, patients again contended that the food was inedible, and that the hospital's Sisters of Charity paid more attention to religious instruction than to medical care. A ward physician asserted that a political disagreement lay behind this charge; the real issue was that patients wanted the hospital to hire secular nurses rather than nurses from a religious order. About fifty patients at the hospital signed a statement expressing their appreciation for the efforts of the ward physician to deal with their concerns; nevertheless, they rejected his assertion that the facility had no problems.[50]

Major demonstrations against the poor quality of food and care erupted at Santa María in December 1919. Family members reported that they had to send relatives food so that they would not go hungry. Patients described a lunch menu consisting of watery soup, stale bread, farina full of dirt and weevils without salt and re-boiled meat; dinner consisted of another watery soup with a small piece of raw cabbage, parboiled beans too hard to chew and a bad stew. The administration punished patients who complained of poor food quality: their rations were cut, and they were given nothing but two eggs and some milk. Because their dissatisfactions were not addressed, patients sent a memorandum to the Minister of Exterior Relations and Culture, the government department that administered public hospitals and sanatoriums. An inquiry was ordered.

According to *La Vanguardia*, the sanatorium management (which worried that a hunger strike might be launched on 25 December) replaced the night watchman with a security force consisting of armed men from Córdoba. The protesters did not view themselves as threatening; instead, they sought only to improve the quality of food and treatment, so as to avoid deaths resulting from the administration's indifference and incompetence. Patients also feared that complaints would result in beatings and expulsions. When patients sent a telegram to the executive committee of the Socialist Party, requesting an investigation, the police arrested the five leaders of the protests and sequestered them. The sanatorium's interim director then met with patients; he was persuaded that their complaints were justified and indicated that he favored radically changing sanatorium policies. Nevertheless, he did not free the leaders. Guards kept the five leaders incommunicado for a week until a new director (Dr. Fernando Gorriti) arrived and freed them. The replacement of the sanatorium director suggests that the newspaper critique of the sanatorium had some credibility.[51]

Although there was a new director, the patients did not see any significant improvements. They complained that they were given too little to eat and that what they were given was indigestible. On one occasion, 100 of 170 patients in a particular ward had upset stomachs. In addition, too many employees were incompetent and poorly trained. Furthermore, one patient was raped. In 1920, the family of a female patient who was expelled held the institution responsible for her poor treatment and pregnancy. The victim was brutally beaten for reporting the rape, and the Sister Superior responsible for the ward denied the abuse.[52] In May 1920, 259 of the 262 patients in the protesting wards sent to Doctor Borda of the Ministry of Exterior Relations and Culture a signed memorandum listing their complaints about Dr. Gorriti (the new director). A day later, the ministry began to investigate. Patients pointed out that they were not revolutionaries but merely wanted digestible food and fair treatment by the nuns and physicians. They denied charges that they were acting at the instigation of Dr. Antonio Cetrángolo, a physician who spent his life working in tuberculosis hospitals, clinics and sanatoriums in Argentina. Their denial is plausible since no protests occurred in the ward directed by Dr. Cetrángolo.[53]

The *La Vanguardia* reporter interviewed several patients who testified to the inadequate care, limited activities, the shortage of food and its poor quality, and the arbitrary expulsions of patients who complained. For example, one of the leaders who signed the memorandum (Lola Denis) was confined in a small-room and provided with only part of her required milk ration; her bedding was not changed in eight days, and the nuns treated her poorly (because she did not want to go to Mass). She was eventually expelled and returned to her family in Buenos Aires. Another patient, Señorita Virginia Garcia, who also signed the manifesto, reported that patients had to bribe the nuns to get food; because she could not afford to do so, she was seldom given milk. When she complained to a physician, he told her that she was free to leave the sanatorium. The library also had been closed for almost six months and there were few activities. The ministry's investigation found that two nurses (who were paid only sixty pesos a month for ten hours per day with leave for only one day a month) were expected to care for 150 patients.[54]

In January 1922, patients again complained about inadequate food and lack of medicine. They also noted that there were only four doctors to care for a thousand invalids, and that patients themselves had to pay for disinfectants and that the administration had not paid sanatorium employees in six months. In March, the protests took on a political dimension, when four patients, four employees and a doctor attended the inaugural meeting of the Radical Civic Union Party (UCR) Committee of Cosquín. Seventy to eighty patients and some sanatorium employees followed up by attending another political meeting in Molinari with sanatorium employees. As conditions worsened, patient representatives sent a telegram on 5 April to Honorio Pueyrredón, Minister of Exterior Relations and Culture in Buenos Aires, restating their complaints.[55]

In October, employees of the national hospitals and asylums (including Santa María) declared a strike. The employees and the director at Santa María disagreed over salaries and work requirements. Córdoba university students declared their solidarity with the strikers and supported sanatorium patient and employee grievances. Patient political influence in the province had increased; for the first time, patients could vote in the province and influence local election. However, only a minority of employees—fifty-nine individuals went out on strike. The strike resulted in no violence and did not interrupt the work of the sanatorium. Nevertheless, the sanatorium's director called for a security squadron from Córdoba to suppress the strike. He accused the striking employees of contributing to disorder within the sanatorium and encouraging patient complaints. Patients supported the strike, even though they acknowledged that their food had improved and admitted that the government had increased financial support for their care. Patients argued that the food was still too expensive and unhealthy—with too many servings of rice without vegetables.[56]

Conflict emerged again in Santa María in 1924, when some patients were playing soccer with a rag ball. Members of the federal police force ordered them to abandon the game and return to their rooms. In the afternoon, when the patients were again playing soccer, policemen armed with colt revolvers challenged the soccer players. This time a soccer player confronted the police: a lieutenant responded by forcing the patient to the ground and began hitting him. A friend of this patient struck the lieutenant with a piece of wood, wounding him. When a third patient protested, the lieutenant imprisoned all three patients in the Cosquín police station. When patients learned of the imprisonment, approximately 250 of them marched solemnly and silently in the direction of the sanatorium exit. The federal police reinforced with soldiers panicked and raised their revolvers and prepared to fire. Fortunately, at that moment the sanatorium director arrived and ordered the guards to put down their arms. Because of the hostile attitude of the police, patients suggested that the sanatorium director fund quality food rather than pay for police protection.[57]

Dr. Cetrángolo, who had thirty years of experience working in tuberculosis institutions, noted that complaints about bad food were common everywhere he worked. He believed that many of the complaints came from individuals who had tuberculosis of the intestines or larynx rather than of the lungs; these patients found eating painful. Cetrángolo advocated placing only six to eight patients in a room rather than placing them in large wards. He further noted that family members tended not to understand how difficult it was to cure tuberculosis. Because personnel failed to explain this, families concluded that the physicians were not providing the necessary medicine and care. In addition, Cetrángolo believed that medical professionals failed to take patient protests seriously, assuming they were never justified. Protests would be reduced, he believed, if patients were given opportunity to engage in a variety of activities, and if supportive friends and families understood that treating tuberculosis is challenging.[58]

To Dr. Cetrángolo's analysis should be added several other issues. Santa María residents (unlike Mont Alto patients) had no magazine in which to express their dissatisfactions, so instead, they turned to group protests and to airing their frustrations in the public press. Wards that offered their patients planned activities and were staffed by concerned physicians were less likely to see patient protests. Furthermore, there was a tradition of successful strikes and work stoppages in Buenos Aires. For example, workers in Buenos Aires bakeries protested against unhygienic conditions in which they worked.[59] Thus, it is not surprising that Santa María also saw strikes and political protests against the sanatorium administrators (who were often inadequately trained, having benefited from political patronage). Particularly in the 1920s and 1930s, many patients thought that they were abused by arbitrary authority in Santa María, which to them seemed more like their jail than their home. The administration's disdain for its patients, suggested by the use of a federal police force, aggravated patient tensions. Santa María administrators in the 1920s were xenophobic; they thought that protest leaders were foreigners, revolutionaries, anarchists and socialists. The authorities punished protesters by prohibiting them from writing letters, confining them to their rooms and denying them library privileges. At times, administrators even used corporal punishment.

Four factors account for group protests at Santa María from the 1920s to the 1940s: the incompetence of the administrators, the large number of patients in the sanatorium, the administration and patient politicization of the institution, and treatment policies that emphasized disciplining patients more than providing them with fresh air, a healthy diet and rest. Yet, in spite of the validity of the protesters' complaints, patient efforts to improve the quality of life at Argentine public sanatoriums were mostly ineffective; trouble makers could be sent to other hospitals and sanatoriums or expelled. Physicians who were committed to improving the treatment of tuberculosis and obtained international recognition for the high standards of Argentine institutions did more to improve patient care than protestors. Conditions did improve by the 1940s.

Collective patient protests in sanatoriums were relatively rare and occurred between 1912 and 1924 when the government underfunded its sanatoriums. Most protests were confined to a few wards, and patients were usually satisfied. One patient, Armando Droz arrived at Santa María in 1924, when he was 19 years old. He expected to die soon but lived past age 96. He spent thirty-six years in the sanatorium working in the machine shop, repairing automobiles and apparatuses used in the clinic, including the pneumothorax machine. Reminiscing in 2000, he fondly remembered the pavilions, the doctors and the countryside. He recalled that he enjoyed playing soccer and working in the machine shop and got along well with doctors (who became his friends). Living in one of the happier wards, he concluded that "we were one family, a great family."[60]

Hospital Sanatorio de Llanura Vicente López y Planes

In addition to the Sanatorio Nacional de Tuberculosos Santa María in the province of Córdoba and the Sanatorium and Municipal Hospital

Doctor Tornú in central Buenos Aires, the Porteño tubercular had another government-supported option. In 1916, the Ministry of Exterior Relations and Culture inaugurated the Hospital Sanatorio de Llanura Vicente López y Planes in the town of General Rodriguez, fifty miles from Buenos Aires. The complex was located-twelve blocks from the railroad station in an 82-hectare park. It was funded by private contributions and the national government, and administered by the Sociedad de Beneficencia. The main building offered 218 beds for poor tubercular women and children. In 1921, the Sociedad dedicated a two-story tubercular maternity pavilion, which was paid for by a generous private donation. By then the complex also included a house for the director, an electric plant, a septic system, laundry facilities and vegetable gardens. In spite of expansion, the number of beds still did not meet the demand. In 1922, the sanatorium had to turn away sick patients, which resulted in complaints in national newspapers.[61]

By 1924, the sanatorium had 803 beds for adult patients and a 304-bed children's section that was privately funded. Two years later, the institution inaugurated a 16-bed section for those who could pay for their room and board. Demands for space in the facility still exceed the supply, so in 1934, a wealthy patron funded construction of two new pavilions to provide a library and to accommodate seventy-two patients. In 1935, another private donor provided a gift for the construction of a chapel and a pavilion for the Catholic Order of Sisters that administered to the ill.[62] The Sociedad de Beneficencia determined the salaries of all personnel and chose the manager who administered the sanatorium. The director was responsible for assigning doctors to various positions, resolving patient and personnel problems, deciding on admissions and departures, assuring appropriate hygiene, reviewing reports on patients and preparing an annual report. The sanatorium purchased an X-ray machine in 1927 and added odontological services in 1928. In 1929, it ordered a modern operating table from Paris.[63]

Initially, the Hospital Sanatorio de Llanura Vicente López y Planes was constructed to care for poor but curable tubercular women and children between the ages three and thirteen. But since space was needed for tubercular men, the sanatorium soon accepted adult males as well. When it became apparent that constructing cottages for those who could pay would help sustain the facility, the sanatorium was opened to the middle class. Private patients agreed to pay for their medical treatment and room and board one month in advance. Although by the 1940s, convalescents were asked to pay for part of their medical costs, the government and the Sociedad de Beneficencia still paid for the room and board of destitute patients. The facility emphasized serving patients whose tuberculosis was in the early stages. Although patients at advanced stages were accepted if they could not be accommodated elsewhere, they were to be transferred to Hospitals Tornú, Muñiz or Rivadavia in Buenos Aires as soon as space became available.[64]

Most patients were well enough to dress themselves, make their beds and attend meals in the dining room; they received traditional sanatorium treatment. On entering the institution, patients were given a rigorous medical exam. They were required to take a warm bath, and their clothes had to be washed and disinfected. Patients were required to sleep with all the doors and windows open. Nurses took patient temperatures every morning, and physicians saw those whose temperature exceeded thirty-seven degrees centigrade. Families could visit patients two afternoons a week.[65]

Life at Vicente López y Planes was similar to that at other sanatoriums. Patients received treatment, rested in lounge chairs, and enjoyed leisure activities such as reading, writing, playing games and listening to music. Patients were not allowed to leave the establishment without permission. Violating the rules led to punishment, including confinement in bed or expulsion from the establishment. Nuns cared for the bedridden, were present when patients were visited by physicians, made sure that the ill received appropriate medications and notified physicians of special patient needs. As in other sanatoriums, mortality remained high. Between May 1916 and 31 December 1921, thirty-four or 18.7 percent of the men and seventy-one or 23.5 percent of the 302 women died.[66]

Vicente López y Planes utilized current treatments. Alicia Kenny, a 19-year-old Argentine, arrived at the hospital in 1947 with a cough. She was sweating, had pain in her shoulder and had lost weight. Physicians soon began pneumothorax therapy, which proved ineffective. In the previous year, streptomycin was proven to be an effective cure for tuberculosis. As soon as it became available in Argentina, the hospital administered thirty grams of streptomycin (one gram a day). Alicia's family paid for two-thirds of the drug, while the Sociedad de Beneficencia paid for the remaining third. Thirty more grams were administered to complete the treatment. Three radiographs showed the clearing of the lungs, which demonstrated the effectiveness of streptomycin. Unfortunately, the drug was expensive. Olga del Carmen Villarreal de Perez, a 23-year-old married woman (the mother of five children), began treatment soon after Alicia Kenny. Her husband wrote to the hospital in 1948, noting that he had already paid for forty grams of streptomycin (and that the Sociedad de Beneficencia had paid for another five), but that he could not afford the additional fifteen grams to continue the treatment. He was working extra hours at night to provide for his five children. The Eva Durate de Perón Foundation eventually provided the fifteen extra grams to complete Olga's cure.[67]

Comparisons of Sanatoriums in Argentina and Pennsylvania

Both Argentina and Pennsylvania were part of a worldwide movement to construct public sanatoriums. Private sanatoriums, operating as small businesses in large houses or small hotels, developed before state institutions. By 1945, Vicente López y Planes, Santa María and Mont Alto each had more than a thousand patients. But in spite of sanatorium expansion, there were never enough beds for the tubercular in sanatoriums and private establishments in either Argentina or Pennsylvania. As late as 1935, the Sociedad de Beneficencia observed that there were 200,000 people with tuberculosis in Argentina but only 6,000 beds for them in public institutions—one bed for every thirty-three patients. In the U.S., in 1925, there were 673,338 beds for a tuberculosis population of over twelve million—one bed for every eighteen patients. Although these are only estimates, it appears that more beds were available for Philadelphia patients than for Porteño ones.[68] Eventually, the number of beds in U.S. private and public sanatoriums surpassed the available beds in both Europe and Argentina as the private entrepreneurs invested in U.S. sanatoriums.

From the early twentieth century, the national government operated sanatoriums in Argentina. Soon it provided the working and middle classes better facilities than private hotels. The Argentine national legislature, the Sociedad de Beneficencia, the Anti-Tuberculosis Association and private individuals sought to raise funds to construct more facilities. In contrast, in Pennsylvania, private sanatoriums provided more than half the beds. As long as the Pennsylvania government subsidized private sanatoriums, they flourished, expanding the treatment options available to the middle and upper classes. Lawrence Flick resented the growth of state sanatoriums and sought continued government support for private institutions. (He himself benefited from the success of White Haven.) In contrast, Emilio Coni, in Argentina, emphasized that state financing was needed to deal with tuberculosis and campaigned for state-operated sanatoriums. Once Pennsylvania invested in public institutions, private sanatoriums found it hard to recruit patients. Private sanatoriums gradually went out of business as the number of tuberculosis patients declined.

Sanatoriums in both Argentina and Pennsylvania were remarkably similar because of the international medical consensus on the nature of tuberculosis and how to treat it. Tuberculosis experts agreed that living in fresh air day and night, year in and year out, resting the body and the mind, and eating abundant nutritious food contributed to healing. Sanatorium physicians also performed surgery when needed. Women were more reluctant than men to travel to or reside at sanatoriums, because they did not want to leave their husbands or children. Sanatorium patients were prevented from infecting friends and relations. But since the tubercular chose when to enter and leave sanatoriums, they did not really isolate tuberculosis patients. The sanatoriums also provided patients with treatments that they could follow in their homes with the building of porches or construction of half-tents, eating an improved diet, and using sputum cups.[69]

Sanatoriums in Buenos Aires and Philadelphia provided similar activities for patients. The activities broke the monotony of the daily regimen and helped decrease patient complaints. But the activities failed to meliorate the sadness of separation from family and friends or the stigma associated with tuberculosis. Many who died had not seen family for years and were buried in the sanatorium cemeteries as no one claimed their bodies. Mont Alto was unique, in that the publication of *Spunk* for more than half a century effectively promoted a sense of community among Mont Alto patients. *Spunk* provided an opportunity for sanatorium patients to question physicians and nurses about treatment and whether a stay in a sanatorium really cured patients. And they were right to raise the question: for all but a few, sanatorium treatments extended life by only a couple of years. It is true, though that some individuals' immune systems did "wall off" the bacteria in the lungs, thus forming tubercles that prevented the spread of bacteria and led to "cures." Some patients, even though "cured," rightly feared the return of the disease and preferred to live and work in communities near where they had been treated.

In both Argentina and Pennsylvania, patients complained of poor food, uncaring nurses, incompetent doctors and arbitrary dismissals. Patients were dissatisfied with the strict regimen. It appears that it was hardest to get patients to follow the rules in Argentina than Pennsylvania, so Argentine sanatoriums punished recalcitrant patients more harshly. What distinguished Buenos Aires patients from their counterparts in Pennsylvania was their willingness to lobby the national government and to stage political protests. Since sanatoriums in Argentina were more centrally managed than in Pennsylvania, patients recognized that to improve the system they needed the support of political parties and politicians. Marches, demonstrations and general strikes have been a part of Argentine political history since the late nineteenth century. The lack of medical facilities from which to choose in Argentina may also have encouraged patients and their families to try to change conditions in their current facility, rather than leave to enter another one. In contrast, patients in Pennsylvania complained to the head administrators: when they were dissatisfied, they left, perhaps going to another facility. The sanatorium rule preventing patients from discussing politics was clearly broken in Argentina. The U.S. patients generally seemed to abide by the rule, and instead discussed treatment options and the nature of tuberculosis. However, as the focus shifted from sanatorium care to cure through medications, in both Buenos Aires and Philadelphia the difference between patients' social classes continued to affect the quality of the care that patients received.

Although a stay in a public or private sanatorium in Argentina or Pennsylvania did not ensure a long life, decrease the fear of death or relieve the anguish over the loss of family and friends, it extended the lives of some patients. Often it provided hope of a return to normal life for both the tubercular and their families. Before effective drugs were introduced or the number of sanatorium beds had reached their maximum number for residents of both cities, death rates due to tuberculosis were already declining. By the 1920s, some academic studies indicated that fewer individuals were cured in sanatoriums than in the home. Improved living conditions permitted more tubercular patients to live at home. Although sanatoriums removed some contagious individuals from the community and thus decreased the number of patients spreading tuberculosis germs, sanatoriums were never a major factor in decreasing the tuberculosis mortality rates.[70]

Notes

1 "Carta de un tuberculosos curado en las sierras de Córdoba," *La Lucha Antituberculosa* 5, no. 1 (June 1905): 7–8.

2 Leroy E. Sutcliffe, "Mont Alto Jingles," *Spunk* 9, no. 8 (November 1917): 20–22.

3 For a detailed discussion of Mont Alto and Santa María, see Vera Blinn Reber, "The Sanatorium Age, Pennsylvania and Argentina, 1900–1945," *Pennsylvania History* 73, no. 4 (Autumn 2006): 412–45.

4 Dr. (John H.) Scrivener, "Argentine Republic, Sanitary Character of the Mountains of Cordova [sic.] and the Andine Heights," *Medical Times and Gazette* (30 October 1869): 525–26; Enrique P. Aznárez, "Historia de la Climatoterapia de la Tuberculosis en las Sierras de Córdoba," *Segundo Congreso Nacional de Historia de la Medicina Argentina* (Córdoba, 21–24 October 1970): 417–18; Juan F. Cafferata, "Higiene Social: La vulgarización de la nociones científicas en la lucha contra la tuberculosis," *Revista del Circulo Médico Córdoba* 7, no. 1–2 (January/February 1917), 30; Félix Garzón Maceda, *De los Hospitales en Córdoba* desde 1573 hasta 1916, vol. 2 of *La Medicina en Córdoba: apuntes para su historia* (Buenos Aires: Talleres Gráficos Rodríguez Giles, 1916), 726; Antonio Súnico, *La Tuberculosis en la Sierras de Córdoba* (Buenos Aires: A de Martina, 1922), 134–35. For Flick and Coni see The Historical Medical Library of the College of Physicians of Philadelphia (hereafter CPP), Lawrence Francis Flick, collected reprints (hereafter FCR), F. L. Flick, "Home Treatment of Tuberculosis" (February 1901): 2 and Emilio R. Coni, *Higiene Social: Asistencia y previsión social. Buenos Aires caritativo y previsor* (Buenos Aires: Imprenta de Emilio Spinella, Ed., 1918), 432–34.

5 Flurin Condrau, "Beyond the Total Institution: Towards a Reinterpretation of the Tuberculosis Sanatorium," in *Tuberculosis Then and Now: Perspectives on the History of an Infectious Disease,* eds. Florin Condrau and Michael Worboys (Montreal: McGill-Queen's University Press, 2010), 73.

6 CPP, JWP, vol. 10: *European Trips*, 80–81 and CPP, FCR, Lawrence F. Flick, "Short Talks upon Work for Consumptives delivered by the Medical Staff of the White Haven Sanatorium of the Free Hospital for Poor Consumptive of Pennsylvania," on the occasion of the Free Exhibition and Donation Week in Philadelphia November 28 to December 3, 1904.

7 Georgina Feldberg, *Disease and Class: Tuberculosis and the Shaping of Modern North American Society* (New Brunswick: Rutgers University Press, 1955), 52–53, 91–92; Sandra L. Wheeler, "From Hospital to Sanatorium:

Institutional Care of the Tubercular Poor in Hartford, 1900–1910," *Connecticut History* 38, no. 1 (Fall 1997/Spring 1999): 2–3, 6–7.

8 Katherine Ott, *Fevered Lives: Tuberculosis in American Culture since 1870* (Cambridge: Harvard University Press, 1996), 46–47, 150–53; "Sanatorio Municipal Doctor Tornú," *Lucha Antituberculosa* 4, no. 12 (12 May 1905): 531; Anna L. Drake, "Nursing in Tuberculosis," *Listening Post* 5, no. 4 (July–August 1927): 4.

9 CPP, Joseph Walsh (hereafter JWP), vol. 10, *European Trips*, "Tuberculosis Work in Europe," German statistics, 116; comparison with the United States, 19–20. Walsh describes in detail some twenty institutions that he visited in his private papers; for descriptions of German sanatoria, see CPP, JWP, vol. 10: 103–26; for English sanatoria, *ibid.*, 82–83, 86–102; for French sanatoria, *ibid.*, 81–82; for U.S. statistics, see Wheeler, 2 and Sheila M. Rothman, *Living in the Shadow of Death: Tuberculosis and the Social Experience of Illness in American History* (Baltimore: John Hopkins Press, 1995), 198; Michael Teller, *The Tuberculosis Movement: A Public Health Campaign in the Progressive Era* (New York: Greenwood Press, 1988), 82. For a discussion of African-American facilities, see Samuel Kelton Roberts, *infectious fear: Politics, Disease and the Health Effects of Segregation* (Chapel Hill: University of North Carolina, 2009), 174, 192–98. For statistics, see David McBride, *From TB to Aids: Epidemics among Urban Blacks since 1900* (Albany: State University of New York Press, 1991), 86; Table 3:1 for African-American deaths in Philadelphia.

10 S. Adolphus Knopf, *Tuberculosis: A Preventable and Curable Disease* (New York: Moffat, Yard and Company, 1909), 175, 191.

11 Godias J. Drolet, "Tuberculosis Hospitalization," *Spunk* 18, no. 12 (March 1927): 17. Trudeau decided to open a sanatorium in the Adirondacks as early as 1882 but did not receive his first patients until the fall of 1884; see David L. Ellison, *Healing Tuberculosis in the Woods: Medicine and Science at the End of the Nineteenth Century* (Westport: Greenwood Press, 1994), 23, 65, 77, 171, 177, 180; Eileen Simpson, *Orphans: Real and Imaginary* (New York: Weidenfeld & Nicolson, 1987), 82. For primary material on Trudeau, see the CPP, HKP, 1903–1957, Mss. 2/0254-01 Series 3, Trudeau Sanatorium materials, and CPP, Lawrence Francis, Flick Papers (hereafter LFP), *Tuberculosis Letters*, vol. 13, 1901, pt. 2, 19 September 1901 C. H. Thomas to Flick.

12 CPP, Hugh M. Kinghorn (hereafter HKP), Trudeau Sanatorium Materials, Mss. 2/054-01, Series 3, 3–9–36.

13 William C. White, "The Official Responsibility of the State in the Tuberculosis Problem," in *Transactions of the Eleventh Annual Meeting, Seattle, Washington, June 14–16,* ed. The National Association for the Study and Prevention of Tuberculosis (Baltimore: William & Wilkins Company, 1915), 271; Baron H. Lerner, "New York City's tuberculosis Control Efforts: The Historical Limitations of the 'War on Consumption'," *American Journal of Public Health* 83, no. 5 (May 1993): 759.

14 Emily K. Abel, "Taking the Cure to the Poor: Patients' Responses to New York City's Tuberculosis Program 1894 to 1918," *American Journal of Public Health* 87, no. 11 (November 1997): 1812–13; Ellison, 181.

15 "First Day Camp in Philadelphia," *Spunk* 3, no. 9 (December 1911): 12.

16 "Information for the Public," *Spunk* 9, no. 1 (April 1917): 1; Commonwealth of Pennsylvania Department of Health, Division of Tuberculosis Sanatoria, "Information and Rules for Patients," Harrisburg, [1914]:4–5.

17 CPP, LFP, Miscellaneous, 170, "The Pennsylvania Society for the Prevention of Tuberculosis, Report for the Year Ending April 13, 1898," p. 6. CPP,

LFR, Henry R. M. Landis, "History of Sanatorium Treatment," *Short Talks upon Work for Consumptives*, November 28 to December 3, 1904, 6.

18 CPP, LCR, Lawrence Francis Flick, "A Year's Work at the White Haven Sanatorium of the Free Hospital for Poor Consumptives," *Philadelphia Medical Journal* (8 November 1902), 7; CP, LFP, Tuberculosis Letters, vol. 14, pt. 3, Lawrence Flick to John T. Morris, 18 November 1901; CPP, LFP, Tuberculosis Letters, vol. 33, pt. 4 (1905) Maldwin to Flick, 2 May 1905; CPP, JWP, vol. 1, White Haven Sanatorium, Lawrence Flick to doctors, 28 March 1905; CPP, JWP, vol. 8 Flick to Walsh, 23 December 1918; CPP, JWP, vol. 3, *Letters and Programmes of the National Association for the Study and Prevention of Tuberculosis*, no. 231 (8 May 1907), 1; CPP, FCR, Lawrence Francis Flick, "Work for Patients as an Economic Factor," *Transactions Of the Fifth National Association for the Study and Prevention of Tuberculosis* (London 1909), 4; J. Woodrow Savacool, "Philadelphia and the White Plague," *Transactions and Studies of the College of Physicians*, ser. 5, 8, no. 3 (1986): 147–81.

19 CPP, LFP, Tuberculosis Letters, vol. 14, pt. 3, Flick to William B. Miller, 2 October 1901; CPP, FCR, Flick, "A Year's Work," *Philadelphia Medical Journal* 8 (November 1902): 5–8; CPP, LFP, Tuberculosis Letters, see correspondence for the diversity of requests to enter White Haven, vol. 19, 1903, pt. 2; CPP, LFP, Tuberculosis Letters, vol. 28, 1904, pt. 6 Columbus Ohio, 27 September 1904 C.G. Probst to Flick; CPP, LFP, vol. 50, Hyman Schutz to Flick, 24 June 1908.

20 CPP, HKP Trudeau Sanatorium material, 1903–1957, Mss. 2/0254-01, Series 3, form 5/28/31. For example, E. Klappenbach, "Tuberculosis pulmonar: Inyecciones de Gayacol-iodoformado," *Anales del Circulo Médico Argentino* 15, no. 5 (1892): 231–32; Ellison, 19, 53.

21 CPP, HKP, 1903–1957; Michael E. Teller, *The Tuberculosis Movement: A Public Health Campaign in the Progressive Era* (New York: Greenwood Press, 1988), 25–26; Feldberg, 91–94; Ott, 136. CPP, LFR, Lawrence Francis Flick, "A Year's Work," 9–13; Flick, "Short Talks on Work for Consumptives," 11–12; CPP, LFP, vol. 16, Walter Wood to Flick, 14 January 1908; CPP, JWP, vol. 6 (1925–1936), "The Advantage of Milk," 25 September 1934.

22 CPP, FCR, William H. Hutt, "First Work in America for the Relief of Tuberculosis," 8; CPP, LFP, Tuberculosis Letters, Miscellaneous no. 45; CPP, LFP, Tuberculosis Letters, vol. 13, 1901, pt. 2, 21 September 1901, George Herman Thomas to Flick; Barbara Bates, *Bargaining for Life: A Social History of Tuberculosis, 1876–1938* (Philadelphia: University of Pennsylvania Press, 1992), 56, 69–74. CPP, JWP, vol. 9 (11 March 1919), Secretary to Charles Jacob.

23 CPP, FCR, Lawrence Francis Flick, "The Tuberculosis Situation in Pennsylvania in the Year 1909: Discussion of Mr. J. Byron Deacon's Paper before the Medical Society of the State of Pennsylvania at Pittsburgh, Pa. October 5, 1910 with a preface telling why it was not published in the Pennsylvania Medical Journal," 10–14; Savacool, 155.

24 "South Mountain Restoration Center: and there was Light," unpublished pamphlet on the center, [1968], 1; Chester County Historical Society (hereafter CCHS), Joseph Trimbel Rothrock Collection (hereafter JRC), Box 5, folder 4, June-September, 1904; CCHS, JRC, Box 6, folder 3, autobiographical statement, West Chester, Pa., December 1912; CCHS, JRC, Box 7, folder 27, lectures and speeches read before club in West Chester; R. H McCutcheon; "Mont Alto Sanatorium: Past and Present," *The Listening Post* 1, no. 2 (January 1923): 6–7; R.H. McCutcheon, "Mont Alto," *Pennsylvania's Health* 10, no. 1 (January-February 1932): 66–67.

25 "Information for the Public," 1; William G. Turnbull, "Tuberculosis Sanatoria," *The Listening Post* 3, no. 24–26 (March–May 1925): 27; William G. Turnbull, "County Tuberculosis Needs," *The Listening Post* 4, no. 37 (April 1926): 4; Mary Brady Caverly, "From Cabin to Classic Revival," unpublished paper, 17 October 1994, p. 1; "Battling for Health at Mont Alto," *Pennsylvania Health Bulletin* 39 (October 1912): 1.

26 Fred C. Johnson, "Subdivision of Tuberculosis Sanatoria. Pennsylvania State Sanatorium for Tuberculosis No. 1 Mont Alto," *Eleventh Annual Report of the Commissioner of Health for the Commonwealth of Pennsylvania, 1916* (Harrisburg: J. L. L. Kuhn Printer to the Commonwealth, 1920), 895, 1912–1923. Luigi T. Mastrangelo, "A Patient's View," *Spunk* 1, no. 3 (June 1909): 10.

27 "Battling for Health," 1–3; Knopf, *Tuberculosis: A Preventable and Curable Disease*, 191–92; "South Mountain Restoration Center," 1; Caverly, 4–5; T. W. Burger, "South Mountain's Sickened City," *Public Opinion* 11 December 2015.

28 Quote is from Samuel A. Silk, "Why Do We Give Tuberculin," *Spunk* 6, no. 10 (January 1915): 8–12; interview with Marie Matteucci of Shippensburg, Pennsylvania, 18 October 2004; Johnson, 895.

29 "Battling for Health," 3–6; Karl Schaffle, "The State Tuberculosis Dispensary an Asset to the Municipality, *Spunk* 9, no. 7 (October 1917): 9–10; Commonwealth, "Information and Rules," 8–13; Nevin Werst, "Personal Hygiene of Tubercular Patients," *Spunk* 2, no. 5 (August 1910): 21–22; Historical Society of Pennsylvania (hereafter HSP), Samuel Gibson Dixon, *Papers 1884–1953*, Box 8, "Cases of Tuberculosis Treated by the Biological Method at the Pennsylvania South Mountain Sanatorium for Tuberculosis, Mont Alto, Pa," Read before the Fifth Pan American Medical Congress, Guatemala City, Guatemala, August 5–10, 1908; William G. Turnbull, "Heliotherapy," *The Listening Post* 4, no. 41 (November-December 1926): 6–9.

30 "Battling for Health," 3–6; Caverly, 2–4; "South Mountain Restoration Center," 1–2; "One Lung Minstrel Company," *Spunk* 6, no. 6 (August 1914): 32–33; "Mont Alto Notes," *Spunk* 9, no. 6 (September 1917): 32–33; *Spunk* 18, no. 1 (April 1916): 30–32; Johnson, 899–900; Harris Aubel, "The Mont Alto Business School," *Spunk* 4, no. 12 (July 1920): 10; "Chickens," *Spunk* 14, no. 1 (April 1922): 14.

31 Because many of Mont Alto's records were destroyed in Hurricane Agnes in 1972, *Spunk* is the major primary source and provides the longest record for Mont Alto. See the following issues of *Spunk*: Joseph A. Stockler, "The Contagiousness of Tuberculosis," 6, no. 6 (September 1914): 12–14; quote on Thanksgiving 6, no. 9 (December 1914): 44–45; 6, no. 9 (December 1914), entire issue on Christmas; 18, no. 5 (August 1926): 26–27; "Christmas at Mont Alto," 6, no. 19 (January 1915): 22–23; 18, no. 10 (January 1927): 31–33; "Hospital Chat," 9, no. 7 (October 1917): 40–42. 6, no. 12 (September 1920) provides a good sample of the types of material included.

32 The poem is by J. H. Wilcox, "The Spunk Cure," *Spunk* 1, no. 3 (June 1909): 12; Luigi T. Mastrangelo, 10.

33 "The Question Box," *Spunk* 13, no. 5 (November 1921): 41; 13, no. 6 (December 1921): 53; 13, no. 7 (January 1922): 50.

34 Leroy E. Sutcliffe, 20–22; Stephanie Kirby, "Sputum and the Scent of Wallflowers: Nursing in Tuberculosis Sanatoria, 1920–1970," *Social History of Medicine* 23, no. 3 (December 2010): 613–18; CPP,LFP, White Haven 28 June 1908, Alexander Armstrong, Superintendent White Haven to Flick, vol. 50 (June/July 1909); CPP, LFP, Johnstown, Pa., 22 June 1908, Mary Klunk to Flick, (June/July 1909); CPP, LFP, White Haven 8 August 1909, Armstrong to Flick, vol. 51 (August 1908).

35 Albert P. Francine, "Results on January 1, 1913 in Philadelphia Patients Discharged from Mont Alto in 1909," *Transactions of the National Association for the Study and Prevention of Tuberculosis, Ninth Annual Meeting, Washington D.C.*, May 8–9, 1913 (Philadelphia; William. F. Fell, 1913), 285; Schaffle, 12; Marc Arnold, *Disease, Class and Social Change: Tuberculosis in Folkestone and Sandgate, 1880–1930* (Newcastle upon Tyne: Cambridge Scholars Publishing, 2012), 119 using the *Lancet* estimates that a pulmonary tuberculosis patient's life expectancy increased from around 18 months in 1850s to 3–5 years in the 1890s and 1900s.

36 Barron H. Lerner, *Contagion and Confinement: Controlling Tuberculosis along the Skid Road* (Baltimore: John Hopkins University Press, 1998), 65; "Problems of Irregular Discharge: Sanatorium Patients are Urged to Consider the High Cost of Leaving against Medical Advice," *Spunk* 52, no. 9 (December 1960): 9–10.

37 "How Must You Live after You Are Apparently Well Again so as to Remain Well," *Spunk* 9, no. 3 (June 1917): 20–22; "After the Sanatorium Then What?" *Spunk* 9, no. 11 (February 1918), 34–35; "Let's Get Acquainted," *Spunk*, 18, no. 8 (November 1926): 20; *Spunk* 21, no. 8 (November 1929): 6–19.

38 Caverly, 2–4, 8–9; "South Mountain Restoration Center," 1–2; "Hospital Notes: New Arrivals," *Spunk* 52, no. 2 (May 1960): 18; 54, no. 7 (October 1962): 18.

39 W.H. Gentry, "The Laboratory and the Eternal Verities of Tuberculosis," *Spunk* 52, no. 1 (April 1960): 9–13; W. Duane Jones, "When Surgery Is Recommended," *Spunk* 54, no. 3 (June 1962): 9–12; James E. Perkins, "Isoniazid Effective TB Preventive," *Spunk* 54, no. 3 (June 1962): 13–15; Aaron D. Chaves, "Motivating Patients to Take Drugs," *Spunk* 54, no. 7 (October 1962): 10–12; Sol S. Lifson, "Misunderstanding about TB: To Eradicate TB- These Understandings Must Be Eliminated," *Spunk* 54, no. 10 (January 1963): 9–12.

40 Aznárez, "Historia de la climatoterapia"; Carlos G. Malbrán and Ezequiel Castilla, "Profilaxia de la tuberculosis en las sierras de Cosquín, Córdoba," *Anales del Departmento Nacional de Higiene* 12, no. 8 (August 1905): 391; Emilio R. Coni, "The Antituberculous Campaign in Latin America," *Medical Record* (2 May 1903): 690–91; Garzón Maceda, 727–29. Archivo Histórico de la Provincial de Córdoba (hereafter AHC), Gobierno, 1894, vol. 6, (10 February 1894): 170–72; José D. González, "Climatología; a las Sierras Cordobesas: y el Proyectado Sanatorio para tuberculosis," *La Semana Médica* 1, no. 30 (9 August 1984): 225–26. Emilio R. Coni, "La Lucha antituberculosa en la República Argentina," *La Lucha Antituberculosa* 5, nos. 4–8 (1905): 164–65; Coni, *Higiene Social*, 432–35; "Sanatorio Municipal Doctor Tornú," 531–35.

41 José Mazzini, "Profilaxis de la Tuberculosis en las sierras de Córdoba," *Actas y Trabajos, vol. 3 of Segunda Conferencia Nacional de Profilaxis Antituberculosa, Rosario 6-8 de Septiembre 1919* (Rosario de Santa Fé: Talleres de la Biblioteca Argentina, 1920), 155–56.

42 Garzón Maceda, 730–31; José Antonio Pérez, "La Tisioneumonología Argentina en los ultimos cincuenta años," *Revista Argentina de Tuberculosis, Enfermedades Pulmonares y Salud Pública* 42, nos. 1–4 (1981): 95–105; Antonio Cetrángolo, "Algunas breve consideraciones sobre la climatoterapia de la tuberculosis en nuestro país," *La Semana Médica* 24, no. 8 (22 February 1917): 242–43; Súnico, 548.

43 Antonio Cetrángolo, *Treinta años cuidando tuberculosos* (Buenos Aires, 1944), 25; José Antonio Pérez, "Gumersindo Sayago y el desarrollo de la tisiologia Argentina," in *Segundo Congreso Nacional de Historia de la*

Medicina Argentina, Córdoba 21 al 24, ed. Academia Nacional de Medicina, Universidad Nacional de Córdoba, Círculo Médico de Córdoba (Córdoba, Argentina: *La Semana Médica*, 1970), 44–53. Garzón Maceda, 730–34; Victor Mirelman, *Jewish Buenos Aires, 1890–1930: In Search of Identity* (Detroit: Wayne State University Press, 1990), 190; Cetrángolo, *Treinta años cuidando,* 24.

44 Garzón Maceda, 736–40; Cetrángolo, *Treinta años cuidando*, 176, 625–26.

45 Cetrángolo, *Treinta años cuidando*, 45–46, 101, 155; Sanatorio Nacional de Tuberculosos Santa María. Santa María Punilla (hereafter SNSM), Hospital Colonia, "Santa María," *Sanatorio Nacional de Tuberculosos Santa María, contabilidad de especies, laboratorio, utiles*, 1935.

46 Cetrángolo, *Treinta años cuidando*, 41–46, 67–69, 75–76, 155; Diego Armus, *The Ailing City: Health, Tuberculosis and Culture in Buenos Aires, 1870-1950* (Durham: Duke University Press, 2011), 75–77.

47 Diego Armus, "Historias de enfermos tuberculosos que protestan Argentina, 1920-1940," in *Avatares de la medicalización en América Latina 1870–1970*, ed. Diego Armus (Buenos Aires: Lugar Editorial, 2005), 68–60. I am particularly indebted to Armus's article for drawing attention to newspaper articles on patient protests.

48 "Nuestra asistencia social," *La Vanguardia* (13 March 1912): 1; Armus, "Historias de enfermos tuberculosos," 68–78.

49 "Teoría y práctica de la historia de Sanatorio Santa María," *La Vanguardia* (8 January 1920): 4; "En el Sanatorio de Tuberculosos de Santa María: Una vista del corresponsal de 'La Vanguardia,'" *La Vanguardia* (16 January 1920): 4.

50 "En El Hospital Tornú: Un Caso Grave," *La Vanguardia* (28 August 1914): 2; "En el hospital Tornú la obra de las enfermeras religiosas," *La Vanguardia* (9 June 1918): 1; "Las denuncias sobre el hospital Tornú," *La Vanguardia* (16 June 1918): 1; "Las denuncias sobre el hospital Tornú: deficiencias del sumario," *La Vanguardia* (17 June 1918): 1; "La denuncias sobre el hospital Tornú," *La Vanguardia* (23 June 1918): 1; "En el hospital Tornú," *La Vanguardia* (11 August 1918): 1.

51 "En el Sanatorio Santa María: Extravagancias del doctor Cabred," *La Vanguardia* (28 December 1919): 1; "El Sanatorio de Santa María: Nuevas denuncias," *La Vanguardia* (29 December 1919): 2; Sanatorio Santa María: La comida de los enfermos-Quejas justificadas," *La Vanguardia* (4 January 1920): 1; "En el Sanatorio de Tuberculosos de Santa María," *La Vanguardia* (16 January 1920): 4.

52 "En el Sanatorio de Tuberculosos de Santa María, 4; Armus, "Historias de enfermos tuberculosos," 75–78.

53 "En el Sanatorio Santa María; La Inmoralidad de un capellán—inercia de la comisión asesora-La comida sigue siendo mala-nombramiento excesivo de empleados," *La Vanguardia* (6 April 1920): 8. "En el Sanatorio de Tuberculosos de Santa María: Una visita del corresponsal de 'La Vanguardia'," *La Vanguardia* (14 June 1920): 5.

54 "En el Sanatorio Santa María; La Inmoralidad," *La Vanguardia* (6 April 1920): 8. "En el Sanatorio de Tuberculosos de Santa María," *La Vanguardia* (14 June 1920): 5

55 "Cartas de las Sierras: Los nuevos conflictos del sanatorio 'Santa María,' Causa de las causas: la cuestión económica—Mal a comida. Gastos exorbitantes—el empirismo administrativo. Seis meses sin pagar a nadie. . . .? La debacle?" *La Vanguardia* (7 February 1922): 2; "En el sanatorio 'Santa María," *La Vanguardia* (12 February 1922); "Denuncia de graves irregularidades en el

sanatorio 'Santa María," *La Vanguardia (*7 April 1922): 2; "En el sanatorio 'Santa María,' Ampliando la denuncia de graves irregularidades," *La Vanguardia* (11 April 1922): 6.

56 "En el sanatorio Santa María: se renuevan, los hechos bochornos de otras épocas," *La Vanguardia* (6 October 1922): 1; "La situación Nacional Santa María: Informe de un telegrama del Centro de estudiantes de medicina," *La Vanguardia* (23 October 1922): 5; "Los sucesos del Sanatorio Santa María," *La Vanguardia* (29 October 1922): 6.

57 "Las últimas incidencias en el sanatorio Santa María: Procedimientos abusivos de la 'Policía interna," *La Vanguardia* (26 July 1924): 4.

58 Cetránglo, *Treinta años cuidando*, 189–98.

59 Armus, *Ailing City*, 121.

60 Based on a questionnaire the author developed and completed by Armando Droz in June 2000 at Santa María Puntilla, Córdoba, Argentina with the help of his daughter Irma Droz.

61 Archivo General de la Nación Argentina (hereafter AGN), Fondos de Sociedad de Beneficencia (hereafter SB), Hospital Vicente López y Planes (hereafter HVLP) legajo 123, 14 December 1921, "Pasado mañana se inaugurará una maternidad en General Rodrígues"; legajo 123, 1 December 1919, "Pabellón: Maternidad"; Legajo 123, Acta de Sociedad, 30 November 1921, "Maternidad Hospital Vicente López y Planes: Inauguración"; Legajo 124, 28 November 1922, "Inconveniencia forma de admisión enfermas."

62 AGN, SB, HVLP, legajo 123, "Dinero receibido por el superior Governor para diferentes construcciones"; legajo 126, November 1927, "Isaac Fernández Blanco"; legajo 129, 12 November 1924, "Acta de Sociedad del dia"; Legajo 129, Buenos Aires 4 September 1934, "Construcción del Pabellón 'Mayora'"; legajo 129, Aprobado en la Asamblea del 19 July 1935, "Reglamento del Hospital de Llanura Vicente López y Planes"; legajo 130, Buenos Aires 21 May 1935, "Construcción de una capilla"; Legajo 131, General Rodríguez 3 June 1937, "Propone ampliar la sección pensionistas"; Legajo 133, exp. 16,526, 16 May 1945, "Pedido de un aparato de Rayos-X para radiografías dentales." The substantial private funding is unusual for a government-run-facility.

63 AGN SB, HVLP, legajo 126, 25 August 1928, "Instalación del servicios Odontológicos"; legajo 126, General Rodríguez, 3 September 1917, "Adquisición de aparatos para el Hospital"; legajo 127, General Rodríguez 31 January 1929, Adquisición mesa Guyot de operaciones"; Legajo 129, aprobado en la Asamblea del 19 July 1935, "Reglamento del Hospital de Llanura Vicente López y Planes," 6–13; legajo 133 exp. 15,396, 13 November 1943, "Adquisición de una mesa."

64 AGN, SB, HVLP, legajo 123, General Rodríguez, 4 March 1918, "Vicente López y Planes"; legajo 124, Buenos Aires 28 November 1922, "Inconveniencias forma de admisión enfermas"; legajo 129, Aprobado en la Asamblea del 19 July 1935, "Reglamento del Hospital de Llanura Vicente López y Planes," 33–34, 40–41, 48; legajo 135, exp. 32,867, 2 June 1948, "Vicente López y Planes."

65 AGA, SB, HVLP, legajo 129, Aprobado en la Asamblea del 19 July 1935, "Reglamento del Hospital de Llanura Vicente López y Planes," 33-40; legajo 124. General Rodríguez 20 October 1922, "Vicente López Planes"; legajo 134, exp. 26606, 27 August 1947, "Vicente López Planes."

66 AGA, SB, HVLP, legajo 129, Aprobado en la Asamblea del 19 July 1935, "Reglamento del Hospital de Llanura Vicente López y Planes," 27–28, 33–37; legajo 124, General Rodríguez 19 October 1922, "Defunciones."

67 Rothman, 247–48; AGA, SB, HVLP, legajo, 124, General Rodríguez 14 February 1948, "Adquisición estreptomicina"; legajo 135, exp. 32,867, 2 June 1948, "Vicente López y Planes."

68 AGA, SB, HVLP), Legajo 124; Lucha Antituberculosa," 25 March 1935; AGN, SB, HVLP, Legajo 123, "Dinero recibido por el superior gobierno para diferentes construcciones," for Argentina. For Philadelphia the author used U.S. population figures for 1925, together with statistics provided by Rothman, 198.

69 Most historians have inadequately dealt with patient attitudes toward treatment. The exceptions are Rothman, 168, 226–245 and Vera Blinn Reber "Misery, Pain and Death: Tuberculosis in Nineteenth Century Buenos Aires," *The Americas* 56, no. 4 (April 2000): 497–528. Even in the early twentieth century tubercular patients who went to hospitals expected to die; by contrast sanatoriums offered hope. Emily K. Abel, *Tuberculosis and the Politics of Exclusion: A History of Public Health and Migration to Los Angeles* (New Brunswick: Rutgers University Press, 2007), 14. Jorge Plaza, *Tratamiento higiénico de la tuberculosis pulmonar*, MD diss., Facultad de Medicina, Universidad de Buenos Aires (Buenos Aires: La Semana Medica, 1912), 39–53, 75–76.

70 Gladys Fernández et al., "Los determinantes sociales de la tuberculosis en la ciudad de Buenos Aires, *Medicina y Sociedad* 73 (May/June, 1984): 64; Frank Macfarlane Burnet and David O. White, *Natural History of Infectious Disease* (Cambridge University Press, 1972), 218; Thomas McKeowan, *The Origin of Human Disease* (London: Basil Blackwell, 1988), 81; Dormandy, 302.

6 Poor and Ill

Children of Buenos Aires and Philadelphia

> Case Study Summary: María P., age fourteen months, became ill 20 November 1899 and was first seen by a physician 4 January 1900. She had developed a light cough, and then cold with a fever. María's mother was very thin with continuous metrorrhagia. During thirteen years of marriage, she had seven children. The first two had died in Rosario, Argentina, of pulmonary tuberculosis... María was born in the country and nursed until eight months; two months before her illness she weighed ten kilos. She was precocious, speaking at ten months like a child of two, and began to walk at eleven months. She had no contagious diseases previously.[1]

> About two years ago I was sent to this hospital [Mont Alto] in order to regain my health. But now I am very thankful because I have regained my health and will soon be ready to go home. I am thankful because my father and mother are living and they advised the best way to get along in this world.[2]

The previous statements provide perspectives on problems facing tubercular children. The physician diagnosing the tuberculosis of María of Buenos Aires considered four factors: the child's illnesses, the mother's wellbeing, sibling health and milk quality. Because a cough and weight loss were common symptoms for many childhood diseases, the doctor needed to consider the family's health history. The physician ruled out unpasteurized milk, since María drank safe milk. The physician initially diagnosed whooping cough. However, since other children in the family had died of tuberculosis and the mother was very thin, the physician considered her to be a carrier. In the second quote, a sixth-grade boy had been asked by the Mont Alto Preventorium in Pennsylvania to express thankfulness for his cure. This young boy justified the two-year separation from his family—a long time for a young person—by emphasizing that his parents cared about his health. These two children, different in age, gender and location, represent the challenges that physicians faced globally in their search to prevent and cure tuberculosis. One child was two, the other entering puberty; one was female, the other was male; one was only beginning treatment, whereas the other had completed two years of care; one lived at home in Buenos Aires, and the other lived in an institution in Pennsylvania. Tubercular children faced unique difficulties: the disruption of their education, separation from parents and siblings, the need to bear discomfort and pain, and death at an early age.

During the twentieth century, parents and public officials came to think that children had needs distinct from adults. In 1904, twenty percent of the inhabitants of Buenos Aires were between ages six and fifteen; in 1910, twenty-seven percent of Philadelphia's population was between ages six and twenty. Both Buenos Aires and Philadelphia public health officials shifted their views: having previously ignored children, who were thought rarely to have tuberculosis, they subsequently sought to protect children from being infected by tubercular adults. This new perspective stemmed from the realization that children died from pulmonary tuberculosis and that unhealthy children who lived were likely to become tubercular adults.

Public health officials focused not on the very ill, but on children who were pre-tubercular. This emphasis was part of a broader social effort of "child-saving," which tried to ensure that children would grow up to be healthy productive citizens. Governments directed many programs at children, such as the following: the regulation of custody, the restriction of child labor, reform of the juvenile justice system, the development of institutional child care, services for poor and abandoned children, expanded educational opportunities, and efforts to decrease infant mortality and infectious disease. Changed attitudes toward children in both Buenos Aires and Philadelphia were reflected in increased financial support for new programs and institutions directed at sick and specifically tubercular children—programs that involved both social action and social control.[3]

Children, Families and Tuberculosis in Buenos Aires

Initially, Buenos Aires physicians overlooked tuberculosis in children. But that neglect ended as mortality statistics supported public concerns about the increasing number of children dying of the disease. Table 6.1 provides mortality data on the number of children in age groups of under 2, 2–9, 10–14 and 15–19. A comparison of the total number of pulmonary deaths for all ages with the generally accepted number of pulmonary deaths for children suggests an undercounting of children's deaths from pulmonary tuberculosis from 2.3 to 6.2 percent. From 1902 to 1911, there are too few reported deaths of boy-babies of Argentine parents and too few registered deaths of girl-babies of foreign parents. Diagnosis of children with tuberculosis was problematic. Children under seven were more likely diagnosed with other types of tuberculosis and

Table 6.1 Pulmonary Tuberculosis Deaths of Minors, Age 0–20 in Buenos Aires, 1900–1911

Year	Under 2				Ages 2–9				Ages 10–14				Ages 15–19				TB Deaths 0–19						Deaths Age 0–19	Deaths Age 20–100	Total Deaths 0–100	0–20 % of Total Deaths	Total of GA TB	0–20% of TB
	Arg		Fng		Arg		Fng		Arg		Fng		Arg		Fng		Arg		Fng		Total						Deaths	
	F	M	F	M	F	M	F	M	F	M	F	M	F	M	F	M	F	M	F	M	F	M						
1900	13	23	4	1	14	13	0	2	12	7	3	1	81	51	12	22	120	94	19	26	139	120	259	1143	1402	18.47	1672	15.49
1901	16	25	0	0	46	37	3	3	33	19	4	5	83	55	26	29	178	136	33	37	211	173	384	1291	1675	22.93	1675	22.93
1902	12	4	0	24	21	1	0	28	33	2	3	16	178	22	18	54	244	29	21	122	265	151	416	1310	1726	24.10	1619	25.69
1903	19	0	0	16	28	0	3	22	37	2	5	14	212	27	28	61	296	29	36	113	332	142	474	1291	1765	26.86	1689	28.06
1904	6	0	1	18	29	0	1	38	34	2	3	19	201	26	28	53	270	28	33	128	303	156	459	1392	1851	24.80	1771	25.92
1905	23	0	1	19	28	0	3	26	28	0	4	18	235	26	21	67	314	26	29	130	343	156	499	1518	2017	24.74	1914	26.07
1906	15	2	3	23	36	3	0	23	37	0	4	12	245	22	25	91	333	27	32	149	365	176	541	1574	2115	25.58	2011	26.90
1907	15	0	3	18	27	1	13	39	37	1	3	17	227	17	26	98	306	19	45	172	351	191	542	1661	2203	24.60	2115	25.63
1908	22	1	1	24	23	0	0	39	14	4	5	19	209	30	29	82	268	35	35	164	303	199	502	1648	2150	23.35	2081	24.12
1909	16	0	0	28	33	1	5	25	39	2	4	14	177	31	28	76	265	34	37	143	302	177	479	1531	2010	23.83	1964	24.39
1910	27	0	0	24	28	3	3	27	29	2	8	14	236	38	25	75	320	43	36	140	356	183	539	1717	2256	23.89	2150	25.07
1911	23	0	0	24	35	6	3	26	13	2	1	15	267	12	30	100	338	20	34	165	372	185	557	1816	2373	23.47	2304	24.18

Source: Buenos Aires, Yearbook 1910–1911, 119–20.
Abbreviations: Arg = Argentine; Fng = Foregn; F = Female; M = Male; GA = Generally Accepted Pulmonary

other diseases than with respiratory tuberculosis because of the difficulty of identifying pulmonary tuberculosis in young children.[4] The questionable statistics may also reflect confusion over nationality. In the examination of gender, from 1900 to 1911, female children born to Porteños died in larger numbers than male children. Pulmonary tuberculosis was most deadly for young women born to Porteño families between the ages of fifteen and nineteen. They were 1.5 times more likely to die of pulmonary tuberculosis than were boys of the same age. Between 1900 and 1911, minors represented from 15.5 to 26.9 percent of the generally accepted total pulmonary tuberculosis deaths.[5]

From 1900 to 1911, the proportion of children who died of tuberculosis was relatively constant: 12.6 percent of all childhood deaths each year stemmed from tuberculosis. Between 1912 and 1917, the number of children dying from tuberculosis increased, even though the number of adults dying from it was declining. The number of ten- to fifteen-year-olds dying of tuberculosis was probably even higher than the statistics indicated since many tubercular children were wrongly thought to have died of pneumonia. In 1930, seventy-five percent of infants contracting tuberculosis before the age of six months died. Children under the age of two, who were poorly nourished, died in larger numbers from tuberculosis than older children. Although the actual frequency of tuberculosis in infancy and childhood could be confirmed with autopsies, few were conducted, and too many cases were misdiagnosed and thus not counted. The existing data were incomplete, focusing only on those who died in hospitals; tubercular children who died at home were often not counted. From 1892 to 1901, a comparison between tuberculosis and other diseases demonstrated that tuberculosis was a major killer, particularly of children aged ten to fifteen. By contrast, the number of children dying of whooping cough and measles decreased.[6]

Immigrant children appeared to die in smaller numbers than native Argentine children. However, the statistics may be skewed, since native Argentine parents were more likely than immigrant parents to take their children to hospitals, where they were tested for tuberculosis. Although statistics occasionally pointed to increased deaths due to epidemics of measles, cholera, diphtheria and smallpox, infant mortality among Porteño children below age one steadily decreased from 17.1 percent of childhood deaths (those under age fifteen) in 1880 to 8.4 percent in 1924. Physicians rarely reported tuberculosis in infants. Tuberculosis was more easily diagnosed among older children. Porteño youth between the ages of ten and twenty—tested in the 1930s—showed fifty percent of them were infected with tuberculosis.[7]

It is clear that poor children were more likely to encounter tuberculosis than wealthy children; the latter ate more nutritious meals and lived in homes that were more spacious and less susceptible to airborne diseases.

Affluent children were also less likely to be infected by school friends, with whom they had only limited contact. (Wealthy children instead associated mostly with children in their extended family.) Prosperous parents provided their children with private physicians and could afford to send them to healthy climates. In the summer, parents rented houses outside the heat of the city or went to the beaches of Mar del Plata. That said, the incidence of tuberculosis among wealthy children was probably undercounted since they were less likely than poor children to be sent to institutions that reported tuberculosis cases.[8]

Middle-class children lived with their families in adequate housing, had a healthy diet, used toys bought in the marketplace and enjoyed leisure activities with their families. They played with children of their own age and school friends on the streets and plazas near their homes and were more likely to come in contact with tubercular children than were wealthy children. By the early twentieth century, school programs identified tubercular children. As a result, middle-class children were often treated for tuberculosis when the disease was in its early stages. They were generally cared for at home.[9]

Poor children, who attended school in small numbers (and only in the early grades), were the most likely to contract tuberculosis. They entered the labor force early and lived with families on the margins of society in tenement houses near the center of the city or in the outer suburbs. In the early twentieth century, many poor children lived on the streets of Buenos Aires. Coming from large families and living in overcrowded tenements, these children often had inadequate diets and lived in homes lacking fresh air. Children from poor families also worked to contribute to the family income. Boys often had part-time jobs as sellers of lottery tickets, messengers, and shoe polishers; girls worked in domestic service or might even be forced into prostitution.[10]

In 1904, more than 7,000 Buenos Aires children labored in the textile, burlap, glass, match, carton and cookie factories, comprising between fifteen and sixty percent of the factories' workforce. Children from ages eight to fourteen, working up to eleven hours a day, often did jobs that were too difficult for them. They were paid either by the piece or two to three times less than adults. With rest breaks only every four to five hours, many children toiled in semi-darkness with poor ventilation. Glass factories, in particular, exploited children, who had to avoid being injured by mechanical belts and had no protection against toxic substances such as arsenic and ammonia. At the beginning of the twentieth century, the number of tubercular children in Buenos Aires was increasing, because children lived and worked under conditions that exposed them to the disease. Working-class children were two to five times as likely as middle-class children to have tuberculosis and to be treated for it by charities.[11]

Institutional Services for Poor and Tubercular Porteño Children

Responding to the poor who had difficulty providing for their families, immigrant communities and government organizations developed programs by the late nineteenth century to improve the living and working conditions of abandoned, orphaned and tubercular children and to decrease childhood mortality. Between 1889 and 1900, immigrant birth rates were high; furthermore, between 12.6 and 15 percent of all Buenos Aires births were illegitimate. Although the Catholic Church's influence was declining, social stigma continued to be attached to women who bore children out of wedlock. Poor women often thought that they had no option but to leave their children with the Casa de Expósitos, Casa de Huérfanos or the Hospital de Niños. Employers of domestic servants prohibited children from living with their parents. Foundling homes provided care and burials when relatives could not afford to pay for these services.[12] The Sociedad de Beneficencia—assisted by the government—supported the expansion of orphanages and children's hospitals for the care of abandoned and ill children. By the late nineteenth century, the secularization of Argentina and the financial limitations of the Catholic Church discouraged religious institutions from creating separate orphanages. Catholic lay women and nuns of various orders served in state institutions.[13] From the early nineteenth century, the Sociedad de Beneficencia operated the Casa de Expósitos (founded in Buenos Aires in 1779), which cared for deserted, orphaned and poor children. Up to eighty percent of the children had working-class parents, who were unable to provide for them. As the population of Buenos Aires increased, the number of abandoned children grew proportionally, and the government added facilities. The Sociedad de Beneficencia also administered the Asilo de Huérfanos, which was built by the Porteño government in 1871 to aid children whose parents had died in a yellow fever epidemic. In 1901, this institution cared for 439 boys (including eighteen who were blind) and 217 girls (of whom eleven were blind). Built to provide for about 500 children, the institution could not adequately care for 656 children. Severe over-crowding occurred when the number of children housed at Sociedad de Beneficencia institutions increased from 1,147 in 1881 to 1,817 in 1895.[14]

Contagious illness was a problem for both the Casa de Expósitos and the Asilo de Huérfanos. In 1912, infant mortality in the Casa de Expósitos was three times greater than it was in the general population, with thirty-five percent of children dying before their first birthday. From fifteen to fifty-four percent of the infants died annually.[15] Orphanages sought to bring infectious disease under control, and they occasionally sent some older children to specialized medical facilities.

In 1914, the Asilo de Huérfanos sent several children to the hospital to be tested for tuberculosis. For example, it requested a bed for Salomón David, a minor, at the Sanatorio Nacional de Tuberculosos de Santa María. Three basic problems help explain the high infant mortality and infection rates in government institutions: more infants were sent to the institutions when the availability of wet nurses declined, as women found more lucrative opportunities; more children were also sent to them because mothers (who were alcoholic, syphilitic, tubercular or debilitated) could not care for their sick children; and the institutions' crowded conditions—combined with the absence of efforts to prevent the transmissions of diseases—led more children to contract diseases (including tuberculosis).[16]

During the 1880s, the Defensorías de Menores of Buenos Aires (a provincial council that was established in 1829 and was responsible for orphans, poor and sick children) was overwhelmed by the number of needy children. Since it lacked the facilities to care for so many children, it sent those under age six to the Casa de Expósitos. Initially, the Defensorías de Menores succeeded in locating some relatives to take responsibility for children. But by the beginning of the twentieth century (as the number of vagabond children increased), children above six years of age were sent to the women's jail, Casa Correccional de Mujeres. Although some of the children were imprisoned for prostitution or stealing, the majority were street children. During their residence in the prison, the girls worked in commerce and as launderers, receiving only a meager salary. In 1892, Buenos Aires established the Patronato de la Infancia (which was administered by men of the elite and hygienists) to improve the care offered to the children of the Sociedad de Beneficencia and the Defensorías de Menores. The Patronato de la Infancia also raised money to operate day-care centers, schools and agricultural centers. In 1895, it created a special commission of women to organize guardianship and medical services for poor children. Despite these municipal efforts, the number of children in the women's jail increased from 466 in 1889 to 1,874 in 1917.[17]

During the 1920s, the number of children in prison decreased, as government services to the poor improved and women who found jobs in the expanding textile industry were better able to support their children. The Cantinas Maternale, an association that was founded in 1915, maintained restaurants in worker's districts. By 1927, it operated five. Women who were six or more months pregnant or had nursing children under age two received two meals daily. In the 1920s, institutional care of children improved. Institutions offered more physician care and focused more on preventing diseases, including tuberculosis. By the 1940s, the care of abandoned children was thought to be a responsibility of the state—rather than the responsibility of charities operated by elite women.[18]

Institutions faced difficult challenges in caring for tubercular children. For example, in 1918, sixty-six percent of the children in the Casa de Expósitos were considered pre-tubercular, and 61.1 percent of the four- and five-year-olds tested positive to tuberculin tests.[19] Justo Arévalo, whose parents were both dead, wrote in 1908 to the President of the Sociedad de Beneficencia about his ten-year-old brother, Amaranto. He stated that Amaranto, who had been healthy when he entered the Casa de Expósitos, had recently been sent to the Hospital de Niños with tuberculosis, which he had contracted at the orphanage. Justo wanted to make certain that everything necessary was done to improve his brother's health. An orphanage administrator replied to Justo that Amaranto had tuberculosis when he entered the orphanage and that because of its contagious and serious nature he had been treated as soon as the disease manifested itself.[20] The orphanage had two particular challenges: providing a healthy environment for pre-tubercular children and deciding how to care for tubercular children.

With government assistance, in 1875, the Sociedad de Beneficencia inaugurated the twenty-bed Hospital de Niños: two doctors worked at the hospital, seeing patients at no charge. Within two years, the hospital moved to a new location and expanded to provide surgical and clinical care for both girls and boys. In 1892, the Hospital de Niños provided a hundred beds for sick children. Its efforts were supplemented by the Hospital San Roque and the Hospital de Clínicas, each of which admitted a maximum of twenty children. Thus, the three institutions combined offered only 140 beds—in a city of 550,000 people. The continued demand for health services led the Sociedad de Beneficencia to inaugurate a new children's hospital in December 1896 with an initial capacity to serve 230 patients. This new facility received children up to age fourteen and was served by twelve physicians. In January and February 1911, the Hospital de Niños cared for between 297 and 314 Argentine children and between forty-one and forty-six immigrant children. The Hospital de Niños continued to expand. In 1943, it had 700 beds, dealt daily with 850 out-patients and employed close to 200 physicians and technical staff.[21]

The Hospital de Niños provided medical assistance, surgery and essential items (such as clothes) to children whose parents had limited resources. It also cared for a small number of abandoned children. Because few children entered the hospital with chronic diseases, such as tuberculosis, mortality rates were low. Initially, the hospital did not even tabulate the number of tubercular children and did not provide separate facilities for them.[22] In fact, the Hospital de Niños did not accept children with tuberculosis. Instead, it sent them to the Casa de Aislamiento (the isolation hospital which became the Hospital Muñiz). Nevertheless, in 1901, the hospital performed a hundred autopsies; forty-eight of them indicated tuberculosis.[23] The number of children diagnosed with tuberculosis in the Hospital de Niños increased steadily. By 1914, the Hospital de Niños acknowledged that it had tubercular children, whom it sought to transfer to the Sanatorio Marítimo y Solarium in Mar del Plata or Hospital Sanatorio de Llanura Vicente López y Planes. The Hospital de Niños continued to accept tubercular children, as long as they were diagnosed only after they entered it. Buenos Aires parents preferred their children to stay there since it was nearer their homes than the distant Hospital Vicente López y Planes. The staff argued that the function of a hospital was to care for the sick, and that it was far better to care for tubercular children and isolate them than to send them home. By the 1940s, the hospital focused its efforts on polio rather than tuberculosis.[24]

Orphanages for Poor Philadelphia Children

Before 1830, orphanages were a rarity in the U.S. because relatives cared for orphaned children. From 1820 to 1860, the number of orphanages in the U.S. grew from 33 to nearly 200. The need for orphanages increased due to cholera epidemics that decimated families and increased immigration (since immigrants did not have extended families). Between 1860 and 1890, as the national population doubled, the number of U.S. orphanages tripled to almost 600. By the 1880s, Protestant churches, Catholic parishes, Jewish communities and nonsectarian groups supported orphanages in Philadelphia. As the U.S. population increased from 92 million in 1910 to 125 million in 1933, the number of orphanages also increased from 972 to 1,321.[25]

Philadelphia orphanages included the Catholic institutions St. Joseph and St. Vincent and the Jewish Foster Home and Orphan Asylum. Throughout the nineteenth century, most children in Pennsylvania orphanages had one living parent. Some widows placed their children temporarily in orphanages until they were able to care for them. Although parents sometimes took their children to orphanages so that they could obtain an education, children lived at an orphanage primarily because of family poverty, which was often caused by a parent's illness, unemployment or death. In the late nineteenth century and early twentieth century, more than fifty percent of the children in Philadelphia orphanages had lost a parent due to a disease, particularly tuberculosis. Orphanages did not want to split up families and emphasized the importance of reuniting children with their families. This approach became increasingly common among orphanage administrators after 1900. In many cases, children resided in community orphanages for only a year or two before they returned to their families. The number of children in orphanages decreased, as adult mortality rates declined and social services provided support to poor families.[26]

From the 1830s to the 1930s, the quality of life for children in families and in orphanages improved, as social attitudes toward children changed. Although managers of orphanages initially viewed poor parents as unfit, they came to realize that unemployment and illness were the root causes of parents' failures to provide for their children. While orphanage children did not receive the individual attention that families offered, the food, clothing and housing provided by orphanages generally compared favorably with what they might have received in their impoverished homes. By the twentieth century, play was thought to be important for childhood development; therefore, it was included in the orphanage curriculum. The chores required in orphanages resembled those done by working-class children.[27]

St. Joseph's Orphan Asylum, the first orphanage in the U.S., was founded in Philadelphia in 1798 in response to a yellow fever epidemic. When the population of German Catholic immigrants in Philadelphia grew from 57,500 in 1846 to 215,000 in 1854, more orphanages were needed. St. Vincent opened in 1859 with five girls and six boys whose ages ranged from three to nine. The orphanage subsequently added new buildings and by 1893 provided shelter for 300 orphans. St. Vincent children appeared to be healthier than orphanage children in Buenos Aires. St. Vincent's records indicate that thirty children had diphtheria in 1862, that a few contracted typhoid fever in 1864 and 1869, and that thirty-two developed scarlet fever in 1877. Records indicate that the prime health concern was normal childhood diseases, not tuberculosis. Although the records indicate that some children had inflamed lungs, there is no evidence that orphanages tested children for tuberculosis. By 1910, sanitation had improved and infectious disease cases declined. St. Vincent had only three deaths from the Spanish flu in 1919 out of 164 cases—a surprisingly low number.[28]

In 1855, the Jewish community of Philadelphia established the Jewish Foster Home and Orphan Asylum. In 1909, the home accommodated 177 children (122 boys and 55 girls). By 1919, the home housed 182 of whom nineteen were full orphans, 122 half orphans, thirty-two were deserted by parents, and nine were indigent. The large number of boys at the Jewish Foster Home, in comparison with Buenos Aires, illustrates a greater focus on abandoned and street children. The children appeared healthy, and there were few pre-tubercular and tubercular children. The Jewish community of Philadelphia, like the one in Buenos Aires, provided for poor children. In particular, they were given an appropriate religious education. As the number of orphans decreased, the Jewish Foster Home changed its role to care for children with special needs. It eventually closed its doors in 1950.[29]

Beginning in the 1910s, state governments began providing mothers' pensions that allowed women to care for their own children. The passage of Social Security legislation in 1935 (and amendments to it in 1936 and 1939) helped widowed mothers and orphaned children. The national government program, however, initially discriminated against unmarried mothers and people of color. With the creation of Aid to Dependent Children in the 1940s and 1950s, children could be cared for by their own parents, and orphanages declined in importance. Between the 1920s and 1960s, as increased financial support was offered to poor families, orphanages slowly decreased in number and changed their missions. The institutions then dealt with foster care, adoption and special-needs children.[30]

Children died of tuberculosis in both orphanages and their own homes. Table 6.2 describes the number of children in age groups under 1, 1–2, 2–5, 10–15 and 15–20. There are slight increases of the death of children during periods of recession. From 1870 to 1938, girls consistently died of pulmonary tuberculosis in larger number than boys, by a ratio of 1.04 to 1.85. Pulmonary tuberculosis was most deadly for girls between the ages of fifteen to twenty. Between 1870 and 1928, minors represented 8.97 to 15.60 percent of all pulmonary tuberculosis deaths, and an average of 11.7 percent of total pulmonary deaths. The pulmonary tuberculosis deaths of minors were slower to decline than adults. In 1937, mortality reached a low of 6.89 percent of all pulmonary tuberculosis deaths. Philadelphia adult pulmonary deaths began to decrease rapidly from 9.2 percent of all deaths in 1917 to 5.91 percent in 1920.

Treatment and Diagnosis of Tubercular Children

Philadelphia and Porteño physicians had difficulty treating and diagnosing tuberculosis in children. They diagnosed children with tuberculosis of the bones, joints, glands, meninges and lungs. In the first twenty-five years of the twentieth century, physicians more often diagnosed infants and young children with meningeal than pulmonary tuberculosis.[31] When physicians saw tubercular children, the children often appeared normal in the early stages of the disease. Identifying tuberculosis in nursing babies was particularly hard, although accurately diagnosing children over age seven was easier. Tuberculosis rarely formed a cavity in the lungs among infants but did so more often in older children. Careful examination of tubercular children showed that many lacked appetite, were tired and anemic, lacked muscle tone, coughed and had frequent colds and diarrhea. But these symptoms characterized many diseases. Although an X-ray and a tuberculin test often confirmed the presence of tuberculosis, physicians at times misread the test results.[32] Because twenty to fifty percent of tubercular children had tubercular parents, the best indicators of tuberculosis in children were family histories of the disease, followed by high pulse and respiratory rates.[33]

Parents did not bring the young to see a doctor because they suspected that their child had tuberculosis, but rather because she was ill and her health was not improving. Most Buenos Aires children came to clinics and hospitals because they had gastroenteritis or bronchitis. María P., a

Table 6.2 Pulmonary Tuberculosis Deaths of Minors, Age 0–20, in Philadelphia for Various Years from 1870 to 1938

Year	*Under 1*	*1–2*	*2–5*	*6–9*	*10–14*	*15–20*	*TB Deaths 0–20*			*Ratio of F to M D*	*Total Pul TB Death*	*0–20% of TB Death*
							F	*M*	*Total*			
1870	32	26	26	18	31	170	170	133	303	1.28	2308	13.13
1972	38	23	20	13	40	175	175	134	309	1.31	2330	13.26
1873	40	18	17	12	28	187	185	117	302	1.58	2291	13.18
1875	23	12	16	17	22	189	154	125	279	1.23	2359	11.83
1876	26	19	19	16	25	217	209	113	322	1.85	2676	12.03
1878	27	13	14	15	28	211	194	114	308	1.70	2491	12.36
1880	16	13	24	16	34	196	175	124	299	1.41	2692	11.11
1881	14	16	18	11	32	199	168	122	290	1.38	2768	10.48
1882	30	14	19	22	27	177	165	124	289	1.33	2909	9.93
1884	37	20	28	14	31	208	178	160	338	1.11	2801	12.07
1887	29	18	21	19	36	200	204	119	323	1.71	2800	11.54
1888	22	16	18	19	35	166	159	117	276	1.36	2695	10.24
1889	22	17	21	24	29	181	176	118	294	1.49	2532	11.61
1890	17	15	22	24	42	191	179	132	311	1.36	2764	11.25
1892	29	11	28	30	35	203	186	150	336	1.24	2709	12.40
1893	23	15	27	17	34	201	165	152	317	1.09	2671	11.87
1895	17	15	34	15	30	165	149	127	276	1.17	2449	11.27
1896	25	15	40	26	30	169	176	129	305	1.36	2514	12.13
1899	32	18	28	18	33	205	190	144	334	1.32	2818	11.85
1900	25	24	26	28	32	220	208	147	355	1.41	2717	13.07

1901	39	27	16	32	36	217	214	153	367	1.40	2946	12.46
1902	29	27	24	25	37	240	224	158	382	1.42	2845	13.43
1903	29	20	33	25	31	263	204	197	401	1.04	3053	13.13
1904	30	24	20	31	55	277	249	188	437	1.32	3117	14.02
1905	25	15	22	13	45	258	231	147	378	1.57	2838	13.32
1906	49	27	31	30	47	309			493	–	3161	15.60
1907	48	29	33	27	52	268	258	199	457	1.30	3157	14.48
1910	22	25	21	19	27	223	182	155	337	1.17	2873	11.73
1914	19	7	10	17	31	157	157		241	–	2684	8.98
1915	13	13	11	17	32	161	161		247	–	2754	8.97
1917	30	18	18	18	38	182	182		304	–	3019	10.07
1918	15	19	16	19	46	200			315	–	3257	9.67
1920	10	15	11	11	30	128	121	84	205	1.44	2130	9.62
1923	10	5	7	18	23	126			189	–	1817	10.40
1928	3	9	10	9	21	123			175	–	1509	11.60
1929	9	13	8	9	13	95			147	–	1451	10.13
1932	7	5	6	3	15	71			107	–	1234	8.67
1937	2	10	2	2	11	55			82	–	1190	6.89
1938	1	2	12	2	12	81			110	–	1104	9.96

Sources: Philadelphia, *Annual Message of the Mayor of Philadelphia, 1912*, v. 3: 126–8; 1938, 370–1; various years.
Abbreviations: F = Female; M = Male; T = Total; F to M D = Female to Male deaths; Pul = Pulmonary.

fourteen-month-old (whose case history was provided at the beginning of the chapter), was misdiagnosed in a typical way. Similarly, in 1893, a physician suggested that Enrique B. (another 14-month-old) who vomited, had diarrhea and lost weight—suffered from gastroenteritis. But when he died, an autopsy revealed that he had tuberculosis of the lungs. When a child had a cough, physicians were unsure whether the child had a viral infection, whooping cough or tuberculosis.[34] The difficulty of diagnosing tuberculosis is illustrated by the prominent physician, Emilio Coni. In 1891, he diagnosed only forty-six cases of tuberculosis out of 6,502 children under five. He concluded that most of the children died of gastroenteritis or other infections of the digestive tract. He listed nineteen percent as dying from pneumonia or bronchitis. But he might have wrongly ascribed tuberculosis deaths to those diseases.[35] Physicians thought that children aged six to fourteen, whose bodies were undergoing major transformation were more likely to get measles, diphtheria, influenza, whooping cough or scarlet fever than tuberculosis.[36]

Physicians tended to prescribe the same medications for children and adults. Tuberculosis medicines were usually experimental and determining the proper doses was difficult. Some medications actually caused adverse reactions in children, as when María P. reacted badly to small doses of potassium iodide. A pediatric physician noted that tuberculin should be administered to a child only with great caution. The three initial doses were to be less than 0.00001 micrograms. If the medication seemed effective, the dose could be doubled and repeated every three to four days. (The adult dosage could be as high as 1 cc three times daily for nine months.)[37] Standard adult medications such as phosphates and calcium often did not benefit tubercular children under the age of five. Cod liver oil, cough syrups, common childhood medications, were recommended if coughing exhausted a child. Physicians prescribed fewer medications for children than for adults, because they tended to be ineffective when given to children. On the other hand, the increasing professionalization of the medical profession led to the adoption of more invasive procedures, even for children. By the 1930s, physicians in Buenos Aires were collapsing the lungs of some children in order to rest them. Physicians believed that this procedure worked best for children aged twelve to fourteen. But the procedure sometimes caused death and was of questionable value.[38]

Public health officials and physicians emphasized preventing tuberculosis, specifically by sending children to a healthy environment and giving them nutritious food. In August 1901, the Buenos Aires municipal government made Sra. Gabriela L. de Coni an inspector. Her task was to visit industrial establishments that employed women and children, to report on their conditions and to promote safety regulations. The Protección de la Primera Infancia created in 1908—was responsible for overseeing institutions servicing children and assuring that they received needed services. An office for the inspection of wet nurses was created in 1919, to ensure that wet nurses would not spread disease.[39] In 1924, Argentina implemented a plan to remove infants of tubercular mothers from their families and place them in rural homes for two years. The program may have prevented tuberculosis in a few children, but it also fragmented families—thereby running counter to the era's efforts to decrease the abandonment of infants. Although Philadelphia pediatric physicians also recommended removing infants from their tubercular mothers, it was less common there than in Buenos Aires.[40] The Argentine government sought to reduce both the abandonment of children and children's mortality by imbuing the working-class with middle-class values. But the programs to teach mothers how to care for their infants reflected middle-class bias against the poor and contributed only minimally to making more healthy children.[41]

Between 1870 and 1945, it was more effective to prevent tuberculosis in children (and adults) than to cure. Among the most successful efforts taken to improve children's health in Buenos Aires were the establishment of milk dispensaries, child care centers with free healthcare tuberculosis clinics and school health programs. At the beginning of the twentieth century, clinics opened by the Argentine Anti-Tuberculosis League benefitted children by diagnosing tuberculosis more rapidly and by giving them additional milk. By 1909, the municipality had opened six milk dispensaries; the Sociedad de Beneficencia added one at the Hospital de Niños. It was hoped that tubercular mothers would obtain pasteurized milk and not nurse their infants.[42] However, with no refrigeration mothers faced the challenge of preventing the milk from becoming contaminated.

The Role of Schools in a Changing Society

Public officials increasingly sought to aid children by instituting tuberculosis prevention programs in schools. By the 1890s, the medical inspection of children was commonplace in both Philadelphia and Buenos Aires. It was thought that schools could help many children by promoting good hygiene and teaching them how tuberculosis could be prevented. Schools used pamphlets, courses and drama to teach children about tuberculosis. It was hoped that the children would then educate members of their families about prevention. By 1919, a U.S. health campaign resulted in a program in which three million children competed to gain weight and to develop good personal hygiene. Municipalities built larger, well-ventilated classrooms to prevent crowding children into small rooms. Schools provided food and milk to children with poor diets at home. Charities and public health agencies in both Buenos Aires and Philadelphia provided open-air schools during the academic year and rural or beach vacations during the summer for debilitated or tubercular children.[43]

By the early twentieth century, efforts to prevent tuberculosis were common in Buenos Aires and Philadelphia schools. In 1902, Philadelphia became the first city in Pennsylvania to support a campaign for child hygiene in public schools. In cooperation with the Board of Education, doctors went to public schools to teach hygiene with the expectation that it would reduce tuberculosis among children. The Philadelphia Board of Education also improved ventilation and lighting in the schools. In Argentina, children learned how the body develops and were taught health practices relating to cleanliness.[44]

In 1881, Dr. Emilio Coni began the first medical and hygienic examination of school children in Latin America in several Buenos Aires schools. Seven years later, Argentina's national council of education put this program into practice in all city schools. Beginning in 1892, the program emphasized preventing diseases, including tuberculosis. Spitting on the floor was prohibited, and children were encouraged to bathe weekly and brush their teeth regularly. Of the 10,707 children who received physical examinations in 1904, physicians diagnosed only five with tuberculosis of the bone and none with pulmonary tuberculosis. But 1,633 children were diagnosed as pre-tubercular, because of their poor health.[45] By 1918, public health officials found that five percent of school children between ages six and fourteen had scrofula; 39.5 percent were anemic.[46] These statistics are, however, unreliable because physicians had difficulty identifying tubercular children and there was no agreement as to who was pre-tubercular. It is likely that many of the pre-tubercular and anemic children had tuberculosis because they had symptoms that indicate it. Public health officials apparently did not use the tuberculin test, which would at least have confirmed the children's exposure to tuberculosis. Family histories could also have indicated the disease: as we have seen, children with tubercular relatives were likely themselves to have the disease.

In contrast to Buenos Aires, Philadelphia public officials had better statistical evidence, which documented that tuberculosis posed a major health problem for school children. In 1920, physicians studied 1,219 patients at the Children's Hospital of Philadelphia. Fifteen percent of those less than one year old were diagnosed with tuberculosis; forty-two percent of those aged one to eight, thirty-two percent of those aged eight to twelve, and eighty percent of those above 12 years reacted positively to tuberculin tests. Between 1925 and 1928, the Henry Phipps Institute performed a larger study on the incidence of tuberculosis in four high schools and four elementary schools in Philadelphia. Physicians administered 4,100 physical exams, tuberculin tests and X-ray exams to children. With more advanced technology, the researchers concluded that tuberculosis in Philadelphia's schools was as prevalent as in the larger cities of Europe. X-rays showed that active tuberculosis was twice as common among high school students as in elementary children. They confirmed the earlier hospital study showing that adolescents were more likely than younger children to have tuberculosis; the disease was also more common in girls than boys. One percent of the girls between ages twelve and eighteen had active tuberculosis, while only 0.4 percent of boys were infected. Evidence suggested that girls in puberty resisted the tubercle bacillus less effectively than boys. In the 1928–1929 Phipps Institute survey of healthy black and white school children in Philadelphia, researchers found no difference in the exposure level. Nevertheless, in the 1930s, the tuberculosis death rates for African-American children in grades five through nine were five times higher than those for white children in those grades. Childhood tuberculosis was most common in poor children who drank unpasteurized milk and were repeatedly exposed to infection.[47]

Open-Air Schools and Vacation Colonies

Physicians agreed that preventing tuberculosis among school children could effectively restrict the spread of the disease, but they could not agree on what steps to take. Between 1895 and 1930, open-air schools and vacation colonies that utilized the fresh air/diet regime were opened worldwide. Private charities in Buenos Aires and Philadelphia, the Buenos Aires municipal government and the Argentine national governments accordingly instituted such programs for poor children whose parents had tuberculosis or who needed more nutritious meals and outdoor activities.[48]

Argentines and North Americans learned about open-air schools from the Germans, who established the first program in 1904 on the outskirts of Berlin. The Red Cross transported children daily to the outdoor facility. The children spent eleven hours a day there and received five nutritious meals. England established open-air schools in 1907, the U.S. in 1908 and Argentina in 1909. The schools served anemic, weak and pretubercular children who lived at home. In Europe, governments located open-air schools in forest and rural settings; in the U.S. and Argentina, they were established in cities. Children spent much time outdoors or in buildings with open fronts or open windows, ate nutritious meals, and rested. Theoretically, the curriculum was identical to that taught in the public schools, but the children actually had a lighter academic load than public school pupils and received more individual instructions.[49]

In 1909, the National Council of Education in Argentina inaugurated two schools with open-air buildings for anemic and pre-tubercular children. The children commuted from their homes Mondays through Saturdays. They were weighed regularly and given medical examinations. But the most significant factor improving the children's health was their meals: breakfasts of coffee, bread and milk; lunches of soup, vegetables, potatoes or noodles and dessert; and suppers of bread and milk. By 1919, children in open-air schools routinely also received tuberculin tests.[50]

The open-air schools in the U.S. were an outgrowth of the therapeutic and preventive work of summer day camps. The first open-air school in the U.S. was opened by two women physicians of Providence, Rhode Island. Chicago, Boston, New York and Philadelphia soon followed suit. The Henry Phipps Institute started an open-air school for children in 1911. In the following year, the Pennsylvania Society for the Prevention of Tuberculosis initiated another open-air school. Two years later, the Board of Education took it over. By 1916, there were at least a thousand open-air schools in the U.S. Like the Porteño open-air schools, they emphasized a standard academic curriculum but also provided a nutritious diet and appropriate rest periods. But by the 1930s, most open-air schools closed. That was because they were expensive and served only a limited number of children. Furthermore, specialists believed that they did not successfully prevent tuberculosis. Open-air schools did, however, increase national awareness of malnutrition among urban school children. In the U.S., they also laid the basis for the redesigning of schools and the development of school lunch programs. Schools built in the 1940s and 1950s had many windows and lunch rooms, reflecting the belief that fresh air, sun and nutritious meals would prevent tuberculosis.[51]

The Argentine National Council of Education opened its first vacation colony in Mar del Plata in 1895, providing 384 children with a nineteen-day experience at a beach. The success of this effort, in which the average child's weight increased by two kilograms, led the Argentine Anti-Tuberculosis League to organize a summer camp in 1902 at Claypole (a small town twenty-five kilometers from Buenos Aires). The camp served fifty youths, age seven to fifteen, who had tubercular parents. The association of women supporting schools (Association de Damas Escuelas y Patronas) established two additional vacation colonies in 1907 and 1909. Located close to train routes and less than two hours from Buenos Aires, these summer vacation camps provided a healthy outdoor environment for poor children who were anemic and malnourished and were considered pre-tubercular.[52] The Sociedad de Beneficencia also established an agricultural colony to give orphans a practical experience of working on a farm. Children at the colony planted crops and fruit trees, harvested vegetables and wheat and cared for cattle, horses and chickens.[53]

Preventoriums for Porteño Children

The difficulty of providing year-round care for urban tubercular children led to the development of preventoriums, pediatric institutions for malnourished and physically weak children that provided the services of home, school and sanatorium. Preventoriums became popular for treating children with latent tuberculosis. They were open year around and they accepted children for a stay of at least six months. They enrolled children who had been exposed to tuberculosis in the home, who had non-pulmonary forms of tuberculosis, who frequently had colds or bronchitis and who suffered from malnutrition and tired easily. Preventoriums often began as open-air schools or mountain or seashore camps and were transformed into more permanent facilities. They provided poor children with a healthy diet, information on cleanliness, and opportunities to play and exercise outdoors. Thus, the preventorium directly confronted poverty, inadequate hygiene, substandard nutrition and medical ignorance—all of which were thought to cause tuberculosis in children. Both preventoriums and hospitals increased efforts to diagnose tuberculosis early and standardized treatment in accordance with medical programs in Europe and the U.S.[54]

Preventoriums were built between 1910 and 1930 after the tuberculin test was developed. Until 1908, children were classified as well or ill; subsequently, the category of "pre-tubercular" was added. Tuberculin testing did not simplify determining whether an individual was infected with tuberculosis: instead, it complicated the understanding of the disease. Children above twelve years were more likely to have been exposed to tuberculosis than younger children. They, therefore, tended to test positive, even if they themselves had not contracted the disease. As a result, the tuberculin test did not clearly indicate who had tuberculosis. Public Health officials nevertheless assumed that pre-tubercular children were more likely to develop active tuberculosis and would, therefore, benefit from entering a preventorium.[55]

Public health officials and tuberculosis associations in Buenos Aires and Philadelphia located preventoriums in isolated areas: near the ocean or mountains in rural districts or on the outskirts of urban centers. The institutions treated both poor and immigrant children, who were thought to be at risk of contracting tuberculosis. Preventoriums also provided a home for children for three to six months (or longer), when their parents were at a sanatorium. Porteño and Philadelphia children from wealthy families did not go to preventoriums, even when their parents had tuberculosis. Nurses oversaw the daily needs of the children. Treatment included bed rest, a healthy balanced diet, fresh air, physical care and education in proper hygiene and school subjects. Caregivers also utilized heliotherapy as a means of "curing" tuberculosis. Children gained weight at preventoriums and returned home healthier, but their infected parents often still lived at home.[56]

In 1893, the Sociedad de Beneficencia of Buenos Aires established the Sanatorio Marítimo in Mar del Plata as a preventorium. It operated until the 1940s, caring for children between the ages three and fourteen who were pre-tubercular, had operable tuberculosis or were convalescing. The Sanatorio Marítimo, the first maritime sanatorium in Latin America, located 500 meters from a beach, began with forty beds. By 1902, the facility had expanded to accommodate 125 children of both sexes. Buenos Aires institutions—including the children's hospital (Hospital de Niños), the foundling home (Casa de Expósitos), the orphanages (Asilo de Huérfanos, Casa de Huérfanos and Colegio de la Merced), public clinics and general hospitals—sent children to the Sanatorio Marítimo twice a year, at the beginning of the summer and during the last half of autumn.[57] Girls comprised between forty-nine and sixty-one percent of the institution's patients. The number of foreign-born children varied between two and four percent.[58]

A solarium was added in 1918 to serve primarily pre-tubercular children. By 1921, the sanatorium and solarium together treated 220 children, mostly from the working-class. The institution eventually accommodated 300 patients, many of whom were quite young. In 1938, the Sanatorio Marítimo y Solarium served forty-nine boys under age five. The number of children with tuberculosis of the bones increased in the 1940s, but the Sanatorio Marítimo did not want to treat children with pulmonary tuberculosis because it is highly infectious.[59] Care at the sanatorium was inexpensive: in 1899, the Sociedad de Beneficencia calculated that it cost only sixty centavos a day per child.[60] As the number of children in the sanatorium and solarium increased, so did the staff. In addition to a medical director and an internist, there were several part-time physicians, nurses, nurse's aides and service personnel.[61]

Nurses observed children for ten days before taking them to the solarium because some children reacted unfavorably to sand and sun. If a child's health was deteriorating, he or she was returned to the Sanatorio or to the children's hospital in Buenos Aires. For example, in 1921 a physician recommended that three children, Sara Salma, age 4; Armando Palacios, age 5; and Joséfa Candidi, age 9—be sent to the children's hospital in the capital because the climate had harmed their lungs. Some physicians thought that a maritime climate helped cure tuberculosis of the bones but actually worsened pulmonary tuberculosis.[62] Exposure to the sun does help the body to make vitamin D, which is particularly important for bone calcification, but there is no evidence that the maritime climate caused pulmonary complications.

The Sanatorio Marítimo developed a precise routine. Each day began at 6:30 A.M., when children washed and brushed their teeth and then did several breathing exercises. After a 7:30 breakfast of coffee with milk and bread, weather permitting the children went to the beach to play in the sand and swim. In cold weather, children wore coats; otherwise, they wore wide blouses of light wool and short wool pants. They would play on the beach for many days before going into the sea; when they did so, they immersed themselves for only three minutes. Healthy children might take fifteen-minute baths in warm ocean water, followed by a period of rest on the sand. The sick children would take only three baths a week. They spent most of their time resting or taking sand baths (that is being covered with dry sand). In March 1926, for example, the boys spent an average of six hours and twenty-six minutes per day in the sun.

Before lunch at 11:00 o'clock, children again did five to ten minutes of breathing exercises. The major meal of the day was lunch, which included soup, a fish or meat entree, vegetables, bread and dessert. For an hour after lunch, the children rested in the dormitory; from 1:30 to 2:00 P.M., they played in the patio of the preventorium. Nurses made certain that the spontaneous play and directed exercises were age-appropriate and that children did not get tired. From 2:00 to 3:30 P.M., patients attended class or performed chores, followed by a snack of milk and bread before returning to the beach from 4:00 to 5:30. Children washed their hands before eating an evening meal of soup, vegetables or pasta, bread and fruit. The dining hall personnel instructed the children to chew their food well and to drink plenty of water. The regimen prescribed a balanced diet of 2,400 calories in the summer; in the winter children received 3,000 calories, to increase body fat and to protect them from the cold weather. Children then had an hour and a half of recreation before 7:30 P.M., when they again did breathing exercises, washed, brushed their teeth and went to bed. This predictable routine varied only to accommodate winter's shorter days and inclement weather. As children improved in health and grew older, personnel increasingly complained about the children's unwillingness to follow the institution's rules. Those who violated the rules were punished but rarely by expulsion. However, in 1921, two 12-year-olds and one 11-year-old were expelled and sent back to the city because of their bad conduct.[63]

The Sanatorio Marítimo y Solarium and various Buenos Aires orphanages sent tubercular children to the Hospital Sanatorio de Llanura-Vicente López y Planes. The Sanatorio Marítimo did not want children with active tuberculosis, so in the 1930s and 1940s, it sent increasing numbers of children with pulmonary tuberculosis to the Hospital Vicente López y Planes. Although forty hospital beds were reserved for children, aged three to thirteen, they were rarely fully occupied. Children seldom comprised more than fourteen percent at Vicente López y Planes. In 1924, when the hospital had 803 beds, less than five percent of the patients were children. The distance from Buenos Aires discouraged parents from sending their children to the hospital or the children could be sent and ignored.[64] Medical facilities were concerned about dealing with children who had been admitted by a parent but then abandoned. For instance, in 1922, the Hospital Vicente López y Planes reported the cure of Julio Fernandez—a ten-year-old who had had pulmonary tuberculosis for two and a half years. Unfortunately, there was no one to inform of this "happiness." Eventually, the hospital discovered that Julio's mother had died; his father had remarried and did not want to claim Julio. The hospital sent Julio to the Casa de Expósitos and subsequently to the Asilo de Huérfanos.[65]

Vicente López y Planes tested all children for tuberculosis and found that more than forty percent carried the bacteria. Children with the bacteria were then separated into two categories: those who appeared to be pre-tubercular and those with active tuberculosis. Those with active tuberculosis were subsequently divided into three groups (depending on how advanced the disease was) with a fourth category consisting of children who needed surgery. The Hospital Vicente López y Planes specialized in helping children with pulmonary tuberculosis. By 1948, the hospital successfully used streptomycin.[66] Because children resided at the Hospital Vicente López y Planes for months, special activities were provided. In order to develop new skills, patients were taught to weave, embroider, sew, type and to print and bind books (the same skills taught at Santa María). Festivals took place in the hospital's pavilions, but dancing was discouraged: the nurses thought that it tired the patients too much. Mass was celebrated in the chapel at fixed times, and a priest administered to the sick when necessary.[67]

Preventoriums for Philadelphia Children

In the first half of the twentieth century, philanthropists, entrepreneurs, and physicians founded seashore hospitals along the North American Atlantic coast. Children's Seashore House of Atlantic City, New Jersey, opened in 1872 for the summer season; only in 1910 did it offer an annual program. Other seasonal seashore facilities served East Coast children: The Boston Floating Hospital opened in 1894, Sea Breeze Hospital on Coney Island, New York, in 1904 and Crawford Allen Hospital outside Providence, Rhoda Island, in 1906. Just as Porteño children traveled to Sanatorio Marítimo, poor and immigrant children of Philadelphia and New York left their urban environments for a seashore experience which lasted two to twelve weeks. Medical personnel and the public, much as in Argentina, hoped that the children's seaside experience would improve their health.[68]

Sea Breeze initially offered a seasonal experience to pre-tubercular children recommended by New York tuberculosis clinics and eventually developed into a year-around program similar to Sanatorio Marítimo. With stays at Sea Breeze, averaging sixteen months, the New York City' Board of Education provided an on-site open-air school. Although Sea Breeze operated initially as a preventorium, it eventually became a state–of-the-art pediatric tuberculosis institution. Beginning in 1910, the Children's Seashore House concentrated on children with orthopedic condition—bone infections, physical deformities and tuberculosis of the hips, joints and spine. Seashore hospitals generally provided a few beds for pre-tubercular children who were malnourished, in poor physical condition and with non-pulmonary tuberculosis, although increasingly they focused on health conditions that required more intensive intervention and functioned more like hospitals than preventoriums.[69]

Like preventoriums in Argentina, their U.S. counterparts cared for children who had been exposed to tuberculosis and had latent infections. The first preventorium in the U.S. opened in 1909 in Lakewood, New Jersey, for children of poor consumptives from New York City. By the 1920s, public or private funding supported more than forty-five preventoriums with 2,783 beds in the U.S. At least one preventorium was located on the outskirts of most large U.S. cities. Philadelphia supported two preventoriums: one was connected to the Chestnut Hill Sanatorium, and the other was affiliated with the Kensington Dispensary at River Crest. California had at least eight preventoriums, while most of the others were located in the Midwest and Northeast. The construction of preventoriums was endorsed by the Progressive political movement in the U.S. The rationale was as follows: during World War I, army recruiters discovered that many young men were unfit for active duty because they had tuberculosis. The U.S. public health officials, therefore, supported the creation of preventoriums, to lessen the incidence of the disease.[70]

It was hard for physicians to decide which sort of children would most benefit from preventoriums. In 1927, a committee of the U.S. National Tuberculosis Association met and recommended six criteria for admission. Preventoriums should accept children who had been exposed to tuberculosis in their home, who had inactive tubercular lesions, who suffered from malnutrition, who tired easily, who frequently had colds or bronchitis or who suffered from rheumatic diseases. Preventorium administrators clearly did not want children with active tuberculosis. Instead, they hoped to admit children who were in poor physical condition and from working-class backgrounds (but had parents who could still pay for at least part of their care).[71]

Mont Alto also operated a preventorium for children. In 1929, one hundred children were sent to Mont Alto for two summer months, doubling the normal number of children there. It was hoped that Philadelphia or Pittsburgh children who spent time in the country during the summer would improve their health and resist infection. The preventorium initially cared for 150 children of both sexes between the ages of six and twelve; that number increased to 200 by 1929. In spite of the fact that African-American children died of tuberculosis in greater numbers than white children, Mont Alto excluded minority children. But in any case, between 1907 and 1914, children comprised less than five percent of the population of Mont Alto. The state clinics recommended that children be sent to Mont Alto when they were underweight and malnourished; the clinics continued to check on the children after they were discharged from the sanatorium. Most children who came to Mont Alto did not have active tuberculosis, but their parents did. Between 1907 and 1914, fewer than eight percent of the children at Mont Alto were listed as advanced cases. Parents paid nothing for their care, except for haircuts and shoe repair.[72]

Philadelphia children traveled to Mont Alto by train. The trip was long, so few parents visited their children there. Children faced their new experience alone with both apprehension and hope. They wondered what their new residence would be like, what they would eat, and whether they would like the nurses. Physicians examined the children to see if they were tubercular and if they had any other physical problems. Nurses took the children's temperatures and pulses and weighed them. Children were discharged from Mont Alto in three to six months if they did not have tuberculosis; thus, they spent less time at Mont Alto than adults did.[73]

Children were divided into four groups according to age and gender with a fresh-air school providing education for those who were old enough. Life for the children—some of whom were only three—was regulated with military precision with specific meal and activity times. The day began at 7:30 A.M. with breakfast by 8:30. Cinnamon toast and creamed eggs on toasts were breakfast favorites. After breakfast, children made their beds and played quietly in their rooms. The boys' beds were reportedly more untidy than the girls'. Children drank milk at 10 A.M. and had lunch at noon. The children's favorite food was stew, and their least favorite spinach. After lunch, the children rested outdoors in the sun on blankets with no talking or exercise permitted. In chilly weather, the children were wrapped in blankets. After milk time at 3 P.M., there was restricted outdoor time until supper at 5 P.M. In addition to daily showers, children received weekly treatment for head lice. They were allowed to play games until seven, and by the 1940s they could listen to the radio until bedtime. They saluted doctors and nurses and turned in at 8:00 P.M. To alleviate young children's fear, older boys would sit with small children until they went to sleep.[74]

Easter Monday was a particularly joyful occasion with unlimited ice cream and cake at lunch and games and an egg hunt in the afternoon. Children attended picnics and sports events throughout the year and did handiwork that was exhibited to the Mont Alto community. In preparation for a September exhibit, girls did needlework and made baskets and caps; boys collected insects. Children particularly enjoyed the activities at Christmas. They performed plays, danced and sang for residents and listened to carols. The local communities of Chambersburg, Waynesboro and Gettysburg provided a variety of Christmas gifts for the children.[75]

In addition to academic subjects, girls between ages ten and fourteen were taught cooking and sewing; boys received manual training. Children who were cured sometimes remained at Mont Alto for a while, to complete classes that might improve their chances of getting a job. Girl and Boy Scout troops provided activities and opportunities to develop a variety of skills. Children had their own student government under the guidance of teachers and received rewards for good behavior.[76] The boys were always more boisterous than the girls; at times, they were punished for breaking screen doors, shattering light fixtures with rubber balls and dancing on wet grass in their stocking feet. Nurses had difficulty enforcing the strict routine on the older boys. When boys got too noisy after hours, the head nurse required them to line up and asked the offenders to identify themselves. In at least one case, a boy took responsibility for the noise and faced the ire of the head nurse.[77]

As in Argentina, North American physicians recommended that children with tuberculosis of the glands, bones and joints go to seashore preventoriums. Children from Philadelphia went to facilities such as the Children's Seashore House in Atlantic City. The Pennsylvania Society for the Prevention of Tuberculosis taught classes in Philadelphia churches for tubercular children and identified and provided funds for children who they thought would benefit from a seashore or country experience. An eight-year-old girl, who lived with her married sister and depended for support on an out-of-work brother-in-law, attended classes at a local church. Money was provided to send her to the country for six weeks and she returned "strong, fat, rosy."[78]

Children's attitudes and memories of their preventorium experience were basically positive. Eileen Simpson, whose mother died of tuberculosis when she was eleven months old (her father died of ptomaine poisoning before she was seven), reported that her six months in the Farmingdale Preventorium—at age eight— was pleasant. She remembered a quarantine period before she moved in with the other children. She declared that "the two weeks at the lower houses stands out in my memory as a time of pantheistic bliss. Never before had I known such freedom." (The housemother was so occupied with cooking and cleaning that she made few demands on the children.) Although Eileen complained about the group showers in the nude and the amount of mush and milk that she was forced to eat, she found her school work, the many diversions and outdoor activities enjoyable. Wilfert Shipe, who went to Mont Alto in 1944, remembered missing a year of school because the sanatorium offered no classes for his age group. In contrast to Eileen, he found the quarantine particularly lonely, since he had nothing to do. Children recognized that their time at preventoriums improved their health, even though they found the routine monotonous.[79]

Comparisons of Buenos Aires and Philadelphia Institutions

Public health policies in both Buenos Aires and Philadelphia reflected the international consensus that emerged between 1900 and 1910, which focused on preventing disease in children. In both Buenos Aires and Philadelphia, upper-class concern about the proper upbringing of poor children led to new social services to deal with ill and abandoned children. Physicians usually evaluated children as thin, weak and unhealthy rather than tubercular; they were sent to summer camps and preventoriums rather than sanatoriums. Public health officials most certainly failed to include the deaths of many of those children as dying of pulmonary tuberculosis. In both Buenos Aires and Philadelphia, more girls than boys died from pulmonary tuberculosis between the ages of fifteen and nineteen. Young women needed more protein during menstruation and when their bodies were developing. Girls age fifteen to nineteen years of poor working families would have been working hard at home or in sweat shops and often had poor diets. If there was a shortage of food, young women would have received the least. When their diets lacked protein, their resistance to disease declined. The deaths of young women influenced both population growth and economic prosperity. Poor children were more likely to succumb to tuberculosis because they had poor hygiene, insufficient food, and lived in housing that lacked sunlight and fresh air. Public health officials thought that children were in effect victimized by their tubercular relatives.

Both cities developed government-supported programs for pre-tubercular children, including many initiatives that were jointly supported by the government and the private sector. In Argentina, the state—co-operating with the Sociedad de Beneficencia and a number of immigrant groups—cared for orphaned and tubercular children. By 1916, Buenos Aires physicians had established a comprehensive system for caring for children who needed to be institutionalized: abandoned and healthy children went to the Casa Expósitos; sick but curable children to the Sanatorio Hospital de Niños; malnourished, pre-tubercular and non-contagious children under the age of fourteen went to the Sanatorio Marítimo y Solarium; curable tubercular children went to the Hospital Vicente López y Planes. Until 1947, the Sociedad de Beneficencia, which was almost entirely funded by the Argentine government, was the chief organization providing care for children and the tubercular in Buenos Aires. [80] In contrast, private charities in Philadelphia received little financial support from the city. Although Philadelphia did not have a clear policy for dealing with tubercular children, its orphanages, hospitals and private religious charities offered care.

In both Philadelphia and Buenos Aires, class influenced children's opportunities and treatment. When middle- and upper-class families faced economic and medical difficulties, extended families cared for children. Working parents with limited resources used a variety of strategies to care for their children. Sometimes they sent their children to orphanages, made them work at an early age or forced boys to support themselves by living on the streets. Children in Philadelphia remained in orphanages for a shorter time than those in Buenos Aires. Philadelphia orphanages accepted many street children; as a result, the city had fewer problems than Buenos Aires with unruly urchins. Public orphanages in Buenos Aires were more crowded, faced more problems with illness and had less financial support than did orphanages in Philadelphia. Although children in both cities went to orphanages because one or both of parents had died of tuberculosis, Philadelphia children were less likely to contract tuberculosis in orphanages than children in Buenos Aires. As governments developed new programs to support the poor, the need for orphanages in Buenos Aires and Philadelphia declined.

The U.S. and Argentine physicians treated tubercular children similarly. In both Buenos Aires and Philadelphia, children went to open-air schools, mountain preventoriums and vacation colonies. Special school programs sought to identify tubercular children at an early stage of the disease, promoted their isolation from tubercular adults, taught hygiene to children, and encouraged a nutritious diet and exercise. Although the Henry Phipps Institute provided more accurate information on the incidence of tuberculosis in school-age children, the Buenos Aires Department of Health began offering medical exams for the city's school children in 1892, ten years before Philadelphia did. The Buenos Aires municipal government also established open-air schools two years before Philadelphia did. Public services in both Buenos Aires and Philadelphia provided special instructions for teachers, better inspection and control of the milk supply, and free lunches for malnourished children.

From 1915 to 1931, more than 7,000 Philadelphia children received a sponsored week or two in the country in the summer, while 2,000 were cared for in sanatoriums and preventoriums.[81] The summer programs were too short to cure children; often children's health deteriorated after they returned home. As a result, public health officials recommended preventoriums. Most children in both Argentina and Pennsylvania were sent to preventoriums rather than sanatoriums, because it was assumed that children were less likely to contract tuberculosis than adults. Both Argentine and North American physicians utilized seashore preventoriums for children with tuberculosis of the glands, bones and joints; however, neither country's preventoriums wanted children with active pulmonary tuberculosis. When physicians diagnosed children with tuberculosis of the lungs, they were sent to hospitals or occasionally sanatoriums that accommodated both adults and children.

Until the 1930s, preventoriums offered few educational opportunities. But since children could spend several years in an institution, both preventoriums and sanatoriums provided teachers and social activities for the children. But institutional stays often meant that children were separated from family and friends for several years; institutionalized children also needed to adapt to a new environment and to a structured schedule.[82] Pennsylvania preventoriums had more permissive rules governing children than did the Sanatorio Marítimo and Solarium. Food at Mont Alto was more varied and nutritious than in Argentina. In both countries, the institutions sought to teach discipline, religious values and vocational skills to working-class, immigrant and poor children. The seriousness of children's illnesses varied greatly, as did their degree of improvement. Cures were elusive, but most physicians hoped that children who stayed at preventoriums for at least six months would become healthy and develop a resistance to tuberculosis.[83]

In Argentina, parents generally preferred the outpatient services provided by the Patronato de la Infancia, Asistencia Pública, Sociedad de Beneficencia and Hospital de Niños rather than hospital care so that they could continue to care for their children at home. Argentina's neighborhood clinics and the Cantinas Maternales provided parents with another outpatient option. In Philadelphia, families preferred the services of clinics established by religious groups or the state to hospital care. Early in the century, Buenos Aires and Philadelphia clinics had been important treatment centers for tuberculosis; but increasingly they focused, instead, on broader social and medical issues. Although Philadelphia and Buenos Aires clinics continued to emphasize preventive measures and to provide free milk to tuberculosis patients, less than twenty percent of those going to the clinics had tuberculosis. Public education continued to be important. By the 1920s, modern public health campaigns, adequate sewage and potable water reduced childhood mortality in both Buenos Aires and Philadelphia. By the 1940s, increased social services for poor families (including single-parent families) in Argentina and the U.S. decreased the number of abandoned children.[84]

Between 1870 and 1945, the government health programs and private charities for the poor in both the U.S. and Argentina remained limited, and facilities were often overcrowded. But in both countries, health professionals expanded programs in response to growing demands. It was often easier to justify expenditures for children (as opposed to adults), since their health seemed to improve more quickly. The Argentine and U.S. government policies continued to reflect the belief that charities and governments should support programs to develop healthy children. The goal was for them to develop into vigorous, patriotic adults who could serve in the military and contribute to the national economy. The declining number of adults with tuberculosis led to fewer tubercular children—and hence, to fewer preventoriums. But since young men failed to pass physicals exams to enter the army in World War II, there is some evidence that government health programs to improve the health of poor children were not altogether effective. The eventual decline of tuberculosis among children stemmed from the decrease of tuberculosis among adults and the improvement in living standards.

Notes

1 Francisco Ragno, "Manifestaciones anormales de las tuberculosis infantiles," *La Semana Médica (Buenos Aires)* 8, no. 20 (16 May 1901): 285–86.
2 "Why I Am Thankful," *Spunk* 19, no. 10 (January 1928): 43, written by a sixth grader in the Children's infirmary at Mont Alto.

3 The papers presented in 1908 at the Sixth International Congress on Tuberculosis in Washington, D.C., acknowledged the large number of children with tuberculosis. See, for example, Wood Hutchinson, "The Localization of Tuberculosis in Children," in *Transactions of the Sixth International Congress on Tuberculosis Washington, September 28 to October 5, 1908* (Philadelphia: William F. Fell Company, 1908), 2, 417–21; Theodore B. Sachs, "Children of the Tuberculous," *Transactions* 2: 479–86 and Cleveland Floyd and Henry I. Bowditch, "A Clinical Study of the Transmission and Progress of Tuberculosis in Children through Family Association," *Transactions* 2: 493–502. Also see, Richard A. Meckel, "Open-Air Schools and the Tuberculous Child in Early 20th Century America," *Archives of Pediatric and Adolescent Medicine* 150 (January 1996): 91–96 and T. N. Kelynack, "Tuberculosis in Infancy and Childhood: The Problem Stated," in *Tuberculosis in Infancy and Childhood: Its Pathology, Prevention, and Treatment*, ed. T.N. Kelynack (London: Bailliere, Tindall and Cox, 1908), 2–9; Leticia Acosta, "Defensa de la infancia contra la tuberculosis," MD diss., Facultad de Medicina, Universidad de Buenos Aires, 1918 (Buenos Aires: Imp. Vitullo Osurio Hnos., 1918), 49, 66–70; Eugene L. Opie, "Infection with Tuberculosis in Children and in Adults, and the Relations of One to the Other," *Transactions of the College of Physicians*, Third Series, 49 (1927): 25–27, 46–47; Cynthia Connolly, "Pale, Poor and 'Pretubercular' Children: A History of Pediatric Antituberculosis Efforts in France, Germany, and the United States 1899–1929," *Nursing Inquiry* 11, no. 3 (2004): 140 and Cynthia A. Connolly, *Saving Sickly Children the Tuberculosis Preventorium in American Life, 1909–1970* (New Brunswick: Rutgers University, 2008), 15, 22, 26–27.

4 Buenos Aires, *Year-Book of the City of Buenos Aires, 1910 and 1911* (Buenos Aires: Centenário Alegre, 1912), 122.

5 Buenos Aires, *Year-Book, 1910–1911*, 119–20; The Buenos Aires statistics for pulmonary tuberculosis deaths of minors 0–19 and adults 20–100 from 1900 to 1911 did not equal the generally accepted number of tuberculosis deaths; the total number of tuberculosis deaths was 93.8–97.1 percent (except in 1901) of the sum of minor and adult pulmonary deaths.

6 Henry Koplik, "Tuberculosis in Infancy and Childhood," *John Hopkins Hospital Bulletin* 23 (April 1912): 113–14; Vera Blinn Reber, "Poor, Ill and Sometimes Abandoned: Tubercular Children in Buenos Aires, 1880–1920," *Journal of Family History* 27, no. 2 (April 2002): 2, 134, 135. Generoso A. Schiavone, "La Tuberculosis en la primera infancia," *La Semana Médica* 37, no. 14 (3 April 1930): 868–69, 875–78.

7 Victoria Mazzeo, *La Mortalidad infantil en Buenos Aires, 1856–1986* (Buenos Aires: Centro Editor de América Latina, 1993), 32–33; Antonio D'Angelo Anzorena, *Tuberculosis de la Primera Infancia* (MD diss., Facultad de Medicina, Universidad de Buenos Aires, Buenos Aires: Imp. Bossio & Bigliani, 1917), 77–81. José M. Borkowski, "Tuberculosis en el escolar" (MD diss., Facultad de Medicina, Universidad de Buenos Aires, 1919), 16; Ricardo L. Hansen and Leonardo P. Repetti, "La Tuberculosis de la segunda década," *La Prensa Médica Argentina* 29 (23 September 1942): 1518–20.

8 Eduardo O. Ciafarado, *Niños en la ciudad de Buenos Aires, 1890–1910* (Buenos Aires: Centro Editor de América Latina, 1992), 46–47; Gregorio Aráoz Alfaro, *La tuberculosis infantil en la República Argentina, Relación presentada al 2 Congreso Médico Latina América* (Buenos Aires: Imprenta Liberia y Casa Editora de A. Etchepareborda, 1904), 22; U. S. Department of Commerce, Bureau of the Census, *Thirteenth Census of the United States Taken in the Year 1910* (Washington, DC: Government Printing Office, 1923), 3, 605.

9 Ciafarado, *Niños en la ciudad*, 9, 34.

10 Ciafardo, *Niños en la ciudad*, 8, 13–15, 18–20; Héctor Recalde, *La higiene y el trabajo: 1870–1930* (Buenos Aires: Centro Editor de América Latina, 1988), II, 77.

11 Augusto Bunge, "El trabajo industrial en Buenos Aires: Informe presentado al Departamento Nacional de Higiene," *Anales del Departamento Nacional de Higiene* 11, no. 9 (September 1904): 404–6 and 11, no. 10 (October 1904): 446–47; Ciafardo, *Niños en la ciudad*, 18.

12 See Donna J. Guy, "Niños abandonados en Buenos Aires, 1880–1914 y el desarrollo del concepto de la madre," *Mujeres y Cultura en la Argentina del siglo XIX*, ed. Lea Fletcher (Buenos Aires: Feminaria Editorial, 1994), 217–26 for an excellent discussion of the problems of abandonment and state efforts to deal with the problem. See also Mazzeo, *Mortalidad infantil*, 72; Donna J. Guy, "Mothers Alive and Dead: Multiple Concepts of Mothering in Buenos Aires," in *Sex and Sexuality in Latin America*, eds. Daniel Balderston and Donna J. Guy (New York: New York University Press, 1997), 160 for illegitimate births.

13 Donna J. Guy, *Women Build the Welfare State: Performing Charity and Creating Rights in Argentina, 1880–1955* (Durham: Duke University Press, 2009), 50, 60–61, 74–78.

14 Archivo General de la Nación Argentina (hereafter AGN), Fondos de Sociedad de Beneficencia (hereafter SB), legajo 121, vol. 8, 1915; Juan A. Alsina, *El obrero en la República Argentina* (Buenos Aires: Imprenta Calle de Mexico, 1905), 137; Norberto Pérez, "Asilo de Huérfanos," *Revista de Higiene Infantil* 1 (1892): 601; AGN, SB, Asilo de Huérfanos, 1 May 1901, legajo 92, vol. 3. See various documents indicating that the number of children at the Huérfanos was smaller; for example, AGN, SB, Asilo 19 August 1909, vol. 6; 31 December 1911, vol. 7; and 31 December 1912, vol. 7.

15 Ubaldo Fernandez, "La Mortalidad infantil," *La Semana Médica* 25, no. 24 (13 June 1918): 659; Guy, "Niños abandonados," 220; Cynthia Jeffress Little, "Society of Beneficence in Buenos Aires, 1823–1900" (PhD diss., Temple University, 1980), 109–10, suggests that the mortality generally varied from 15 to 32 percent with a high of 54 percent and a low of 10.5 percent.

16 AGN, SB, Asilo de Huérfanos, 21 March 1885, legajo 92, vol. 1; 18 November 1914, vol. 8.

17 Guy, "Niños abandonados," 222–24; Donna J. Guy "Mothers Alive and Dead: Multiple Concepts of Mothering in Buenos Aires," in *Sex and Sexuality in Latin America*, eds. Daniel Balderston and Donna J. Guy (New York: New York University Press, 1997), 160; Donna J. Guy, "Niñas en la cárcel; La Casa Correccional de Mujeres como instituto de socorro infantil," in *Historia de las mujeres en la Argentina*, eds. Fernando Gil Lozano, Valeria Silvina Pita, María Gabriela Ini, vol. 2 (Buenos Aires: Aguilar Altea Taurus Alfaguara, 2000), 27–32; for the number of minors in prison, 30.

18 Donna J. Guy, "Niñas en la cárcel," 35, 41; Mazzeo, *Mortalidad infantil*, 73; Guy, "Niños abandonados," 220; S. Madrid Paez, "Asistencia preventiva de la infancia en la lucha antituberaculosa," *Primer Congreso Pan América de la Tuberculosis Córdoba, Octubre 10–16 de 1927*, Tomo 3 (Córdoba: Imprenta de la Universidad, 1927), 166.

19 Little, 122–24; Genaro Sisto, "La escuela preventiva de mar para niños débiles y su importancia en la profilaxis antituberculosa," *La Semana Médica* 26, no. 11 (13 March 1919): 264–69.

20 AGN, SB, Asilo de Huérfanas, 6 October 1908, legajo 92, vol. 68 and 19 October 1908. The administration's explanation was probably correct, because tuberculosis usually has an extended gestation period.

21 AGN, SB, Hospital de Niños, legajo 119, vol. 1, "Acta adicional sobre la fundación e inauguración de Hospital de Niños" and 11 June 1896, vol. 2; Emilio Coni, "La asistencia de niños enfermos en Buenos Aires," *Revista de Higiene Infantil* 1 (1892): 597–98; Oscar R. C. Vogliano, *Hospital de Niños* (Buenos Aires: Colophon, 1975), 37–44, 97; Caupolicán R. Castilla, "Hospital de Niños: en el cincuentenario de la fundación de su actual edificio," *La Semana Médica* 50 (9 December 1943): 1331–32. AGN, SB, Hospital de Niños, 31 January 1911 and 28 February 1911, legajo 120, vol. 6.

22 José M. Jorge, "Estadística del Hospital de Niños correspondiente al año 1878," *Anales del Círculo Médico Argentino* 2, no. 5 (July 1979): 324–29; Alsina, *Obrero*, 137–38; AGN, SB, Hospital de Niños, 25 November 1904, legajo 119, vol. 3.

23 "La tuberculosis como enfermedad popular; causas; medios de prevenirla y curla," *La Revista de la Tuberculosis* 1, no. 3 (August 1901): 82; AGN, SB, Hospital de Niños, 1906–1907, legajo 120, vol. 4 and 2 November 1908, legajo 120, vol. 5.

24 AGN, SB, Hospital de Niños, 1906-07, legajo 120, vol.4, 23 November 1906; ibid., 31 December 1908; ibid., 20 May 1914, ibid 10 March 1915; ibid., 27 November 1916, legajo 121, vol. 7. AGN, SB, Hospital de Niños, 1943–1949, legajo 114, exp. 9355/3.

25 Timothy A. Hacsi, *Second Home: Orphan Asylums and Poor Families in America* (Cambridge, MA: Harvard University Press, 1997), 50–53.

26 Michael E. Teller, *The Tuberculosis Movement: A Public Health Campaign in the Progressive Era* (New York: Greenwood Press, 1988), 36–37; Hacsi, *Second Home* 1–4, 195, 213–20.

27 Timothy Hacsi, *Second Home: Orphan Asylums and Poor Families in America* (Cambridge: Harvard University Press, 1997), 28, 49–50, 195, 211, 219, 221–28, 249–50.

28 Francis Xavier Roth, *History of St. Vincent's Orphan Asylum, Tacony, Philadelphia: Memoir of Its Diamond Jubilee, 1855–1933* (Philadelphia: Nord-Amerika Press, 1934), 13–15, 17–19, 35, 45–46, 61, 71, 778.

29 Jules Doneson, *Deeds of Love: A History of the Jewish Foster Home and Orphan Asylum of Philadelphia: America's First Jewish Orphanage* (New York: Vantage Press, 1996), 5–6, 15, 44, 169. For a discussion of Jewish orphanages in Buenos Aires see Donna J. Guy *Women Build the Welfare State*, 50–51.

30 S. J. Kleinberg, *Widows and Orphans First: Family Economy and Social Welfare Policy 1880–1930* (Urbana: University of Illinois Press, 2006), 162–66.

31 League of Nations, Health Organisation, *Tuberculosis Statistics: Summary of the Report Addressed by Dr. S. Rosenfeld (Vienna) to the Health Committee of the League of Nations, April 1925* (Réunies, Chambéry: Health Section, 1926), 22.

32 Zacarías Gutman, "Diagnóstico de tuberculosis infantil y sus dificultades" (MD diss., Facultad de Medicina, Universidad de Buenos Aires, 1904, Buenos Aires: Imprenta Librería y casa editor de A. Etchepareborda, 1904), 33; "Algunas formas clínicas especiales de tuberculosis pulmonar en el niño," *La Semana Médica* 24, no. 17 (26 April 1917): 504–5; Juan P. Garrahan and Octavio M. Pico, "La escuela para niños débiles en la profilaxis antituberculosa, los niños débiles," *La Semana Médica* 27, no. 23 (20 May 1920): 698–99; Acosta, 50–62; Koplik, 119–20; Frank A. Craig, "The Prognosis in Pulmonary Tuberculosis in Children under Fifteen Years of Age (USA)," in *Transactions of the Sixth International Congress*, vol. 2, 668; L. Emmett Holt, "A Report Upon One Thousand Tuberculin Tests in Young Children,"

in *Transactions of the Sixth International*, vol. 2, 557–58; Frederic Maurice McPhedran, "The Diagnosis and Classification of Pulmonary Tuberculosis in Childhood and Adolescence," *American Review of Tuberculosis* 20, no. 4 (October 1929): 536.

33 For Buenos Aires see Ciafarado, *Los Niños en la ciudad*, 9 and Donna J. Guy, "The Politics of Pan-American Cooperation: Maternalist, Feminism and the Child Rights Movement, 1913-1960," in *Feminism and Internationalism*, eds. Mrinaline Sinha, Donna Guy and Angel Woolacott (Oxford: Blackwell, 1999), 112.

34 Ragno, 286–89; Gregorio Aráoz Alfaro, "Tuberculosis difusa de los niños," *Revista de la Sociedad Médica Argentina* 3, no. 15 (May/June 1894): 157–60.

35 Emilio R. Coni, "Mortalidad infantil en 1891," *Revista de Higiene* 1 (1892): 21.

36 J. Claxton Gittings, Frank Crozer Knowles and Ashley P. C. Ashhurst, *Tuberculosis in Infancy and Childhood: Lectures Delivered at the Children's Hospital, Philadelphia, under the Auspices of the Philadelphia Pediatric Society* (Philadelphia: J.B. Lippincottt Company, 1922), 262–63; Craig, "The Prognosis in Pulmonary Tuberculosis," 668; Schiavone, 868–69, 875–81.

37 José D. Terán, *Pre-Tuberculosis: Contribución a su estudio* (Buenos Aires: Arsenio Guidi Buffarine, 1905), 61–66, 73–77; Garrahan and Pico, 699; Aráoz Alfaro, "La Tuberculosis infantil," 25; Gittings, Knowles and Ashhurst, 229–68. For a discussion of the use of tuberculin with adults, see Chapter 4.

38 Pedro Cantonnet, "La Frenicectomía en la tuberculosis pulmonar del niño," *La Semana Médica* 39, no. 15 (14 April 1932): 1191; Paride T. Panza, "Sobre profilaxis de la tuberculosis," *La Semana Médica* 28, no. 12 (24 March 1921): 37–38; Sisto, 265–66.

39 Mazzeo, *Moralidad infantil*, 63–64, 70–72; Acosta, 66–7.

40 Gittings, Knowles and Ashhurt, 233–34.

41 Eduardo Ciafardo, "La práctica benéfica y el control de los sectores populares de la ciudad de Buenos Aires, 1889–1910," *Revista de Indias* 54, no. 201 (May/August 1994): 383–408, contends that charity associations sought not only to alleviate social problems of the poor but also to implement capitalist effort to regulate, organize and disciple them with the religious objective of converting the poor to Catholicism and teaching Christian morality, the moral imperative to work, and the failing of socialist and anarchist thinking.

42 Coni, *Higiene Social: Asistencia y previsión social: Buenos Aires caritativo y previsor* (Buenos Aires: Imprenta de Emilio Spinella, Ed., 1918), 432–34; "Liga Argentina contra la tuberculosis," *Alianza de Higiene Social* 9, nos. 8/9 (January/February, 1910): 229–32; Aráoz Alfaro, "La tuberculosis infantil," 22.

43 Ramón Iribarne and Juan M. Hitache, "La educación antituberculosa," in *República Argentina, Primer Congreso Nacional de Medicina, vol. 5, Actas y Trabajos: Biología y patología: higiene y medicina pública* (Buenos Aires: Imprenta y Casa Editora de Flaiban, 1918), 492–93; Genaro Giacobini, "La medicina escolar en la lucha contra la tuberculosis," in *República Argentina, Segundo Congreso Nacional de Medicina, 1 al 8 Octubre de 1922, vol. 5, Actas y Trabajos* (Buenos Aires: Las Ciencias, 1927), 260–62; Borkowski, 72–73, 106, 126; Heather Munro Prescott, "The White Plague Goes to College: Tuberculosis Prevention Programs in Colleges and Universities, 1920–1960," *Bulletin of the History of Medicine* 74, no. 4 (Winter

2000): 753; Teller, 110, 119; Knopf, *Tuberculosis: Preventable and Curable* (1909), 252–59.

44 Genaro Giacobini, "La tuberculosis pulmonar en el niño escolar," *Primer Congreso Pan-Americano de la Tuberculosis, Córdoba 10–16 Octubre 19223* (Córdoba: Imprenta de la Universidad, 1922): 284–85; John Molitor, "Educational Hygiene as Applied to School Children," *Spunk* 12, no. 2 (May 1920): 5–10.

45 "Inspección escolar en la República Argentina, Uruguay, Chile y Brasil," *Alianza de Higiene Social* 9, no. 7 (December 1909): 218–20; Coni, "La lucha antituberculosa," (1905): 137–39.

46 Sisto, 265.

47 Gittings, Knowles and Ashhurst, 13; American Philosophical Society (hereafter APS), Eugene Opie Papers (hereafter OP), "Tuberculosis in School Children in Philadelphia," Box 50, Tuberculosis no. 4; David McBride, *From TB to Aids: Epidemics among Urban Blacks since 1900* (Albany: State University of New York Press, 1991), 64, 87.

48 Meckel, 95; Teller, 111.

49 Meckel, 91–99; H. W. Hetherlington, "Open-Air Schools for the Treatment of Tuberculosis in Children," in *Tuberculosis in Public School Children* (Philadelphia: Henry Phipps Institute, University of Pennsylvania, 1929), 512–18; Teller, 114–16; Connolly, "Pale, Poor and 'Pretubercular' Children," 142.

50 "La escuela para niños débiles," *Alianza de Higiene Social* 9, no. 7 (December 1909): 198–99; Garrahan and Pico, 700; Teodoro A. Tonina, "Las escuelas al aire libre," *La Semana Médica* 30, no. 3 (18 January 1923): 104–5; Emilio R. Coni, "Asistencia de tuberculosos en la Capital Federal," *Revista de Ciencias Médicas* 8, no. 92 (1925–26): 214–15.

51 Teller, 82, 113–14; Sherman C. Kingsley, ed., *Open Air Crusaders: A Report of the Elizabeth McCormick Open-Air School together with a General Account of Open Air School Work in Chicago and a Chapter on School Ventilation* (Chicago: United Charities of Chicago, 1910); James H. Cassedy, *Charles V. Chapin and the Public Health Movement* (Cambridge: Harvard University Press, 1962), 130; Meckel, 92, 95; Historical Society of Pennsylvania, pamphlet, "Day Camp for Tuberculosis," (Philadelphia: William F. Fell Company, 1912); Historical Society of Pennsylvania, Pennsylvania Society for the Prevention of Tuberculosis, *Annual Report 1913* (Philadelphia: William F. Fell Company, 1913), 28–29.

52 Emilio R. Coni, "La lucha antituberculosa en América Latina," *Alianza de Higiene Social*, 9, nos. 3–4 (August/September 1909): 76; Emilio R. Coni, "Colonia de vacaciones de Bella Vista," *Alianza de Higiene Social* 9, no. 7 (December 1909): 195; Coni, "La lucha antituberculosa" (1905): 140.

53 AGN, SB, Casa de Huérfanas, November 1918, legajo 39, exp. 631–32.

54 Meckel, 95; Cynthia Anne Connolly, "The TB Preventorium," *American Journal of Nursing*, 100, no. 10 (2000): 62.

55 Cynthia A. Connolly, "Nurses: The Early Twentieth Century Tuberculosis Preventorium's 'Connecting Link'," *Nursing History Review* 10 (2002): 130–31, 141.

56 Connolly, "The TB Preventorium," 62–64; Connolly, "Pale, Poor and 'Pretubercular,'" 143; José M. Jorge, "Sanatorio Marítimo y Solarium de Mar del Plata," *La Semana Médica* 28, no. 35 (1 September 1921): 258–59.

57 "Sanatorio Marítimo de Mar del Plata," *Revista de la Tuberculosis* 1, no. 8 (January 1902): 285; Coni, "La lucha antituberculosa" (1905): 159–60; Jorge, "Sanatorio Marítimo," 261–62.

58 AGN, SB, Sanatorio Marítimo, Hospital y Asilo Marítimo, legajo 103, vol. 3; "Sanatorio Marítimo de Mar del Plata, 288.

59 AGN, SB, Sanatorio Marítimo, legajo 100, exp. 7988, Mar del Plata, 21 November 1938; AGN, SB, Sanatorio Marítimo, legajo 102, exp. 1034, 8 January 1946 and "Ingreso de menores," 1946–48; Jorge, "Sanatorio Marítimo," 266; Jorge R. Dietsch, "Sanatorios marítimos: sus importancia y necesidad en la asistencia social," *Revista de la Asociación Médica Argentina* 56 (January 1942): 36.

60 AGN, SB, Sanatorio Marítimo, 15 November 1899, legajo 103, vol. 1, "Promedio del costo diario de asilados;" AGN, SB, Solárium Mar del Plata, legajo 96, exp. 7103, "informes," Mar del Plata, 4 February 1926.

61 For example see, AGN, SB, Solárium Mar del Plata, 5 June 1920, legajo 95, exp. 6; AGN, SB, Sanatorio Marítimo, 30 September 1920, legajo 98, exp. 2894. AGN, SB has extensive material on personnel.

62 Coni, "La lucha antituberculosa" (1905): 159–60. Jorge, "Sanatorio Marítimo," 266, 292–95; AGN, SB, Sanatorio Marítimo, 21 October 1921, legajo 98, exp. 4794; AGN, SB, Sanatorio Marítimo, 7 November 1921, exp. 4907; AGN, SB, Sanatorio Marítimo, legajo 102, exp. 1034, "Ingreso de menores," 1946–48, 24 July 1946 and 29 October 1946.

63 For a discussion of the children's schedules, meals, and activities, see Jorge, "Sanatorio Marítimo," 262–64, 269–83, 288–91, 295; AGN, SB, Sanatorio Marítimo, legajo 98, exp. 7109, Mar del Plata, March 9, 1926. AGN, SB, Sanatorio Marítimo, 21 October 1921 and November 1921, legajo 98.

64 AGN, SB, HVLP, General Rodríguez 15 March 1918, legajo 123; AGN, SB, HVLP, 28 November 1922, legajo 124, "Inconveniencias formas de admisión enfermas;" AGN, SB, HVLP, legajo 124, "Movimiento de niños comprendidos entre los 3 y 13 años habido durante los años de 1916–1921"; AGN, SB, HVLP, legajo 123, "Dinero recibido por el superior gobernador para diferentes construcciones;" legajo 126, November 1927, "Isaac Fernández Blanco"; AGN, SB, Asilo de Huérfano, legajo 87, exp. 8486, "Asilo de Huérfanos respecto a niños enfermos, Asilo General Martin Rodríguez," 1927; AGN, SB, Sanatorio Marítimo legajo 102, exp. 1034, Buenos Aires 1946; AGN, SB, HVLP, legajo 135, exp. 26360.

65 AGN, SB, Hospital de Llanura Vicente López y Planes, 20 October 1922, legajo 124; ibid., 28 October 1922; ibid., 9 November 1922; ibid., 14 November 1922; ibid., 16 January 1923; ibid., 30 January 1923.

66 AGN, SB, HVLP, legajo 123, General Rodríguez 22 September 1917 (sent to) Señora Inspectora de turno de Hospital Vicente López y Planes; AGN, SB, HVLP, legajo 123, General Rodríguez, 15 March 1918; AGN, SB, HVLP, Asilo de Huérfanos, legajo 87, exp. 8486, "Asilo de Huérfanos;" AGN, SB, HVLP, legajo 135, exp. 22849, 16 June 1948.

67 AGN, SB, HVLP, legajo 126, 24 January 1928, "Se la Hace saber que deber prohibir bailes"; AGN, SB, HVLP, legajo 127, 23 May 1929, "Solicitan la banda de música del Instituto 'Ángel T. de Alvear'"; AGN, SB, HVLP, legajo 129, 19 July 1935, "Reglamento del Hospital de Llanura Vicente López y Planes."

68 Meghan Crnic, "Seeking the Salubrious Sea: The Health and Environments of Urban American Families, 1870–1930" (2013), Publicly Accessible Penn Dissertations, 4–5, 94.

69 Crnic Meghan and Cynthia Connolly, "'They Can't Help Getting Well Here': Seaside Hospitals for Children in the United States: 1872–1917," *The Journal of the History of Childhood and Youth* 2, no. 2 (Spring 2009): 221, 223–28; Jacob A. Riis, "The Story of Sea Breeze," *The Outlook* 197 (May 1914): 85–88.

70 There is a question as to which was the first preventorium: Sea Breeze or Lakewood. Although Sea Breeze opened earlier it operated first as a seashore camp and then as a hospital. For statistics see Connolly, *Saving Sickly Children*, 2–3; for information on Lakewood, 55–59; Farmingdale, 60–79; Teller, 110; "Tuberculosis Work in Philadelphia," *Monthly Bulletin of the Department of Public Health and Charities of the City of Philadelphia* 4, no. 6 (June 1919): 86.

71 Connolly, *Saving Sickly Children*, 101–2; APS, OP, "River Crest, 1930," Tuberculosis Prevention, #4, Box 50, which includes a good deal of material on preventoriums nationally.

72 For statistics, see Fred C. Johnson, "Subdivision of Tuberculosis Sanatoria. Pennsylvania State Sanatorium for Tuberculosis No. 1 Mont Alto," in *Eleventh Annual Report of the Commissioner of Health for the Commonwealth of Pennsylvania, 1916* (Harrisburg: J. L. L. Kuhn Printer to the Commonwealth, 1920), 912–13 and R. H. McCutcheon, "Mont Alto Sanatorium: Past and Present," *The Listening Post* 1, no. 2 (January 1921): 6–9; A. J. Bohl, "Testing for Tuberculosis," *Pennsylvania's Health* no. 5 (September-October, 1930): 20–21; "Tuberculosis in the Young," *Spunk* 12, no. 12 (March 1921): 24.

73 "Children's Hospital: Notes: Wonder of a Child Patient," *Spunk* 18, no. 10 (January 1927): 31; Mary Brady Caverly, "From Cabin to Classic Revival," unpublished paper, 17 October 1994, 7–8; Wilfert Shipe, Jr., "First Hand Account: Life in the Children Preventorium, Mt. Alto, Pa. 1944–45," unpublished paper, 23 June 1998, Mt. Alto Archives.

74 Karl Schaffle, "The State Tuberculosis Dispensary an Asset to the Municipality," *Spunk* 9, no. 7 (October 1917): 9; "Children's Home," South Mountain Restoration Center, privately produced, 1935, videocassette, Mt. Alto Archives. Caverly, "From Cabin to Classic Revival," 4–8; Wilfert Shipe, Jr., "First Hand Account," *Spunk* 9, no. 7 (October 1917): 33–34; *Spunk* 4, no. 7 (October 1912): 27; "Children's Hospital Notes: Wonders of a Child Patient," 31–32.

75 "Christmas at the Preventorium," *Spunk* 18, no. 10 (January 1927): 31; "Mont Alto Notes," *Spunk* 9, no. 7 (October 1917): 33; *Spunk* 15, no. 2 (May 1923): 25; *Spunk* 19, no. 9, (December 1927): 43.

76 "Occupational Therapy," *Spunk* 12, no. 6 (September 1920): 51; "Children's Hospital Notes," *Spunk* 19, no. 4 (July 1927): 37; *Spunk* 19, no. 11 (February 1927): 44; *Spunk* 20, no. 2 (May 1928): 43.

77 "A Visit to the Children's Home," *Spunk* 4, no. 7 (October 1912): 27; Shipe, "First Hand Account."

78 University of Pennsylvania (hereafter UP), Visiting Nurse Societ of Philadelphia Records (hereafter VNS), Records MC5, Box 4, pp. 11–13, *Twenty-Third Annual Report of the Visiting Nurse Society of Philadelphia for Year Ending February 18, 1909*, "Report of Special Nurse on Tuberculosis," no. 2, vol. 20, 1 May 1908 to 28 February 1909.

79 Eileen Simpson, *Orphans: Real and Imaginary* (New York: Weidenfeld & Nicolson, 1987), 3–4, 47–61 (quote 51); Shipe, "First Hand Account."

80 AGN, SB, Hospital de Niños, 10 May 1915, 22 July 1915, 22 July 1915, 9 August 1915, legajo 121, vol. 8; Guy, *Women Build the Welfare State*, 134, 164–68.

81 Lawrence F. Flick, "The Crusade against Tuberculosis in Philadelphia," presented to the Philadelphia County Medical Society on 23 November 1932 (privately printed), 7–8.

82 For one of the few collections of childhood experiences, see Ann Shaw and Carole Reeves, eds., *The Children of Craig-y-nos: Life in a Welsh*

Tuberculosis Sanatorium, 1922–1959 (London: Wellcome Trust Centre for the History of Medicine, 2009), which provides oral interviews from adults who spent time as children or teenagers in a sanatorium; Connolly, *Saving Sickly Children*, 64–66, 69–71, 93–95, 118–22, details the attitudes of parents and children toward U.S. preventoriums.

83 Jorge, "Sanatorio Marítimo," 293–95; José Vallis, "Sanatorios Marítimos," *Revista de la Asociación Médica Argentina* 56, no. 477–78 (15–30 January 1942): 24–28; AGN, SB, Sanatorio Marítimo, 22 May 1893, legajo 103, vol. 1, "Informe sobre el resultado de la asistencia de este hospital de los niños expósitos" and 19 January 1921, legajo 98, exp. 1339.

84 Alejandro Raimondi, "Colocación familiar del recién nacido hijo de padres tuberculosis," *Archivos de Tisiología* Tomo 5, no. 2 (January–June 1928): 58–59; Guy, "Mothers Alive and Dead," 157–58, 166–69; Coni, "La lucha antituberculosa en América Latina," 75–77; Schiavone, 868.

7 Tuberculosis in Global and Comparative Perspective

> Consumption is caused by the inhalation of a very minute germ, the so-called tubercle bacillus, visible under high magnification.[1]
>
> Two Important Facts about Tuberculosis:
> Tuberculosis is preventable.
> Tuberculosis is curable.
>
> Tuberculosis is prevented by doing two things:
> 1 Killing the germs that cause the disease.
> 2 Having people become healthy, so that they will not be predisposed to the disease.[2]

Between 1870 and 1945, tuberculosis infected people in every region of the globe. Agreement on the nature and prevention of tuberculosis is reflected in the quotations above from the 1908 international tuberculosis conference. Government policies affecting tuberculosis shaped the exchange of ideas about the disease, efforts to prevent it and the search for a cure. Physician disagreements over the contagiousness of tuberculosis continued into the early twentieth century. However, patients were slower than health experts to accept that tuberculosis is infectious. Public health officials sought to improve working-class living conditions, personal hygiene and social habits through legislation and social pressure. Although cultures, medical traditions and individual choices influenced how local physicians and public health officials dealt with the disease, a worldwide consensus was emerging on the prevention and treatment of tuberculosis.

Formal international exchange of ideas concerning disease existed by the eighteenth century. Thus, U.S., British and West Indian physicians and scientists argued in their medical journals as to whether yellow fever was contagious or caused by the peculiarities of local climate. However, these discussions tended to emphasize national rather than international approaches to explanations of disease.[3] The international efforts at consensus on the nature and treatment of disease began unsuccessfully at the International Sanitary Conferences between 1851 and 1885; conference delegates could not agree to standardize quarantine and sanitation regulations against the spread of cholera and yellow fever. In contrast, by 1890, the international consensus on tuberculosis led to similar government policies and public health campaigns in many countries, including the U.S., Argentina, Great Britain and Japan.[4]

Tuberculosis physicians and public health specialists were among the first to promote global approaches to disease. Philadelphia and Buenos Aires physicians utilized medications and medical procedures developed in Europe. Public health experts adapted programs used by other cities. Globally, states built sanatoriums to treat tuberculosis patients. In the Americas and Europe, the fumigation of houses and other hygienic measures, such as the isolation of infected individuals and the safe disposal of sputa, were implemented to prevent infection and improve health. Such policies also focused on changing the morals of the poor and sought unsuccessfully to decrease alcoholism, prostitution and public rowdiness. With increased global contacts, public health officials worried about physical and moral contagion, since individuals were exposed to more germs and new ideas which undermined the patriarchal family and traditional religious values.

In the early twentieth century, western physicians and public health officials in all populated areas increasingly agreed on how to treat tuberculosis. Globally, as was seen in Buenos Aires and Philadelphia, treatments fell into two broad categories: medications/surgical procedures and fresh-air/diet regimens. Yet, in one sense, the agreements on treatment were possible because the fresh-air/diet regimens allowed flexibility and could include practitioners of folk medicines as well as homeopathic and osteopathic medicines. Physicians, who experimented with tuberculin injections, artificial pneumothorax or thoracoplasty reported on their results at national and international conferences. Governments and entrepreneurs built class-specific sanatoriums in the mountains and by seashores to treat patients.

Because European values and beliefs shaped Argentina and the U.S., differences over patient treatments and government policies were less varied than they were in Japan and India. Developments in France and Spain were extremely important in shaping tubercular programs in Buenos Aires. Spain's early acceptance of tuberculosis as contagious shaped colonial policy, while the French focus on the separation of babies from tubercular mothers influenced a similar policy in Buenos Aires. England, where physicians were members of the elite, distinct from those in the trade guilds such as surgeons and apothecaries, served as the model for Philadelphia doctors; at the same time, the U.S. never developed a national health service as comprehensive as Britain's. Koch's discovery of the tuberculosis bacillus in Berlin gave Germany the prestige to attract international tubercular experts. His laboratory focused on finding a cure for tuberculosis and attracted tuberculosis experts from all over the world. The advanced state of German research on tuberculosis assured

Germany's dominant influence on medical policy decisions in the U.S., Argentina, France and Great Britain.

Great Britain's Encounters with Tuberculosis

Great Britain was among the first nations attempting to counter tuberculosis. Several factors contributed to this early focus: the rise of industrialization, which saw an increase in the number of the tubercular poor; government statistics on mortality, which drew attention to tuberculosis; and the professional influence of physicians in shaping medical policies toward tuberculosis. By the first decade of the twentieth century, tuberculosis was the single greatest killer in Great Britain and responsible for one death in eight. Based on the number of deaths and the chronic nature of tuberculosis (patients suffered for four to five years before death), at least one in every forty adults between the ages of twenty and sixty had an active case of tuberculosis. Given the difficulty of diagnosis, the numbers were likely much higher.[5]

After Robert Koch's 1882 announcement that tuberculosis was contagious, the understanding of tuberculosis as a hereditary disease had to be revised. Yet six months after Koch's announcement, thirty-four of the thirty-six members of the Cambridge Medical Society viewed tuberculosis as hereditary. Michael Worboys maintains that Koch's importance in Great Britain rested on his new theory about germs, which created the discipline of bacteriology and research programs that sought to prevent and cure tuberculosis. Thus, Koch's greatest influence stemmed from the fact that germ theory persuaded physicians and the public that tuberculosis could be cured and prevented. If tuberculosis was not inherited, physicians could develop new procedures to cure it; and if it was contagious, public health officials needed to focus on prevention.[6]

British physicians reacted more quickly to the contagious nature of tuberculosis than their Buenos Aires and Philadelphia colleagues. The British formed the National Association for the Prevention of Consumption and other forms of Tuberculosis (NAPT) in 1898, six years before their counterparts in the U.S. took action. NAPT sought to educate the public about prevention methods, promote sanatoriums for the poor and terminate tuberculosis in cattle. By 1913, English physicians were required to report patients with tuberculosis; but general practitioners notified government officers only erratically. Whether in London, Philadelphia or Buenos Aires, patients often avoided doctors who notified government officials; the result was that only poor tuberculosis patients who utilized public services were consistently identified. The British campaign against tuberculosis between 1880 and 1914 was also linked to efforts to shape the morality of the poor, specifically men's alcoholism and vagrancy, women's work in prostitution and the failure to meet middle-class standards of hygiene; these endeavors preceded later reforms in Buenos Aires and Philadelphia. Because middle-class British women developed a feminist consciousness before their counterparts in either Argentina or the U.S., they played an active role in shaping British reform movements.[7]

Britons seemed less willing to accept public tuberculosis dispensaries than either Porteños or Philadelphians. British citizens resented paying taxes, while local medical practitioners believed that the public dispensaries were taking their patients. County medical health officials preferred financial support for public sanatoriums, rather than public clinics; they had no control over clinics and they received no additional funding for them. Furthermore, public dispensaries were primarily administrative and diagnostic centers. They did not treat patients, but instead only referred them to general practitioners. Without physician support, dispensaries which served the poor were often substandard. In spite of physician opposition, the number of public dispensaries increased in the 1930s, and tuberculosis prevention and treatment were included in public health services. As in the state tuberculosis clinics in Philadelphia, nurses weighed and took patients' temperatures, gave them sputum tests, and told them to eat more eggs and milk, to use separate utensils and to sleep in a room alone. Visiting health nurses occasionally told families to disinfect bedclothes by laundering with bleach and fumigating rooms. When tuberculin tests and X-rays became available, public dispensaries employed them to identify the tubercular.[8]

In the 1890s, British entrepreneurs sponsored small, private, nursing-home sanatoriums. It was expensive to travel to the continent, so when climate was deemphasized as part of the cure, opportunities opened for local British investors. By 1900, there were twenty-three private sanatoriums with some 400 beds located primarily in the British coastal resort areas. These sanatoriums served the middle class. The first two public sanatoriums opened in 1900 as part of a national anti-consumption campaign. Charitable sanatoriums were organized or operated by existing consumptive hospitals, a local branch of the NAPT, or prominent physicians supported by public funding. The British government took five years to build the Kings Sanatorium at Midhurst, Sussex; in 1905, it cost the equivalent of one million dollars and accommodated 100 patients. Due to high costs and individuals' preference for home treatment, sanatorium treatment in Britain, as in the U.S. and Argentina, remained limited. By 1913, only four percent of those diagnosed with tuberculosis went to sanatoriums for an average of a three-month stay.[9]

As in Buenos Aires and Philadelphia, tuberculosis contributed in Britain to the declining income of the poor. Based on the annual admissions to workhouse infirmaries in which sixty percent of patients had consumption, F.B. Smith argues that tuberculosis was a fundamental cause of pauperization in nineteenth-century England. The impoverished tubercular tended to be identified at the late stages of the disease, which diminished even further their slim chance of recovery. Tuberculosis mortality was as much as fifty percent higher in lower-class neighborhoods than upper-class districts. In the 1930s, in England and Wales, unskilled male laborers were almost twice as likely to be diagnosed with tuberculosis as were upper- and middle-class men. Private charities created sanatoriums for the underprivileged, but many poor people could not afford to stop working. British middle-class consumptives often went to small private nursing homes or sanatoriums in Britain or in southern Europe. Beginning in 1900, wealthy sufferers might enter one of London's hospitals specializing in tuberculosis treatment. Education and efforts to isolate tuberculosis patients characterized health policy in Great Britain as it did worldwide.[10]

Between 1850 and 1940, large-scale postmortem surveys in Great Britain revealed that tuberculosis in children was largely undiagnosed and under-reported. All parents focused on the health of their children, but for the poorest families, inadequate wages and housing and the parents' own health issues made paying for medical treatment difficult. Working-class parents' strategies for obtaining welfare were often limited by the availability of public infirmaries and their unwillingness to use them. Beginning in the 1890s, open-air schools and preventoriums treated underweight, anemic children. Public health officials supported preventive methods, including the boarding of poor children in foster homes in the country or their attendance at open-air schools. Middle-class parents utilized child-rearing manuals that taught them how to provide a clean healthy home. Fresh air and plenty of milk and meat were recommended for both girls and boys. Because elite parents could afford to provide for their children, they easily avoided tuberculosis prevention regulations. As in Buenos Aires and Philadelphia, class determined the type and availability of health care for children.[11]

During the first two decades of the twentieth century, national funding for both tuberculosis treatment and preventive efforts directed by the NAPT increased. The government began to license dairies in 1923. In 1925, owners had to notify the government of tubercular cattle; the owners were compensated when the cattle were slaughtered. Initially, these regulations did little to reduce bovine tuberculosis: in the 1930s, thirty percent of non-pulmonary and two percent of pulmonary tuberculosis deaths originated from the consumption of meat or milk from tubercular cattle. With advances in surgery during World War I, sanatorium and general hospital physicians used new techniques including thoracic surgery; but British physicians were less inclined to operate than their counterparts in the U.S. In 1942, seventy percent of the patients discharged from a New England sanatorium had some form of pneumothorax, while in the 1930s, in Britain only ten percent of patients had the same procedure. The Second World War changed tuberculosis practices in Great Britain. The increase of tuberculosis during the war years and the need for military recruits raised interest in the National Tuberculosis Service and encouraged mass radiography campaigns to identify early tuberculosis cases. The government paid allowances to patients and their families, and there was growing support among health professionals for BCG (Bacillus Calmette-Guérin) vaccinations to prevent tuberculosis. After the war, tuberculosis programs were reorganized under the new National Health Services.[12]

In the first half of the twentieth century, Britain provided training and employment opportunities at sanatoriums. Although it was usual for the lower and working classes to work in sanatoriums to help pay their expenses, the British placed a heavy emphasis on work therapy. Unique to Britain was the village settlement movement. The Papworth Village Settlement was the best-known example. Founded in 1917, it consisted of a hospital and sanatorium for those with tuberculosis and a village where former patients lived with their families and worked in industries at union pay rates. With the decline of tuberculosis in Britain after the war and the closing of sanatoriums, former patients continued to have difficulty finding work. When recovered, patients found jobs, these often paid less than those held before the patients became ill.[13]

The French Approach to Tuberculosis

In the early part of the nineteenth century, the French viewed consumption as hereditary as had the English, North Americans and Argentines. But an examination of French literature and opera suggests they also initially romanticized the disease. For example, the intellectual and artistic community viewed consumptive women as having heightened sensibilities and emotions. The Western European respect for French authors spread the image of the sensual consumptive woman widely, even when the charitable and medical communities viewed tuberculosis as contagious and female mortality was high. David Barnes points out that in the 1830s, in Paris, nearly two-thirds more women died of tuberculosis than men, whereas by 1890, when tuberculosis was more generally viewed as contagious, more men than women died. In the 1860s, Jean Antoine Villemin's research showed that tuberculosis was an infectious disease. This made it easier for the French to accept Koch's 1882 discovery, although there was disagreement as to how contagion occurred and what policies should be implemented. In the last half of the nineteenth century, many French people moved from the country to the city. This migration led to increased sanitary problems in the cities, as well as the spread of tuberculosis from cities to the home villages since infected individuals often returned home to benefit from the country air or to die.[14]

In all European countries and the U.S., public health professionals blamed the poor and working class for the large number of tuberculosis cases. In line with this reasoning, French public health programs were directed at the poor and campaigns against spitting, disinfection and prostitution were initiated to prevent the spread of tuberculosis. As in Argentina, the French women worked in charitable organizations to teach the working class to adopt middle-class family values and ideas of healthy living. The bourgeoisie particularly criticized the lack of sunlight, poor ventilation, filth and overcrowded working-class housing. Both the French government and private enterprise disinfected rooms of those who died of a contagious disease. Although the number of properties disinfected rose during the early twentieth century, too often disinfection simply meant cleaning and deodorizing. David Barnes argued that in no other country was venereal disease and prostitution linked with tuberculosis as they were in France. Alcoholism and syphilis combined with prostitution and sexual excesses were commonly cited by physicians to explain tuberculosis among the poor in France and in Argentina. Furthermore, tubercular prostitutes were not viewed as victims or potential patients but as the source of contagion. However, in spite of the efforts of French social services, there is no evidence that either disinfection or decreased alcoholism lowered the number of tuberculosis patients.[15]

The wealthy did not want dispensaries in their neighborhoods, so they were instead established in poor districts. Dispensary personnel educated families on how contagion occurred and provided food, clothing and medication for those who chose not to go to sanatoriums or those who were not offered sanatorium beds because they were considered terminal cases. In 1919, the government supported the creation of sanatoriums and contributed to patient support, but beds were limited. The French government did not introduce the BCG vaccination until 1925 because of concerns about its safety, even though the French developed the BCG vaccination in 1908.[16]

French socialists denounced the disproportionate incidence of tuberculosis among the working class as well as middle-class efforts to blame the poor for the spread of tuberculosis. The French Left pointed to the significance of contagion before Koch offered evidence to support that view. Because socialists accepted the medical establishment's view of tuberculosis as contagious, they sought to absolve workers of the blame for tuberculosis by focusing instead on their limited income and poor working conditions. The French Left saw tuberculosis as a side effect of industrial capitalism and economic exploitation. Syndicalists made working-class health an important political issue. They emphasized that tuberculosis resulted from diminished resistance due to malnutrition, overwork, long hours, poor housing and low wages. The Left also pointed to the lower tuberculosis mortality rate that stemmed from wage increases and reduced working hours. In addition, it argued for public-supported sanatorium care for workers. Because the government came to view tuberculosis as an occupational disease, French workers with tuberculosis received medical treatment analogous to that of industrial accidents. In contrast, the Philadelphia socialist and labor movements focused on organizing labor unions, actions to increase wages and reduce numbers of working hours, and electing individuals to political office; there is no evidence that they had any interest in tuberculosis prevention policies. The Argentine socialist movement did seek to improve living conditions of patients in sanatoriums and working conditions in the "dusty" trades where poor air circulation led to a variety of respiratory diseases including tuberculosis. However, the labor movement in Buenos Aires devoted little effort to an anti-tuberculosis campaign.[17]

French physicians resisted the required reporting of tuberculosis cases to local authorities as a violation of patient confidentiality. As in Buenos Aires and Philadelphia, French public health physicians most consistently reported tuberculosis among the poor and working classes. When wealthy individuals became infected with tuberculosis, they tended to blame their female domestic servants. As in other countries, French physicians lacked the ability to provide a cure, and the best private physicians could do was to assure that their wealthy patients died in more comfort. Although it is always difficult to prove the significance of cultural influences, French attitudes toward tuberculosis agreed with those of Argentina. In particular, the Porteño and the French held similar attitudes toward prostitution and alcoholism as causes of tuberculosis. The Argentine elites respected French culture, generally understood French and preferred to study at the Institut Pasteur rather than in Berlin.

Germany's Impact on Global Policies

Of the European countries, Germany had the most impact on the development of global tuberculosis policies because physicians and researchers worldwide looked to German research to understand the cause of tuberculosis and for a cure. In the 1860s, Germany initiated the sanatorium regimen, which emphasized fresh air, diet and rest. In the 1890s, Robert Koch developed and tested tuberculin, which failed as a cure but became a useful diagnostic tool. However, German physicians could not agree on which treatment was most useful and split into two groups: those who advocated rest, fresh air, improved nutrition and exercise, and those who recommended Koch's tuberculin. Germans also advanced arguments for the use of artificial pneumothorax, so both U.S. and Argentine physicians went to Germany to learn the procedures for using it. German government policy encouraged the building of sanatoriums. As a result, by 1900, Germany had sixty sanatoriums. (In 1900, France had only 6 sanatoriums; by 1925, France had 127 sanatoriums, but Argentina had only 3.) German sanatoriums accepted tuberculin as a cure;

after being used on only twenty-nine percent of patients in 1905, it was used on seventy percent in 1910.[18]

Alexander Spengler, a German doctor who fled to Switzerland after the 1848 revolution in Germany, transferred the concept of the sanatorium to Switzerland. He noted that Swiss residents of Davos seemed unaffected by tuberculosis and popularized Davos as a health resort. In 1900, he constructed a hotel sanatorium. Wealthy Europeans went to Davos to seek a cure for tuberculosis and contributed to Switzerland's reputation for a healthy environment. Swiss sanatoriums, which were hotels more than hospitals, were owned by private investors and sanatorium doctors offered rooms whose prices varied with the view. Although the First World War decreased visitors from Buenos Aires, Philadelphia and London, the more benign regimen and the clear air of the Alps continued to attract wealthy international tuberculosis patients until after World War II. The Swiss investment in tuberculosis treatment resorts encouraged their continued existence until the late 1950s. Some of the tuberculosis resort facilities remain as hotels and conference centers.[19]

Although dispensaries were not a German invention, Germany rapidly increased the number of tuberculosis clinics; it had twenty-six in 1904, 321 in 1910 and 1,145 by the beginning of World War I in 1914. In comparison, France had twenty-six in 1902, fifty-two in 1917 and 508 in 1925. England operated sixty-four by 1911 and nearly 400 in 1918, while the U.S. had 450 clinics in 1915. In 1909, when both Buenos Aires and Philadelphia had a population of over a million, each operated six state, municipal or charity clinics that provided free care in working-class neighborhoods. Pennsylvania continued to increase the number of clinics, and in 1941, Philadelphia alone operated twenty-seven tuberculosis clinics. The rapid increase of German sanatoriums and clinics illustrates Germany's commitment to seeking both to prevent and cure tuberculosis among all classes in order to assure a productive workforce. At the same time, Germans blamed the poor living in slums with poor hygiene and alcoholism for the increased incidence of tuberculosis.[20]

Spain Shapes Latin American Policies

Spain shaped Latin American medical practices in the early independence era. Unlike northern Europe, the Spanish in the early nineteenth century held tuberculosis to be contagious, and after Koch's discovery implemented prevention efforts. Between 1901 and 1930, tuberculosis contributed to at least 30,000 deaths annually in Spain: eighty percent of those who died were workers between fifteen and thirty-five years old. Spanish hygienists and physicians came to believe that malnutrition, unhealthy housing and long working days created the tubercular environment of the working class. Government hygienists also blamed alcoholism, immorality, illiteracy, sexual promiscuity and masturbation for the spread of the disease. Thus, public health campaigns, rather than seeking to improve living and working conditions, emphasized changing the values of the working class. Local state dispensaries and private charities emphasized education and assistance to the tubercular and became the major institutions to fight tuberculosis in Spain. Spain opened its first sanatorium for the wealthy in 1897 and two years later inaugurated a poorly funded sanatorium for the general public. The limitations of government and voluntary measures against tuberculosis led a 1912 group of Madrid doctors, politicians and aristocratic women to organize the Popular League against Tuberculosis (Liga Popular contra la Tuberculosis), which through an annual street collection, raised funds for a tuberculosis prevention campaign and support of a sanatorium in Madrid. The socialist parties and newspaper, *El Socialist*, unimpressed by street collections, suggested that the wealthy and middle class could more effectively benefit the poor and decrease tuberculosis if they supported increased workers' wages and lower rents, did not sell bad food and gave up their second homes. Between 1901 and 1931, legislation required physicians to have training in the treatment of tuberculosis, protected children from working in factories, limited the working day for women and regulated the purity of milk.[21]

Buenos Aires medical personnel, who were influenced by Spanish practices in the eighteenth century, had initially viewed tuberculosis as contagious. But with independence, Argentina sought to break away from Spain's influence. The result was a heated debate in Argentine medical journals between those who thought tuberculosis was contagious and those who thought it was hereditary. The elite and middle-class Porteños believed that changing the values of the working class was the key to preventing tuberculosis. However, because Buenos Aires physicians went to Berlin and Paris to study tuberculosis in the nineteenth century, German and French medical practices influenced Argentine discussions more than Spanish ones. Argentine socialist parties emphasized that higher wages and shorter working hours were critical to assuring that the working class had good health. Thus, global influences, including socialist ideas and the perceived superiority of French and German research rather than Spanish historical tradition shaped later tuberculosis policy and practices in Buenos Aires.

Tuberculosis Policy and Practices in Africa and Asia

Tuberculosis policy and practices in Africa and Asia largely stemmed from European influences. For example, in South Africa, the poverty in which Africans lived, their lack of access to medical attention, British labor policies and the Eurocentric perspective that viewed Africans as easily susceptible to disease contributed to the rapid spread of tuberculosis and high mortality rates. European imperialism shaped colonial health policies within Africa as it had in the Americas. However, British imperialism emerged in Africa after Britain had lost her empire in the Americas at a time when tuberculosis was receiving global attention. Thus, British colonial policies more directly influenced tuberculosis policies in South Africa than in Philadelphia and also demonstrated that low standard of living along with malnutrition and poor hygiene contributed to high mortality from tuberculosis.[22]

The South African case also shows that the increased incidence of tuberculosis does not stem from the movement of people to cities per se, but from concentrations of populations and internal migrations. The discovery of diamonds in South Africa in 1867 and gold in 1886 led to the increase of African populations at mine sites and the growth of large coastal and industrial towns. By 1912, tuberculosis was three times more common in large coastal and industrial towns than in rural areas. Seasonal migration in which the infected moved from the urban and mining areas to rural South African villages assured the onset of tuberculosis among the rural population. As a result, in the 1920s, over ninety percent of the black adult population of parts of Ciskei and Transkei contracted tuberculosis. Legislation that limited African access to land and worker recruitment, which attracted rural laborers to work in the mines, further aided the spread of tuberculosis. By the beginning of the twentieth century, tuberculosis patients were concentrated in mining areas, because of the size of the labor force and the difficult working and living conditions there. The workers' crowded sleeping arrangements (beds were in constant use because of double shifts in the mines), poor nutrition, long working hours, and the dust and silicosis that workers inhaled activated the disease.[23]

Beginning in 1916, mine owners improved working and living conditions in the gold mines and excluded workers who might be tubercular. As a result, by 1935, morbidity declined among gold miners. Slum clearance and sanitary improvements provided some success in decreasing tuberculosis deaths in the urban areas. Nevertheless, by the late 1930s and early 1940s, the mine owners and municipal governments no longer effectively prevented those with tuberculosis from moving to industrial areas. However, racial policies forced workers to live in overcrowded African townships on inadequate diets and without clean water or sewage removal. The result was increased tuberculosis in South Africa at the time when fewer than ten percent of deaths in Argentina, the U.S. and Western Europe stemmed from tuberculosis.[24]

In part because of racism, South Africa had no interest in instituting health reforms, implementing progressive housing and nutrition policies, or developing sanitation and medical services for the greater part of its population. The majority of South African black workers, like the poor in Philadelphia and Buenos Aires, had no power to pressure either their employers or the state to reform the system. In contrast with the

U.S., no debates occurred between white and black community leaders as to whether the high levels of tuberculosis among Africans resulted from poor living conditions or racial inferiority or whether communities should develop policies that decreased tuberculosis in the African areas. Just as nineteenth-century, white Philadelphian and Porteños blamed tuberculosis on southern African Americans and provincial Argentines, white South Africans believed that black Africans' race, ignorance and culture were responsible for tuberculosis. But, in fact, Africans could not afford nutritious foods and were forced to live in overcrowded districts.[25]

Although British disdain for India's culture was not as strong as British belief in the inferiority of Africans, by the end of the nineteenth century, British colonial rule had pushed the traditional Indian medical practitioners underground: the European medical corps dismissed them as ineffective. Colonial policies supporting urbanization and industrialization in India led to population concentrations and the expansion of tuberculosis, but the British colonial government failed to implement public health practices that were accepted in the West. A great famine, which killed five million Indians between 1895 and 1901, initially distracted the British from developing tuberculosis prevention policies. Because of concerns about cholera and the widespread occurrence of tuberculosis, the colonial government eventually fostered limited sanitation in a few towns and villages and promoted mass education campaigns on hygiene. Independent countries such as the U.S. and Argentina did more to implement global policies than did colonies subject to exterior political power. Racial attitudes and cost led to the slow implementation of the globally accepted tuberculosis policies in India and in colonies generally. For example, the establishment of tuberculosis hospitals and sanatoriums remained controversial, because of the cost and disagreements about whether these institutions would help those viewed as culturally and biologically inferior. By the time of independence in 1947, tuberculosis was the second greatest cause of mortality in India but failed to receive as much attention from the government as malaria and cholera. The low priority accorded tuberculosis prevention programs meant that the British government passed on a major public health issue to an independent India.[26]

The acceptance of policies on tuberculosis depended on recognition of the effectiveness of modern medicine. Only as Asian countries came to accept western medicine did they implement global policies regarding tuberculosis. Argentina, the U.S. and India, colonized by Europeans, replaced most populist medical practices with western ones. By contrast, China and Japan remained independent from Europe, and their populations continued to utilize their traditional medical systems and to reject many western ideas regarding tuberculosis. Yet, before the advent of streptomycin, traditional Japanese and Chinese remedies offered chances for recovery as great as those offered by western medicine and also provided tubercular patients with additional choices. Of course, traditional medicines, which encouraged the use of herbal mixtures and patent medicines, were popular in all societies, including in Buenos Aires and Philadelphia.[27]

The Japanese government only slowly developed measures to prevent tuberculosis because of the reluctance of their medical establishment to accept Koch's discovery, the Japanese view that health was a personal and not a governmental issue, and the high cost of public health measures. However, beginning in 1858, the Tokugawa government endorsed western medicine, thereby increasing the Japanese acceptance of European interpretations of consumption. After the Meiji government (1868–1912) sent representatives to Paris in 1899 to learn about disease classification, the Japanese accepted more aspects of the European system. Between 1862 and 1912, at least 763 Japanese doctors trained abroad in western universities. However, the Japanese absorbed western medicine in fragments, without paying attention to the differences among the various schools of medical thought. Although many practitioners continued to include Japanese and Chinese theories and treatment of tubercular disease, physicians acknowledged many western ideas about tuberculosis. The first sanatorium established in Kobe in 1889 preceded both the Mont Alto State Sanatorium in Pennsylvania (1901) and the Sanatorio Nacional de Tuberculosos Santa María in Argentina (1900); physicians familiar with western ideas increasingly recommended that the tubercular improve their diet and go to the seashore or mountains to improve their health.[28]

The Japanese Anti-Tuberculosis League founded in 1913 (later than those in Buenos Aires and Philadelphia), focused on education with an emphasis on prevention. Most ordinances, including the requirement to not hire those with tuberculosis and to disinfect the premises of tuberculosis patients who died, were unenforced. Although the Japanese government had begun collecting medical statistics in the nineteenth century, the under-reporting of tuberculosis limited the value of the statistics, as it did in Buenos Aires and Philadelphia. Nevertheless, it was clear by the beginning of the twentieth century that tuberculosis was widespread in urban areas. Young women in the textile industries, who labored long hours in dust-filled rooms and consumed little protein, often became infected. After working for only a year or two, they spread tuberculosis to isolated villages when they returned home.[29]

The general Japanese population believed that pulmonary tuberculosis was hereditary and stigmatized a patient's entire family. On 21 May 1938, Toi Mutsuo, a twenty-two-year-old resident of the isolated mountain hamlet of Kaio, killed himself and thirty-one others and injured three. His suicide note stated, "I am dying to get revenge on my neighbors for the oppressive hardheartedness they have towards someone with a disease they believe is incurable." It is important, though, to recall that Porteños and Philadelphians returning from sanatoriums also worried about ostracization and preferred to keep their illness a secret.[30]

Tuberculosis began declining in Japan by 1930; but the rate of infection began to rise with the wartime strain on the economy. Beginning in the 1930s, the state implemented public health prevention programs in order to develop a vigorous military. Japanese physicians also began to utilize bacteriological exams, tuberculin tests, X-rays and vaccinated those under age thirty with BCG. Land reform, which improved the economic situation of farmers, contributed to a decline of tuberculosis deaths after World War II. The Japanese case demonstrates the significance of good nutrition to prevent tuberculosis, and the impact of efforts to advance military capability in spurring tuberculosis prevention programs.[31]

This brief examination of African, Asian and European tuberculosis policies reveals that in spite of differing cultures and medical systems, Western-educated health professionals broadly agreed as to the cause and treatment of tuberculosis. Although a few physicians were skeptical, sanatoriums, rest, fresh air and diet became the basis of tuberculosis cures. In spite of the value of BCG, its cost and questions about it safety limited its use until after World War II. Racial and cultural attitudes in western nations influenced tuberculosis policies toward minorities. For example, the incorrect assumption in Philadelphia that African Americans were racially predisposed toward tuberculosis initially led to limited treatment for them.[32] Although Western governments recognized the importance of supporting prevention policies in their colonies, high costs and racial attitudes discouraged their implementation. The tuberculosis problem was primarily left to postcolonial independent governments, when Asian and African physicians and health officials followed the western medical practices.

Patients understood that the sanatorium extended life, but that it did not necessarily cure. However, the continued popular belief that tuberculosis was hereditary led to discrimination against the ill and their families. The stigma of tuberculosis remained an issue for the general population in Argentina and U.S. through the 1950s. Thus, individuals might try to hide the fact that they had contracted tuberculosis and spent time in a sanatorium. In the first half of the twentieth century, tuberculosis patients were often absent from their neighborhoods for long periods. Their absences aroused neighbors' suspicion, and illnesses impoverished those who were unable to work.[33]

Tuberculosis Mortality

Table 7.1 indicates that early in the twentieth century, pulmonary tuberculosis mortality rates began to decline gradually and erratically in

Year	1911	1920	1925	1928	1930	1932	1934	1936	1938	1940	1942	1945	1947
Asia													
China													
Guanghzhou					85	70	72						
Hong Kong				105		139	158	158					
India													
Chennai			284	260	146	123	147	140	159				
Delhi				213		254	240	232					
Kolkata			228	213	207	172	222	268	271				
Mumbai			194	111	109	106	141	150	155				
Japan	215	224	194	191	186	171	193						
Kobe				288	217	211	220	259					
Tokyo				198	151	158	278	292					
Yokohama				280	192	179	193	224					
Pakistan				189									
Karatchi				196	206	110	177	186	145				
Philippines	302												
Manila			368	435	601	525	453	284	315				
Middle East													
Ankara				90	102	78	131	90	117				
Baghdad				218	246	186	147		96				
Beirut				277	59	48	46	22	57				
Istanbul				312	217	213	202	186	184				
North Africa													
Alexandria			146	85	66	71	83	67	63				
Algiers				214	165	153	170	123	168				
Cairo			118	71	68	64	65	79	77				
Casablanca				154	77	73	123	97	100				
Tunis				274	234	233	201	140	204				
South Africa			53	51	47	42	40						
Cape Town				79	74	69	76	55	76				
Durban				51	49	49	37	29	54				
Johannesburg				53	76	60	33	24	22				

(Continued)

Year	1911	1920	1925	1928	1930	1932	1934	1936	1938	1940	1942	1945	1947
Europe													
Austria	322	282	171		138	130		101	101	142	154	151	85
Vienna	260			189	134	128	102	87	109	132	133	257	121
Belgium	129	116	101		92	83	73	72	69	68	95	78	63
Antwerp					90	75	63	63	49				
Brussels			136	82	68	62	54	54	55	93	111	94	71
Czech Republic		260	192		161	150	138	129	123	135	156		96
Prague	355		174	173	133	123	124	114	122	133	176	170	99
Denmark		106	91		71	69	55	47	41	35	35	32	30
Copenhagen	176		108	95	73	74	62	47	51	44	43	40	38
Eng./Wales	147	113	104		90	84	76	57	62	70	66	61	55
Birmingham				159	89	84	72	71	70	84	86	76	70
Bristol				187	99	73	74	71	56				
Liverpool				93	122	113	101	85	81				
London	124		117	105	87	82	76	69	72	97	102	87	69
Manchester				82	119	100	101	90	86				
Finland	281		248	180	240	211		210	199	212	220	187	167
Helsinki				211	192	177	150	176	138	168	180	169	156
France	217	185	159	74	158	139		118	143	137	154	111	81
Le Havre				91	262	210	208	198					
Lyon	247		261	168	148	112	45	33	92				
Marseille				220	122	114	93	80	120				
Paris	341		280	229	196	170	149	145	155	194	198	119	72
Toulouse					150	104	121	115					
Germany	160	154	107		79	75		71	63	68	76	83	73
Berlin	194		121	101	82	78	78	76	75			239	223
Cologne			121	98	67	70	57	64	61				
Frankfort				83	65	58	50	51	44				
Hamburg	159		114	93	61	67	56	64	57				
Munich	197		117	91	69	68	69	55	53				
Greece			160	165	162	162	145	128	116	230	456		
Athens				406	316	375	370	353	361				
Hungry	367	316	256	224	199	194	152		142	133	153	120	106
Budapest	352		291	279	144	138	115	109	118	120	139	246	101

Ireland	212	163	[illegible]	183	120	124	117	117	109	123	147	124	124
Dublin	258		185	173	144	134	128	129	117	163	187	164	165
N. Ireland		201	167	229	128	112	112	103	92	98	97	80	73
Belfast	201		172	148	113	103	96	92	103	114	113	93	76
Italy	172	160	153	88	112	104	93	87	80	74	102	91	77
Milan			191	143	78	78	57						
Naples				89	95	92	93						
Rome	192			158	114	116	66	106	99	119	173	176	138
Venice			207	181	118	90	69						
Netherlands	157	147	99	77	75	64	55	50	45	44	61	86	37
Amsterdam	136		97	79	53	38	35	37	41	37	71	116	36
Utrecht				91	53	46	42	45	26				
Rotterdam			110	84	55	46	43	37	39				
Norway	218	210	189	279	149	136		102	88	82	73	65	56
Bergen				117	117	120	73	88	60				
Oslo			167	155	135	121	87	77	79	76	60	61	53
Poland				140									
Kraków			432	206	155	131	106	116	115				
Warsaw				128	171	152	147	130	135			266	158
Portugal				133	192	168	166	159	153	152	160	152	153
Lisbon				469	456	317	351	310	397	370	342	370	356
Romania				158					167	177	191	178	182
Bucharest				206	212	212	196	225	284	208	204		
Russia				84									
Moscow	270		157	172									
St. Petersburg	376	510	284	237									
Scotland	177	124	111	84	89	84	75	74	69	81	82	79	80
Edinburgh	88		133	105	76	70	66	62	61	92	84	69	
Glasgow			134	123	80	87	78	87	85	143	140	133	
Spain	157	176	150	138	124	117	111	101	129	113	122	112	124
Barcelona			135	167	119	106	97	79	165				
Grenada				176	116	138	144	127	87				
Madrid	247		253	218	145	129	106	99	169	92	133	106	108
Seville			406	397	301	227	238	214	209				
Valencia			180	156	116	114	96	82	152				
Sweden	191	163	146		126	114	102	93	82	71	68	65	56

(Continued)

Year	1911	1920	1925	1928	1930	1932	1934	1936	1938	1940	1942	1945	1947
Stockholm	193		154	157	124	116	96	86	92	76	72	60	51
Switzerland	216	180	154	165	125	116	101	95	82	78	83	83	67
Berne				144	106	88	49	71	78				
Geneva				164	129	118	62	80	81				
Zurich				111	73	72	66	57	47				
North America				172									
Canada		75	67	237	79	68	59		55	51	51	46	43
Montreal				142	109	91	70	76	69	67	80	64	59
Ottawa				195	58	60	53	49	51	37	43	40	34
Quebec				123	108	80		75	60	119	113	85	86
Toronto				45	32	22	16	17	17	30	33	29	30
Vancouver				181	68	58	54	57	56	68	70	52	48
Winnipeg				273	45	30	31	29	20	29	28	29	27
U.S.	138	101	75	70	63	56	51	51	45	42	40	37	31
Baltimore		139		216		77	69	92	77	82	80	73	72
Boston		116	98	82	69	60	67	55	46	60	64	62	58
Chicago	166	85	83	86	57	50	55	49	47	62	52	50	49
Los Angeles				130		81	69	67	39	56	52	48	46
New Orleans	215		133	166	135	113	106	124	109	81	67	66	61
New York	176	109	87	89	64	55	53	57	47	51	48	44	43
Philadelphia	187	121	94	83	71	71	70	58	54	65	60	56	54
Saint Louis		87	90	75	59	59	53	60	53	56	56	44	32
San Francisco		125	103	92	75	67	55	60	49	67	56	54	58
Seattle		71				50	56	52	40	49	47	46	41
Washington DC		127		80		107	105	93	62	83	67	66	67
Central Amer.				142									
Havana			266		157	144		146				145	
Mexico City	321			130	97	84	80	77	73				71
Panama City					263	250	194	234	233			182	
San Salvador				336	278	258	295	295	355			395	341
South America													
Argentina				79						85			
Buenos Aires	167	169	176	150	148	140	125	108	109			80	78
Bolivia												47	
La Paz					63	91	197					68	

Brazil							268					292	273
Belém				370	353	450		245			274		
Manaus				378	361		239	319			255		
Recife				362	430	428	322	288			402		
Rio de Janeiro				254	261	271	268	269	300		317	323	
Salvador			313	344	356	337		331	362		507		
Santos			229	246	239	213		261	244				
São Paulo			108	104	99	108		114	121		137		135
Chile	264	249	233	245	256	255	262			235		236	207
Santiago				378	385			366	374				280
Valparaiso				589	413	398		313	364				
Colombia												43	42
Barranquilla					93	135		171	195				
Bogota				154	83	101	114	111	117				120
Ecuador												72	73
Guayaquil				461	638	519							514
Quito				141	165	139		200	161				125
Peru												99	
Callao				503	528	528	529	506	465				
Lima				590	345	386	334	370	376				340
Uruguay	150	158	157	138	139	132		116		109		103	93
Montevideo			272	259	214	191	203	177	193				180
Venezuela													86
Caracas				375	380	380	428	378	286				143
Oceania													
Australia	83	67	58	485	50	46	44						
Brisbane					47	37	46	43	40				
Melbourne				67	58	51	47	50	44				
Perth				81	66	48	56	60	46				
Sidney				54	49	49	44	43	44				
New Zealand	73	71	51	50	46	42	42						
Christchurch					44	26		43	28				
Wellington				65	54	37		41	55				

Sources: Buenos Aires, *Yearbook 1910–1911*, xxix; "Tuberculosis Mortality in Europe," 666–2; League of Nations, Health Section, "Corrected Statistics of Notifiable Diseases," for various years.
Mostardini, 137, 139, 144; Tuberculosis Reference Statistical Yearbook, various years.

European and American cities. (Globally, other forms of tuberculosis deaths were low.) A comparison of statistics of various cities suggests that pulmonary tuberculosis deaths peaked in the Americas and Europe from 1911 to 1913. Tuberculosis deaths in Philadelphia and other U.S. cities continued a slow decline. However, the decline of tuberculosis deaths in European cities was interrupted by World War I. During the war, the number of tuberculosis civilian and military deaths increased most dramatically in those cities where there was population displacement and direct fighting. London, indirectly affected by war, had lower tuberculosis mortality than cities in continental Europe. However, during the early years of World War I, there was a disproportionate increase in mortality among females, fifteen to forty-four, in British coastal port towns and cities.[34] Tuberculosis deaths also increased in Buenos Aires between 1914 and 1919 when basic necessities became more expensive. The limited availability of meat and other nutritious foods contributed to tuberculosis mortality.

Political instability and civil conflicts lead to the displacement of people and increased poverty. At the same time, labor shortages and financial stringency decreased public health programs. World War I military conscription led to better diagnosis of young men infected with tuberculosis as initially only the healthy were drafted. The influenza pandemic of 1918 also increased tuberculosis mortality. After the war and influenza pandemic, tuberculosis mortality continued to decline in American and European cities. At the same time, pulmonary tuberculosis mortality increased erratically in Asian, African and Middle Eastern cities through the 1930s. The wealth and size of districts included in a city affect the mortality data. For example, it is clear that African townships were not included in the urban South African data as tuberculosis mortality is too low.

City governments faced a challenge in their efforts to decrease tuberculosis mortality. Philadelphia and Buenos Aires witnessed a gradual decline in tuberculosis among all groups even before the introduction of effective medications. Thus, in Philadelphia in 1904 tuberculosis accounted for twelve percent of total deaths; in 1938, it claimed only 4.54 percent of all deaths. In Buenos Aires, tuberculosis mortality rates declined from 1886 to 1895 and then began to increase again between 1896 and 1918; by 1938, tuberculosis accounted for 9.48 percent of all death.[35] It is also of interest that the number of recorded pulmonary tuberculosis deaths declined at the same time that physicians were identifying the disease more accurately and life expectancy was increasing.[36]

In the U.S., particularly in those cities with large African-American populations, Baltimore and New Orleans, and in Brazil in Recife and Salvador, pulmonary tuberculosis deaths remained high and declined more slowly; the poor had a deficient diet and limited health facilities.

There was higher pulmonary tuberculosis mortality in port and industrial cities probably due to the influx and concentration of diverse populations. There was also higher mortality in tropical lowland cities than in high altitude cooler cities. National data which includes both urban and rural deaths show rural deaths to be lower than the urban ones, which were generally more accurate. At the same time, the numbers of tuberculosis deaths in various cities of a specific country were more similar than the number of deaths between countries. Examining tuberculosis statistics for entire countries provides a comparison and broad picture of tuberculosis mortality. However, data on cities convey the understanding of specific causes and effects of tuberculosis.

Central to an understanding of tuberculosis deaths are two issues: the accuracy of diagnosis and the validity of the reporting. From 1870 to 1912, public officials undercounted tuberculosis deaths in both Buenos Aires and Philadelphia because of the difficulty of diagnosing the disease. In the nineteenth century, only an autopsy verified that a person had died of tuberculosis. By the early twentieth century, physicians in Buenos Aires and Philadelphia were successfully testing patient's sputum for the tuberculosis bacteria. However, diagnosing tuberculosis at the beginning stages remained difficult. Even in 2018, a tuberculosis skin test only indicates that a person was infected with *Mycobacterium tuberculosis*; it does not clarify whether an individual has latent tuberculosis or the disease. The WHO (World Health Organization) stated that skin and blood tests were often erroneous; and X-rays detected only advanced lung damage. Sputum tests are needed to prove that an individual has tuberculosis.[37]

From 1861 to 1880, physicians did not agree as to how to report tuberculosis. Moreover, to placate families the causes of many tuberculosis deaths were intentionally hidden and instead ascribed to diseases such as asthma, dropsy, inflammation of the lungs or chest, bronchitis or pneumonia. Given the stigma surrounding tuberculosis, families thought that pneumonia was a more acceptable cause of death than tuberculosis. In Philadelphia, from 1895 through 1906, there were eight years in which the pneumonia death rate was higher than the tuberculosis death rate. In Buenos Aires, the pneumonia rate was higher than the tuberculosis death rate in every year from 1887 through 1911.

Table 7.2 reveals that Buenos Aires from 1887 to 1911 had a differential of 0.62 to 9.07 percent between pneumonia and tuberculosis deaths. From 1880 to 1912, there was an average of 2.64 percent differential between Buenos Aires and Philadelphia tuberculosis deaths. Since reported pneumonia deaths were greater than tuberculosis deaths in Buenos Aires, and Philadelphia suffered from a greater number of tuberculosis deaths than Buenos Aires, tuberculosis deaths were undercounted in Buenos Aires. Tuberculosis deaths were at least 2.64 percent higher than

Table 7.2 Pneumonia and Tuberculosis Deaths in Philadelphia and Buenos Aires, 1880–1912

Year	*Phila Total Pop*	*BA Total Pop*	*Phila Total Deaths*	*BA Total Deaths*	*Phila No PN Deaths*	*BA No PN Deaths*	*Phila No Pul TB Deaths*	*BA No Pul TB Deaths*	*Phila PN Deaths% of Tot D*	*BA PN Deaths% of Tot D*	*Phila TB Deaths% of Tot D*	*BA TB Deaths% of Tot D*	*BA DIF Bw PN & TB*	*TB DIF Bw BA & Phia D*
1880	847,170	286,700	17,711	7,073	995		2,692	774	5.62		15.20	10.94		4.26
1882	886,539	325,000	20,259	7,196	1,429		2,809	808	7.05		13.87	11.23		2.64
1885	849,432	394,700	21,392	9,295	1,519		2,821	1,017	7.10		13.19	10.94		2.25
1886	971,362	421,600	20,005	9,994	1,456		2,834	853	7.28		14.17	8.54		5.63
1887	993,801	450,500	21,719	12,938	1,703	1,179	2,800	1,041	7.84	9.11	12.89	8.05	1.07	4.85
1888	1,016,758	481,000	20,372	12,367	1,587	1,199	2,695	1,069	7.79	9.70	13.23	8.64	1.05	4.58
1889	1,040,245	514,200	20,536	14,736	1,582	1,755	2,532	1,245	7.70	11.91	12.33	8.45	3.46	3.88
1890	1,046,964	526,900	21,732	16,417	2,015	1,795	2,764	1,168	9.27	10.93	12.72	7.11	3.82	5.60
1891	1,069,264	516,880	23,367	14,332	2,111	1,547	2,624	1,024	9.03	10.79	11.23	7.14	3.65	4.08
1892	1,092,168	550,080	24,305	14,692	2,209	2,410	2,709	1,078	9.09	16.40	11.15	7.34	9.07	3.81
1893	1,115,562	583,280	23,655	14,290	2,555	1,872	2,671	1,103	10.80	13.10	11.29	7.72	5.38	3.57
1894	1,139,457	616,480	22,680	13,702	2,142	2,311	2,513	1,283	9.44	16.87	11.08	9.36	7.50	1.72
1895	1,163,864	649,680	23,796	14,947	2,572	2,260	2,449	1,166	10.81	15.12	10.29	7.80	7.32	2.49
1896	1,888,797	682,880	23,982	13,645	2,705	1,734	2,514	1,268	11.28	12.71	10.48	9.29	3.42	1.19
1897	1,214,256	716,080	22,735	14,216	2,723	2,028	2,388	1,411	11.98	14.27	10.50	9.93	4.34	0.58
1898	1,240,266	749,280	23,790	13,533	2,480	2,258	2,590	1,490	10.42	16.69	10.89	11.01	5.68	-0.12
1899	1,266,832	782,480	23,796	13,567	2,424	2,050	2,818	1,450	10.19	15.11	11.84	10.69	4.42	1.15
1900	1,293,697	815,680	25,078	16,504	2,959	2,499	2,717	1,672	11.80	15.14	10.83	10.13	5.01	0.70
1901	1,321,408	840,880	24,137	15,807	2,577	2,020	2,946	1,675	10.68	12.78	12.21	10.60	2.18	1.61
1902	1,349,792	885,080	23,847	14,097	2,976	1,917	2,815	1,619	12.48	13.60	11.80	11.48	2.11	0.32
1903	1,373,414	924,480	25,510	13,996	3,191	2,608	3,053	1,689	12.51	18.63	11.97	12.07	6.57	-0.10
1904	1,399,268	967,280	25,976	14,313	2,970	1,860	3,117	1,771	11.43	13.00	12.00	12.37	0.62	-0.37
1905	1,425,122	1,013,680	24,807	15,916	2,297	2,280	2,838	1,914	9.26	14.33	11.44	12.03	2.30	-0.59
1906	1,450,976	1,063,880	27,768	17,916	2,669	2,350	3,161	2,011	9.61	13.12	11.38	11.22	1.89	0.16
1910	1,554,902	1,306,680	27,045	20,968	2,840	3,267	2,873	2,150	10.50	15.58	10.62	10.25	5.33	0.37
1911	1,583,190	1,378,880	26,276	22,869	2,612	3,049	2,960	2,304	9.94	13.33	11.27	10.07	3.26	1.19
1912	1,611,478	1,456,080	25,660	22,982	2,193		2,654	2,253	8.55		10.34	9.80		0.54

Sources: Gache, *Climatologia*, 181, 219; *Buenos Aires, Year-Book 1910–1911*, 61; Besio Moreno, 405–6, 430–31.
Philadelphia, *Annal Message of the Mayor*, 1912, vol. 3:109; 1920: 482; 1938: 450 and various years.
Abbreviations: Pop= population; PN= pneumonia; No= number; Pul TB= Pulmonary Tuberculosis; Tot= Total; Deaths= Deaths; Dif= Differential; Bw= Between.

the reported number of deaths. Although physicians in Buenos Aires diagnosed pneumonia, rather than tuberculosis, the misattribution of tuberculosis to bronchitis or pneumonia was a global problem.[38]

Dr. S. Rosenfeld (Vienna) provided an excellent analysis in a report to the Health Committee of the League of Nations of the problems related to the collection of tuberculosis statistics. He found three major types of errors in the League of Nations health statistics. Inaccuracies occurred because the initial official regulations governing the collection of statistics in different countries resulted in various interpretations of the regulations. Errors also occurred due to the limits of medical science or practice, particularly, misdiagnosis and lack of medical death certificates. Finally, misunderstanding occurred due to the mode of presentation of the statistics such as age and disease categories.[39] To this analysis must be added two further points. Health experts regularly undercounted minority populations; they failed to diagnose the tuberculosis of African Americans in U.S. cities and of indigenous residents in Latin American cities. Finally, tuberculosis deaths per 100,000 in given cities, varied according to the published year of the report and fluctuated according to the sources utilized.

Decline of Tuberculosis

The slow global decline in tuberculosis deaths occurred at the beginning of the development of national public health policies and before the development of antibiotics. The timing of the tuberculosis decline has led to debates among demographers, medical historians, public health officials and medical professionals: which factors explain the decrease in the number of individuals who contracted tuberculosis before the development of an effective cure? An analysis of the debates relating to the causes for the decline of tuberculosis provides insight into past global tuberculosis policies and current efforts to deal with the recent return of tuberculosis in more virulent forms.

Thomas McKeown, author of *The Modern Rise of Population* and *The Origin of Human Disease*, is the strongest exponent of the argument that tuberculosis diminished because of increased resistance brought about by improved nutrition and a rising standard of living. He claimed that in Great Britain, tuberculosis mortality began to decline in the seventeenth century and certainly by 1838, well before public health policies were established or an extensive number of sanatoriums built. He also concluded that better nutrition was the prime reason for the reduction of infectious diseases because of the link between malnutrition and infection and the evidence that an improved diet led to better health. F.B. Smith agreed that an improved diet explained the decline of tuberculosis, further noting that tuberculosis increased during World War I and in regions where food was inadequate. Smith also suggested that mortality declined because of increased immunity and because the most susceptible people had already died.[40]

Michael E. Teller agreed that tubercular mortality rates began to fall before the sanitary reforms of the late nineteenth century. Although sanatorium treatment removed some infectious cases from homes and better protected families, it at best alleviated the disease for only a small minority. Similarly, Allen K. Krause, the director of the Johns Hopkins University tuberculosis laboratory, noted that as early as 1830 tuberculosis began to decline in countries that were advancing industrially and increasing in wealth even before efforts were made to combat the disease. He agreed with Teller that more sanatoriums did not solve the tuberculosis problem because individuals would infect others before entering the institutions. Krause believed that the environment (that is, people's living conditions) provided the setting for tuberculosis. He also recognized that physical trauma (pregnancy, accidents and illness) could activate tuberculosis. When working and living conditions improved, tuberculosis morbidity decreased; when recessions and World War I increased poverty, tuberculosis increased. Krause favored a radical reordering of society to improve the quality of life for the poor and working classes. He also supported increased expenditures to cure those with tuberculosis. He argued that rather than enacting regulations to prevent tuberculosis, the emphasis should be on education, persuasion, medical training and research. For Krause, "The solution of the tuberculosis problem is, therefore, partly dependent on the removal of other evils and inequalities which constitute, no doubt, a more fundamental social problem than does tuberculosis itself."[41]

The most substantial challenges to McKeown's focus on improved diet as the cause of the decline of tuberculosis are Leonard Wilson's "The Historical Decline of Tuberculosis in Europe and America: Its Causes and Significance," Anne Hardy, *The Epidemic Streets: Infectious Disease and the Rise of Preventive Medicine, 1856–1900* and Greta Jones, *'Captain of All These Men of Death': The History of Tuberculosis in Nineteenth and Twentieth Century Ireland.* Wilson began by questioning McKeown's evidence and argued that the available data were too limited to prove that medical and public health measures did not influence the decline in tuberculosis mortality. Indeed, recent historians examining McKeown's evidence agree that the inaccurate diagnosis of tuberculosis and the limits of tuberculosis mortality statistics make it impossible to prove that the tuberculosis decline began early in the nineteenth century. In fact, the data from Buenos Aires and Philadelphia suggest that a steady decline of tuberculosis began only in the first quarter of the twentieth century. Although tuberculosis might have decreased among the upper classes in England, Wilson also pointed out that the upper classes did not change their diet nor suffer from a lack of nutritious food. After Wilson dissected McKeown's arguments, he asserted that tuberculosis declined "because of reduction in the opportunities for patients with pulmonary tuberculosis to spread their infection," not because of a rising standard of living or the innate tendency of the disease to decline. Thus, Wilson utilized comparative data from various countries and cities to show that the decrease of tuberculosis was linked to the isolation of patients and efforts to prevent the spread of tuberculosis. He contended that the public health movement played a significant role in the decline of tuberculosis. He concluded that the rest treatment was effective for many patients at the early stages of pulmonary tuberculosis and that medical and public health policies to prevent tuberculosis after 1882 successfully accelerated the rate of tuberculosis decline in England, Wales, Prussia, Massachusetts and New York City. Anne Hardy, using additional British evidence, asserted that beginning as early as the 1850s, national health reforms and local sanitary measures contributed to the decrease of tuberculosis.[42]

Greta Jones, who studied nineteenth- and twentieth-century tuberculosis (focusing on the rise and decline of tuberculosis in Ireland), further challenged McKeown's thesis. She argued that the industrialization and urbanization of Ireland between 1880 and 1900 were central to the rising number of tuberculosis cases at the turn of the century. Here, she took issue with Krause, who thought that urbanization and industrialization in the U.S. improved the standard of living. By contrast, Jones argued that the beginnings of industrialization created large numbers of poor people who endured crowded living and working arrangements in cities. Tuberculosis mortality intensified further when rural immigrants returned home to die. Even if nutritional standards improved, overall tuberculosis may still have increased, because a higher per capita GNP may disguise the deterioration of living standards of some groups within the society. In effect, the industrial environment rather than income explains tuberculosis mortality numbers. Jones further suggested that although the limited resources of the public health campaign in Ireland between 1899 and 1914 had little influence on the decline of tuberculosis mortality, it laid the basis for a more effective campaign in both the Republic of Ireland and Northern Ireland. The greatest decrease in tuberculosis mortality in Northern Ireland followed the establishment of its Tuberculosis Authority and implementation of mass radiography efforts between 1946 and 1951. The new tuberculosis services in the Republic of Ireland ensured that drug therapy would be effective by developing a system for tracking and monitoring those who had tuberculosis. Thus, Jones agreed with Krause on the significance of poverty on tuberculosis mortality. But she disagreed with Anne Hardy and Leonard Wilson, who emphasized the importance of the national health reforms and local sanitary measures. Jones argued, instead, that the public health campaign was too narrow in focus and its resources too limited. She concluded that factors unique to the socio-economic environment of a region will influence the groups most affected and the level of tuberculosis mortality.[43]

When examining the decline of tuberculosis in Britain from 1880 to 1930, Michael Worboys noted that in those years five different groups offered explanations of the decline. Insanitationists stressed the role of general sanitary improvements (such as improved provision of running water and sewage treatment); infectionists emphasized the control of the spread of disease resulting from decreased overcrowding; hygienists focused on the need for health education and lifestyle changes and called attention to the role of diet within the context of changing behavior; diathesians argued that the disease had eliminated those most susceptible to it; and tubercularisationists thought that the population had acquired immunity to the disease. The debates among these experts were linked to specific policy efforts to control tuberculosis both nationally and internationally. British infectionists and hygienists remained influential in shaping British policy until the 1950s, while tubercularisationists shaped colonial tuberculosis policy in the 1930s and 1940s.[44] In the case of both Buenos Aires and Philadelphia, hygienists and insanitationists came to dominate.

Public officials preferred explanation for the decline of tuberculosis deaths in Buenos Aires and Philadelphia is directly connected to the policies that they put in place and the amount of influence those officials had on a nation's tuberculosis policy. In effect, if an official worked on sanitary improvements, it is the improvement in the provision of running water, sewage treatment and housing that led to a decline in tuberculosis deaths. However, mortality rates from Buenos Aires and Philadelphia support McKeown's and Krause's focus on the importance of the standard of living and improved nutrition. Patients and their families in Buenos Aires and Philadelphia understood that better housing, increased wages, shorter working hours and sound nutrition contributed to their health. The timing and rate of industrialization and urbanization also suggest reasons for the increase in the number of tuberculosis deaths in both Buenos Aires and Philadelphia. The population expansions in both Buenos Aires and Philadelphia made public health efforts with limited budget support difficult to enforce. Nor was an emphasis on improving of the morals of the poor an effective public health initiative. Since sanatoriums treated only a minority of those with tuberculosis, their impact on the decline in tuberculosis deaths was minor. The Buenos Aires and Philadelphia cases cannot prove that tuberculosis declined because of the population's increased immunity to tuberculosis.

The physician and anthropologist Paul Farmer, writing from contemporary clinical experiences with both drug-susceptible tuberculosis and MDR-TB (multi-drug resistant tuberculosis), in Haiti and Peru, emphasizes that poverty and racism increased the chances of infection: the poor lived together in cramped urban housing, where tuberculosis could be endemic, and where malnutrition decreased the effectiveness of medications. Once infected, destitution and discrimination limited patients' access to effective therapy, decreased the ability of the sick to follow the required regimens and diminished the possibilities for recovery. He argued that what the poor required was both effective clinical intervention and an increase in their standard of living.[45] Interestingly, Farmer's arguments are not much different from those advanced by Allen Krause, 80 years earlier. Recent scientific evidence indicates that resistance to tuberculosis could increase in a given population within a short period of time.[46] Thus, historians who argue that tuberculosis declined because the population became more resistant may have a point.

Public health officials need to take into consideration issues that may be unique to a particular global area. When a nation is at war, the number of tuberculosis cases increases. War spreads disease because combatants are drawn from a diverse epidemiological background, sent to regions to which they are not acclimatized and bring infections to war-zone residents who may have little immunity. The more actively involved the nation is in military conflicts, the more likely the rise in the number of tuberculosis cases among both the military and civilians. The destruction of civilian housing, the close quartering of soldiers in military barracks, and the construction of prison and refugee camps all lead to crowding and provide the environment in which tuberculosis spreads. Malnutrition resulting from the disruption of agricultural production and food rationing contributes to the reactivation of latent tuberculosis. Physical exertion, mental-stress and the increased employment of the population in industries that have dust as a by-product weaken the resistance to infection. Finally, war generally disrupts public health programs, since public health professionals are recruited into the military and funds are appropriated for support of the war. World Wars I and II directly impacted Paris and London, but had only limited influence on Buenos Aires and had an indirect influence on Philadelphia.[47]

While Jones' emphasis on the correlation between urbanization and industrialization and the rise of tuberculosis mortality is relevant to both Buenos Aires and Philadelphia, further factors unique to specific economic and social environments contribute to the numbers of tuberculosis cases and the mortality rate. The decrease of tuberculosis in both Buenos Aires and Philadelphia was based on a combination of factors that decreased poverty and led to a higher standard of living: the availability of pasteurized milk and affordable meat; improved wages with shorter hours and healthier living conditions; and public health policies that promoted legislation to improve housing and build sewage and water purification plants. In effect, Paul Farmer's arguments for contemporary Peru and Haiti—that lessening poverty and providing effective clinical care will decrease tuberculosis—holds true for Buenos Aires and Philadelphia from 1880 to 1945.

However, it is impossible to prove that any one specific factor explained the conquest of tuberculosis. Although Wilson utilized comparative data to show that public health policies caused the decline of tuberculosis, those same data do not preclude the importance of other factors. Furthermore, historians may be focusing on the wrong factors to analyze morbidity and mortality. By focusing more narrowly on cities and even communities within them, historians might understand trends more clearly. Broader national statistics hide differences. For example, Samuel Roberts argued that central to the decline of tuberculosis in the African-American community were improvements in nutrition and the standard of living as well as the public health efforts focused on tuberculosis. David Barnes suggested that the level of material wealth correlates directly with tuberculosis death rates: in effect, the lower the hourly wages and the higher the unemployment, the greater the tuberculosis mortality.[48]

Re-evaluating the historical decline of tuberculosis since the mid-nineteenth century, Matthew Gandy argued against a single-factor explanation and suggested a more complicated picture. He noted that the decline in mortality due to tuberculosis began first in Britain, Germany and Belgium and occurred at a later time in France, Ireland and Norway. In the case of France, for example, mortality rates twice as high as those in Britain persisted into the twentieth century. He further argued that the perceived conflict in the historical literature between the "nutritionists" and "contagionists" "obscured the relationship between public health interventions and broader social and political developments." He indicated that relevant factors include workplace-safety legislation and housing construction that contributed to social and economic improvements.[49]

In conclusion, in order to understand the tuberculosis epidemic of 1993–2003 and any future epidemics, it is important to consider the various actors that influenced the decline of tuberculosis—not a single theory.[50] Isolating and curing those with tuberculosis is certainly central to ending the global spread of the tuberculosis bacteria. Innovative forms of testing for *Mycobacterium tuberculosis* and new medications continue to be important. Strengthening immune systems through high-protein diets and rest contributes to the successful cures of individual patients. However, all these efforts are dependent upon the decrease of poverty. Poverty, limited public health efforts, and failure to isolate patients, in addition to the rise of bacteria resistant to multiple drugs and the AIDS epidemic help explain the global resurgence of tuberculosis. Nevertheless, the general diverse social and geographical incidence of tuberculosis works against a global historical explanation for its rise and the means to reduce it.

Notes

1 Chemnitz Association, "Protection against Consumption," in *Transactions of the Sixth International Congress on Tuberculosis, Washington, September 28 to October 5, 1908 with an Account and Catalogue of the Tuberculosis Exhibition* (Philadelphia: W. F. Fell Company, 1908), 5, 283.

2 George H. Kress, "Facts a Mother Should Know Concerning Tuberculosis," *Transactions of the Sixth International* 5: 304–5.
3 Katherine Arner, "Making Yellow Fever American: The Early American Republic, the British Empire and the Geopolitics of Disease in the Atlantic World," *Atlantic Studies* 7, no. 4 (December 2010): 449–63.
4 Paul, Weindling, "International Sanitary Conference," in *International Health Organizations and Movements, 1918–1939*, ed. Paul Weindling (New York: Cambridge University Press, 1995), 7–15.
5 Michael Worboys, *Spreading Germs: Disease Theories and Medical Practice in Britain, 1865–1900* (Cambridge: Cambridge University Press, 2000), 195. Linda Bryder, *Below the Magic Mountain: A Social History of Tuberculosis in Twentieth-Century Britain* (Oxford: Clarendon Press, 1988), 1, 4 (death rate). Donald S. Harris, who was assigned to consular duties at the U.S. Consulate in Glasgow in 1945, found that tuberculosis was one of the most significant problems in determining whom to admit to the United States.
6 Worboys, *Spreading Germs*, 194, 209, 217; Thomas Goetz, *The Remedy: Robert Koch, Arthur Conan Doyle and the Quest to Cure Tuberculosis* (New York: Gotham Books, 2014), 70, 204–6.
7 Michael Worboys, "The Sanatorium Treatment for Consumption in Britain, 1890–1914," in *Medical Innovations in Historical Perspectives*, ed. John V. Pickstone (New York: St. Martin's Press, 1992), 55; Frank Mort, *Dangerous Sexualities: Medico-Moral Politics in England since 1830* (London: Routledge & Kegan Paul Ltd., 1987), 47, 78–9, 105–6, 149–50; Bryder, *Below the Magic Mountain*, 43; *Marc Arnold, Disease, Class and Social Change: Tuberculosis in Folkestone and Sandgate, 1880–1930* (Newcastle upon Tyne: Cambridge Scholars Publishing, 2012), 110–11.
8 F. B. Smith, *The Retreat of Tuberculosis 1850–1950* (London: Croom Helm, 1988), 69–73; *International Congress on Tuberculosis, Official Report of the Executive Committee for Great Britain and Ireland: Report for England and Wales* (London: William Clowes & Sons, 1908), 10–46; Thomas Dormandy, *The White Death: A History of Tuberculosis* (Washington Square, New York: New York University Press, 2000), 311–12.
9 College of Physicians of Philadelphia (hereafter CPP), Joseph Walsh Papers (hereafter JWP), vol. 10, European Trips, J. Walsh, "Tuberculosis Work in Europe," 82–83, 86–102; Worboys, "Sanatorium Treatment," 53–54, 57, 64–65.
10 F. B. Smith, *Retreat of Tuberculosis* 16, 19–20, 42, 45–6, 103–5 (pauperization), 109, 127, 136–37; Worboys, "Sanatorium Treatment," 57; Bryder, *Below the Magic Mountain*, 142–48, 149–51.
11 Siân Pooley, "'All We Parents Want Is That Our Children's Health and Lives Should Be Regarded': Child Health and Parental Concern in England, c. 1860–1910," *Social History of Medicine* 23, no. 3 (December 2010): 537–45; F. B. Smith, *Retreat of Tuberculosis* 12, 15; Linda Bryder, "'Wonderlands of Buttercup, Clover and Daisies;' Tuberculosis and the Open-Air School Movement in Britain, 1907–39," in *the Name of the Child: Health and Welfare, 1889–1940*, ed. Roger Cooter (London: Routledge, 1992), 74–76.
12 Bryder, *Below the Magic Mountain*, 45, 70–71, 95, 128–33, 184–86, 227–53.
13 F. B. Smith, *Retreat of Tuberculosis*, 79–82; International Congress on Tuberculosis, Official Report, 35–39; Linda Bryder, "Papworth Village Settlement—Unique Experiment in the Treatment and Care of Tuberculosis," *Medical History* 28 (1984): 372–89.
14 David S. Barnes, *The Making of a Social Disease: Tuberculosis in Nineteenth-Century France* (Berkeley: University of California Press, 1995), 12–13 (women), 25–30, 41, 48–51, 74–76, 94–96, 142, 145.

15 Barnes, *Making of a Social Disease*, 105, 117, 166, 250; David S. Barnes, *The Great Stink of Paris and the Nineteenth-Century Struggle against Filth and Germs* (Baltimore: Johns Hopkins University Press, 2006), 148–50, 156, 158.

16 Barnes, *Making of a Social Disease*, 105, 119–20, 248; Bryder, *Below the Magic Mountain*, 139.

17 Barnes, *Making of a Social Disease*, 139–40, 215–46, 250; Mark H. Haller, "Recurring Themes," in *The Peoples of Philadelphia: A History of Ethnic Groups and Lower Class Life, 1790–1940*, eds. Allen F. Davis and Mark H. Haller (Philadelphia: Temple University Press, 1973), 286–88; Nathaniel Burt and Wallace E. Davies, "The Iron Age, 1876–1905," in *Philadelphia a 300-Year History*, ed. Russell F. Weigley (New York: W.W. Norton & Company, 1982), 428–29, 495; Lloyd M. Abernethy, "Progressivism in 1905–1919," in *Philadelphia A 300-Year History*, ed. Russell F. Weigley (New York: W.W. Norton & Company, 1982), 528–30; "En el Sanatorio Santa María; de un capellán—inercia de la comisión asesora-La Comida sigue siendo mala-nombramiento excesivo de empleados," *La Vanguardia* (6 April 1920): 8; "En el Sanatorio de Tuberculosos de Santa María; Una vista del corresponsal de 'La Vanguardia.'" *La Vanguardia* (14 June 1920): 5.

18 F. B. Smith, *Retreat of Tuberculosis* 97–99; Bryder, Below the Magic Mountain, 26 (statistics for use of tuberculin); Barnes, Making of a Social Disease, 248–50; Emilio R. Coni, "Armamento antituberculosos francés y argentino," *Revista de Ciencias Médicas* 7, no. 82 (February 1925): 260 for numbers of sanatoriums and dispensaries.

19 F. B. Smith, *Retreat of Tuberculosis* 97–103; Mitya New, "Silent Heroes of Past Not Forgotten in Switzerland's Davos," *North American News Report*, (16 January 1993); visit by author to Davos in October 2006. Thomas Mann made Davos internationally known with his novel Magic Mountain translated by H.T. Lowe-Porter (New York: Vintage International, 1992) that described the treatment in 1912 of his wife Katja.

20 Barnes, *The Making of a Social Disease*, 248–49. For Buenos Aires and Philadelphia clinics see Emilio R. Coni, "La Lucha antituberculosa en la América Latina," *Alianza de Higiene Social* 9, nos. 3/4 (August/September 1909): 75–77 and "Tuberculosis Work in Philadelphia," *Monthly Bulletin of the Department of Public Health and Charities of the City of Philadelphia* 4, no. 6 (June 1919), 85; David McBride, *Integrating the City of Medicine: Blacks in Philadelphia Health Care, 1910–1965* (Philadelphia: Temple University Press, 1988), 129 (for 1941).

21 María José Báguena Cervellera, *La Tuberculosis y su historia* (Barcelona: Fundación Uriach, 1992); Jorge Molero-Mesa, "'The Right not to suffer consumption:' Health, Welfare, Charity, and the Working Class in Spain during the Restoration Period," in *Tuberculosis Then and Now: Perspectives on the History of an Infectious Disease*, eds. Flurin Condrau and Michael Worboys (Montreal: McGill-Queen's University Press, 2010), 171–80.

22 Randall M. Packard, *White Plague, Black Labor: Tuberculosis and the Political Economy of Health and Disease in South Africa* (Berkeley: University of California Press, 1989), 5, 12, 33–38, 43, 125; C. Metcalf, "A History of Tuberculosis," in *A Century of Tuberculosis: South African Perspectives*, eds. H. M. Coovadia and S. R. Benatar (Cape Town: Oxford University Press, 1991), 24–25.

23 C. Metcalf, 22, 28; Packard, *White Plague*, 9–12, 68–86; Gillian Burke and Peter Richardson, "The Profits of Death: A Comparative Study of Miners' Phthisis in Cornwall and the Transvaal, 1876–1918," *Journal of Southern African Studies (Great Britain)* 4, no. 2 (April 1978): 147–71.

24 Packard, *White Plague*, 193, 211–31; Randall M. Packard, "Tuberculosis and the Development of Industrial Health Policies on the Witwatersrand, 1902–1932," *Journal of South African Studies* 13, no. 2 (January 1987): 204–6.
25 Packard, *White Plague*, 14–16; 49–57, 61–65, 158; Samuel Kelton Roberts, *Infectious Fear: Politics, Disease and the Health Effects of Segregation* (Chapel Hill: University of North Carolina, 2009), 52–54.
26 Ira Klein, "Death in India, 1871–1921," *Journal of Asian Studies* 32, no. 4 (August 1973): 642–43; Mark Harrison and Michael Worboys, "Disease of Civilization: Tuberculosis in Britain, Africa, and India, 1900–1939," in *Migrants, Minorities and Health: Historical and Contemporary Studies*, eds. Lara Marks and Michael Worboys (London: Routledge, 1997), 111–12, 117.
27 Bridie J. Andrews, "Tuberculosis and the Assimilation of Germ Theory in China, 1895–1937," *Journal of the History of Medicine and Allied Sciences* 52, no. 1 (January 1997): 118, 129–30, 132–33, 140, 149–51.
28 William Johnston, "A Genealogy of Tubercular Disease in Japan," *Social History of Medicine* 7, no. 2 (August 1994): 248, 257–58, 260–67; William Johnston, *The Modern Epidemic: A History of Tuberculosis in Japan* (Cambridge: Harvard University Press, 1995), 116, 195; Pierre-Yves Donze, "Studies Abroad by Japanese Doctors: A Prosopographic Analysis of the Nameless Practitioners, 1862–1912," *Social History of Medicine* 23, no. 2 (August 2010): 248–54.
29 Johnston, *Modern Epidemic*, 69, 84.
30 Johnston, *Modern Epidemic*, 107–8 and quote 116.
31 Johnston, *Modern Epidemic*, 96–99, 163–64, 208, 214, 245–49, 253–54, 283–87.
32 See Roberts, infectious fear, 42–66 for a fine discussion of racialized public policies and tuberculosis.
33 Interview with Marie Matteucci, Shippensburg, Pennsylvania, 18 October 2004; David S. Barnes, "Targeting Patient Zero," in *Tuberculosis Then and Now: Perspectives on the History of an Infectious Disease*, eds. Flurin Condrau and Michael Worboys (Montreal: McGill-Queen's University Press, 2010), 53–4; Flurin Condrau, "Beyond the Total Institution: Towards a Reinterpretation of the Tuberculosis Sanatorium," in *Tuberculosis Then and Now: Perspectives on the History of an Infectious Disease*, eds. Flurin Condrau and Michael Worboys (Montreal: McGill-Queen's University Press, 2010), 84–85.
34 Matthew R. Smallman-Raynor and Andrew D. Cliff, *War Epidemics: an Historical Geography of Infectious Diseases in Military Conflict and Civil Strife, 1850–2000* (New York: Oxford University Press, 2004), 652–58.
35 See Table 2.1: Comparative Demographics, Buenos Aires and Philadelphia 1870–1938.
36 "Laetare Medal Conferred on Lawrence F. Flick M. D. in the Hall of the Society 5 May 1920," *Records of the American Catholic Historical Society of Philadelphia* 31, no. 2 (1920): 117–20.
37 Donald G. McNeil, Jr., "New Tuberculosis Test May Soon Be Possible," *New York Times* 2 (January 2018), D6.
38 League of Nations, Health Organisation, *Tuberculosis Statistics: Summary of the Report Addressed by Dr. S. Rosenfeld (Vienna) to the Health Committee of the League of Nations, April 1925* (Réunies, Chambéry: Health Section, 1925), 21.
39 League of Nations, Tuberculosis Statistics: Summary of the Report, 12–30 provides a thorough discussion on the accuracy of the League's tuberculosis statistics.

40 Thomas McKeown, *The Modern Rise of Population* (New York: Academic Press, 1976), 68, 93, 135; Thomas McKeown, *The Origin of Human Disease* (London: Basil Blackwell, 1988), 81–85; Smith, *Retreat of Tuberculosis* 173: 236–47.

41 Michael E. Teller, *The Tuberculosis Movement: A Public Health Campaign in the Progressive Era* (New York: Greenwood Press, 1988), 95–96, 134–37; Allen K. Krause, *Environment and Resistance in Tuberculosis* (Baltimore: Williams & Wilkins Company, 1923), 7–10, 20–22; Allen K. Krause, *Rest and Other Things: A Little Book of Plain Talks on Tuberculosis Problems* (Baltimore: Williams & Wilkins Company, 1923), 71–73, 87–88, 100–103, 113, 142, 158–59 quote 100–101.

42 Leonard G. Wilson, "The Historical Decline of Tuberculosis in Europe and America: Its Causes and Significance," *Journal of the History of Medicine and Allied Sciences* 45, no. 3 (July 1990): 366–96, quote 395; Anne Hardy, *The Epidemics Streets: Infectious Disease and the Rise of Preventive Medicine, 1856–1900* (Oxford: Clarendon, 1993), 264–66.

43 Greta Jones, *'Captain of all These Men of Death:' The History of Tuberculosis in Nineteenth and Twentieth Century Ireland* (Amsterdam, Netherlands: Rodopi, 2001), 2, 38, 63, 82–83, 119, 227, 229–34.

44 Michael Worboys, "Before McKeown: Explaining the Decline of Tuberculosis in Britain, 1880–1930," in *Tuberculosis Then and Now: Perspectives on the History of an Infectious Disease*, ed. Michael Worboys (Cambridge: Cambridge University Press, 2000), 159–64.

45 Paul Farmer, *Infections and Inequalities: The Modern Plagues* (Berkeley: University of California Press, 1999), 13–14, 206–208; Paul Farmer, *Pathologies of Power: Health, Human Rights, and the New War on the Poor* (Berkeley: University of California Press, 2005), 146–47, 151.

46 Sébastien Gagneux, "Host-pathogen co-evolution in human tuberculosis," *Philosophical Transactions of the Royal Society B. Biological Sciences* 367, no. 1590 (19 March 2012): 54–55.

47 Matthew Smallman-Raynor and Andrew D. Cliff, "War and Disease: Some Perspective on the Spatial and Temporal Occurrence of Tuberculosis in Wartime," in *The Return of the White Plague: Global Poverty and the 'New' Tuberculosis*, eds. Matthew Gandy and Alimuddin Zumla (London: Verso, 2003), 74–76, 82–92; Gastone Mostardini, "L'evoluzione della mortalità tubercolare in Europa," *Lotta contro la Tuberculosi* 21, nos. 3–4 (March–April, 1951): 135–57 argues that World War I increased tuberculosis mortality in Europe to a greater extent than did World War II; those countries with better health services were least affected.

48 Roberts, *infectious fear*, 32–39; David S. Barnes, "The Rise or Fall of Tuberculosis in Belle-Époque France: A Reply to Allan Mitchell," *Social History of Medicine* 5, no. 2 (1992): 279–90; Farmer, *Infections and Inequalities*, 42–43, 48–49.

49 Mathew Gandy, "Life without Germs: Contested Episodes in the History of Tuberculosis," in *The Return of the White Plague: Global Poverty and the 'New' Tuberculosis*, eds. Matthew Gandy and Alimuddin Zumla (London: Verso, 2003), 26–27.

50 Matthew R. Smallman-Raynor and Andrew D. Cliff summarize seven theories that explain the causes of epidemic disease decline in War Epidemics: an Historical Geography of Infectious Diseases in Military Conflict and Civil Strife, 143–50. The theories are: the Crisis Hypothesis, the Urbanization Hypothesis, the Economic and Nutritional Hypothesis, the Medical Hypothesis, the Environmental Hypothesis, the Treatment Hypothesis and the Prevention Hypothesis.

Epilogue

Tuberculosis Developments and Patient Experiences

> To the Donald Meadows family, tuberculosis was just something nobody seemed to get much anymore. That was a year ago. Their education began last May, when their 3-year old daughter, Penny, became ill... the doctors...found Penny had tuberculosis. On the advice of doctors, Donald Meadows, 26, and his wife Betty, 24, had chest x-rays taken. They also had tuberculosis. A few weeks later Mrs. Meadows' brother... had a chest x-ray that showed that he too had tuberculosis.... Another brother...developed tuberculosis in the army. [In addition a sister-in law and another brother also developed tuberculosis. This made seven cases in the same family in the 1960s.][1]

> Two years ago (2014) a hospital administrator confirmed that my brother Gary had tuberculosis.... 'It's worse than we thought,' she said. 'There might not even be any medication to help him.'.... Gary didn't have just multi-drug-resistant TB: He had 'extensively drug-resistant' TB.[2]

By 1945, medications appeared to cure tuberculosis successfully. However, as the previous quotes indicate, some U.S. families were severely harmed by the disease. New medications, although effective initially, were in short supply. Eventually, new strains of drug-resistant tubercle bacilli emerged. Between 1945 and 1955, patients continued to enter sanatoriums. In 1955, Chuck Felton, 17, traveled to Cresson. On arrival his clothing were "fumigated" and sent home with his parents. Chuck lived the next year in a ward with fifteen older men. Sometimes he woke up in the night to patient coughing and in mornings found an empty bed. Each patient had a radio on his bedside table. Cresson had a store, library, school for children and vocational training for older patients. When "cured," college-age patients received scholarships to Penn State.[3]

Marie K. Matteucci, 18, arrived at the South Mountain Sanatorium in Mont Alto in early 1955. Since her father had died of tuberculosis and black lung disease in the 1940s, she was required to regularly visit a tubercular clinic to be X-rayed and have sputum checked. When a lesion was found on her lung, Marie first went to the state sanatorium in Hamburg, which was closer to her home town of Tunkhannock, near Scranton. She intensely disliked this sanatorium because of its large patient wards and frigid rooms, which required a hat and gloves even in bed. After four months, she transferred to Mont Alto. Here, she first shared a room with five others of similar age before eventually receiving her own room in one of the Dixon cottages. When her health improved, Marie began working for two hours a day as a hospital photographer taking pictures of newly arrived patients as well as autopsies. Eventually, working eight hours a day, this job also gave her freedom of movement throughout the grounds. After eighteen months, new medications, including para-aminosalicylic acid (PAS) and isoniazid (INH), and pneumoperitoneum treatments, cured Marie and she left in 1956 to attend college, although she continued treatments. The Department of Vocational Rehabilitation provided a scholarship which paid for her books, tuition and housing; Marie graduated from Shippensburg State College in 1960.[4]

Routine life in the sanatorium was little changed from an earlier era. But once patients could be treated with antibiotics at home, cities and states closed preventoriums and sanatoriums. Those individuals who survived the disease to return to their home communities often preferred that no one know they once had the disease because tuberculosis was contagious and associated with stigma. Some former patients faced job discrimination, and those who had lived in sanatoriums often chose not to discuss their experiences. Nevertheless, fear of tuberculosis was declining. With the availability of an effective medicine, tuberculosis began to resemble curable diseases like pneumonia and meningitis.[5]

In spite of the discovery of streptomycin in 1943 and the hope that tuberculosis would soon be defeated, tuberculosis continued to be a challenge to public health officials in developed countries and a major infection in third-world countries in which diagnosis and treatment were not readily available. Between 1945 and 1947, little streptomycin was available and physicians needed to decide who would receive the treatment and how it was financed. By 1953, nine U.S. companies were producing the needed medications. After World War II, thoracic surgery became common-place in part because surgeons gained experience treating traumatic chest injuries during the war. Furthermore, the availability of antibiotics made operating on infected tissues relatively safe. From 1947 to 1953, the U.S. public health services used X-rays to screen large urban populations, so as to detect active cases early. By the mid-1950s, physicians standardized the treatment of tuberculosis with three drugs: para-aminosalicylic acid (PAS), isoniazid and streptomycin. New treatments and technology increased the medical influence of physicians who administered these new medications and controlled access to them. It was commonly believed that tuberculosis had been conquered.[6] By the 1960s, heart disease, cancer and strokes surpassed tuberculosis as major causes of death in the western world.[7]

However, tuberculosis did not completely disappear from poor neighborhoods in Buenos Aires and Philadelphia as poverty limited the access to health care. Furthermore, discriminatory attitudes toward African Americans persisted in the U.S. Popular beliefs accepted the genetic origin of disease but presumed the cultural, social and psychological inferiority of African Americans. Segregation supported unhealthy neighborhoods. Health care providers continued to deny the existence of a tuberculosis crisis within Black communities. Social rather than biological factors contributed to the resurgence of tuberculosis.[8] Tuberculosis remained a contagious disease transmitted to those who came in contact with individuals with active tuberculosis, and it continued to infect individuals of all ages.

The reappearance of tuberculosis as a major news item during the 1980s challenged popular belief that tuberculosis was successfully cured. The easy movement of individuals across national borders and the failure to recognize that tuberculosis continued to exist in poor communities, complicated medical treatment, while the most effective treatments were only partially available to the poor. Thus, there is a clear relationship between poverty and disease. Ninety-five percent of tuberculosis cases and ninety-eight percent of tuberculosis deaths occurred in developing countries. On the other hand, "Among the developed countries it is not the richest societies that have the best health but rather those with the smallest income differentials between rich and poor."[9] Race, age, social class and geography determine who contracts tuberculosis, who receives medications and how effective the treatment will be.

Medical experts were completely caught off guard in the 1980s when the number of reported cases of tuberculosis began to arise rapidly around the world. Public health officials failed to consider disease historically and failed to realize that social changes can cause old diseases to occur. They had focused only on humans and did not consider how plants and other animals contribute to disease development. Public health officials paid little attention to how parasites evolved or species interacted. They wrongly thought that economic development would ensure global prosperity and that increased resources would be devoted to improving public health. Western medical organizations viewed technology as a panacea; they failed to realize that poor and minority groups were not benefiting from economic prosperity and more effective medications.[10]

End of the 1870–1945 Tuberculosis Institutions

Between 1946 and 1956, physicians thought of sanatoriums as the ideal environment for monitoring patients on drug therapy. Nevertheless, sanatoriums began to close or were converted to other uses as the number of tuberculosis patients decreased. In Philadelphia, White Haven was transferred in 1946 to Jefferson Medical College. It continued to operate as a sanatorium until it was sold in 1956 to the Commonwealth of Pennsylvania to be used to care for the mentally retarded. In November 1954, the last tuberculosis patient left the Trudeau sanatorium. In Pennsylvania,

Hamburg closed its doors in 1959, Cresson in 1964 and Mont Alto in 1968. As the number of tuberculosis patients dwindled, state mental hospitals in need of additional space took over institutions that had previously housed tuberculosis patients. In 1965, the Pennsylvania Office for Aging acquired the Mont Alto facilities; it soon accepted older adults from mental hospitals to provide treatment that would lead to their returning to their communities. By 1968, the South Mountain Restoration Center provided long-term nursing care for geriatric mental patients in what had been a tuberculosis hospital. The rise of drug-resistant tuberculosis gave new life to some tuberculosis facilities especially as the need for residential mental health facilities has decreased.[11]

Santa María, Vicente López Planes and Hospital Doctor Tornú confronted similar changes. During the 1960s, most former sanatoriums became general medical centers, mental health establishments, regional hospitals, research institutions or drug treatment centers. Some buildings were torn down or simply vacated. Santa María followed Mont Alto's pattern: buildings vacated by tubercular patients were used for mental health and drug rehabilitation treatment programs. Other buildings on the ground were abandoned. In 1987, the Hospital Dr. Enrique Tornú had many unused buildings in disrepair and was transformed into the Hospital General de Agudos Dr. E. Tornú to offer general medical care. With the revival of tuberculosis, it once again began to offer tuberculosis care. The age of tuberculosis sanatoriums ended, even although the disease itself remained in existence.[12]

Preventoriums faced the same restructuring as sanatoriums. They began to decline in significance in the 1930s, because of the lack of evidence that they were effective, the decrease in the number of tubercular children and the institutions' financial problems. The increase in child welfare agencies in both Buenos Aires and Philadelphia devoted to family assistance—and the U.S. Social Security Act of 1935, which supported widows and their children—diminished the need for preventoriums for sickly children. Preventorium facilities were converted to other uses. For example, Rest Haven (an important California preventorium) opened in 1913 and enjoyed its greatest period of growth between 1920 and 1942; without adequate funding it shut down in 1951. In 1955, River Crest near Philadelphia redirected its focus to serve those with mental retardation and other disabilities.[13]

Studies of out-patient treatment in Madras, India, from 1956 to 1959 illustrated the continued importance of global cooperation in combating tuberculosis. The study also contributed to sanatorium closings in both Argentina and the U.S. In the Madras studies, patients were randomly chosen to be treated with a combination of isoniazid and PAS therapy for twelve months in either their homes under very unfavorable conditions or in the controlled sanatorium environment. The results demonstrated that home treatment was as effective as sanatorium or hospital care. Although adequate healthy food is important for those with tuberculosis, the Madras research indicated that patients did not require an improved standard of living but instead an adequate supply of medicine and supervision in administering it. Patients preferred out-patient treatment—which also had the advantage of being cheaper. Thus, an increasing number of patients left sanatoriums. The Madras study globally impacted the treatment of tuberculosis patients as out-patient treatment centers began efforts to ensure that those under care took their required medications. This approach encouraged developed nations to provide medications for people in poorer societies. In western nations, a new issue related to civil liberties emerged when social service agencies threatened patients with confinement if they failed to take their medications. The Madras study also deemphasized the role of poverty in ensuring that patients follow their drug regimen; it assumed that improved supervision would guarantee that patients took their medications correctly. However, unpredictable housing, unhealthy food and erratic work make routine difficult and impeded the ability of the poor to take their scheduled medications.[14]

New Global Tuberculosis Outbreak

Although the world standard of living had been rising since the late 1940s and was still improving in the 1980s, tuberculosis nevertheless broke out again in the late twentieth century. Four factors explain the outbreak: the emergence of new tuberculosis bacteria strains (MDR-TB and XDR-TB) that do not respond to the standard medications; the rise of HIV/AIDS (Human Immunodeficiency Virus/Acquired Immunodeficiency); the poverty of those contracting the disease; and cutbacks in public funding for tuberculosis prevention and cure. The escalating number of tuberculosis cases lead to more infected individuals. The World Health Organization dosage recommendations for rifampicin and isoniazid may be too low for HIV patients with the result that patients are contagious for longer than necessary. MDR-TB develops when the tuberculosis bacteria resist the two most powerful anti-tuberculosis drugs, isoniazid and rifampicin. XDR-TB is even more dangerous because it also resists second-line fluoroquinolone medications. MDR-TB and XDR-TB epidemics occurred because resistant bacteria strains developed when patients failed to complete prescribed treatment or received insufficient or substandard medication. The new strains of bacteria became particularly deadly when associated with AIDS. HIV/AIDS patients with weakened immune systems are susceptible to multi-drug-resistant strains of the disease. Not only did tuberculosis increase the death rate of AIDS patients, but unlike AIDS it easily spread through coughing.[15] Before HIV, eighty-five percent of tuberculosis cases were pulmonary tuberculosis. But with the AIDS epidemic, non-pulmonary tuberculosis has become more common. A weakened immune system, inadequate housing and unhealthy food created an environment in which individuals could contract MDR-TB or XDR-TB.[16]

Between 1945 and 1954, the U.S. reports of new tuberculosis cases decreased by fourteen percent, and tuberculosis deaths decreased by seventy percent. However, tuberculosis in comparison with other diseases killed at a younger age; in 1947, the median age of death for cancer was sixty-four and for heart disease, sixty-nine.[17] By 1976, tuberculosis was statistically the twenty-first cause of death and accounted for only one out of every 550 deaths.[18] Tuberculosis again became prevalent in the U.S. between 1985 and 1992; the number of cases increased by sixteen to twenty percent annually. In this era, the resurgence of tuberculosis disproportionately affected racial and ethnic minorities. Tuberculosis increased by twenty-seven percent among Blacks, seven percent among Hispanics and forty-six percent among Asian/Pacific Islanders, but decreased by ten percent among non-Hispanic Whites and twenty-three percent among Native Americans. This increase occurred not only because of the AIDS epidemic and the rise of drug-resistant strains, but also because of a cutback in public health programs. Cities ended mass X-ray screening programs, and public clinics were unprepared for the large number of new tuberculosis cases. The growth of urban poverty—leading to more individuals in homeless shelters—revealed the relationship between tuberculosis and poverty. The poor were at greater risk; their immune systems were often weaker, due to poor health and repeated exposure to tuberculosis. Furthermore, often they could not afford medications, health services or even basic food and housing.[19]

In the early 1990s, an intensive national campaign in the U.S. attempted to bring tuberculosis under control; the federal government spent more on the disease and paid medical personnel to utilize directly observed therapy (DOT) to ensure that patients took their drugs. The number of new tuberculosis cases began falling in 1993. There were 12,904 new cases in 2008, which marked the sixteenth year of decline in the reported U.S. tuberculosis cases. By 2014, only 9,421 new tuberculosis cases were reported; this represented the lowest rate on record since the beginning of national reporting in 1953. Pennsylvania reported 214 cases in 2013 and 209 in 2014. However, in 2015 the number of U.S. tuberculosis cases increased to 9,563 indicating that U.S. efforts to eliminate tuberculosis had stalled. Pockets of tuberculosis continue to emerge. (Since 2014 in Marion, Alabama, poverty and mistrust of medicine led to late diagnosis and treatment of twenty people and three deaths, nearly all African-Americans.) Moreover, throughout the U.S., fewer doctors are familiar with tuberculosis leading to misdiagnosis. Devastating state budget cuts in public health gutted prevention programs. The U.S. government's failure to screen temporary visa holders also contributed to an increase in tuberculosis cases.[20]

In 1988, Philadelphia confronted the resurgence of tuberculosis by opening a publicly funded tuberculosis clinic, the Lawrence F. Flick Memorial Center. The Philadelphia Department of Public Health sought to reduce the number of tuberculosis cases through prevention, diagnosis and treatment. It offered free tuberculosis testing and case management of those with latent and active tuberculosis infection through DOT and patient care in the Flick Center. HIV patients who became tubercular, those with drug-resistant tuberculosis, and tubercular immigrants posed the greatest challenges to Philadelphia's public health efforts. Between 1994 and 2004, Philadelphia accounted for thirty-nine percent of all Pennsylvania cases, but only twelve percent of its population. Beginning in 1996, however, the reported tuberculosis cases in Philadelphia began to decline. In 1995, the Philadelphia Tuberculosis Control Program reported 309 new cases. By contrast, in 2007, only 133 new cases were reported: of these 100 (seventy-five percent) were classified as pulmonary tuberculosis, twenty-three (seventeen percent) as extra-pulmonary tuberculosis and ten (eight percent) as both. Between 1997 and 2007, tubercular cases among the foreign-born doubled, exceeding those among the U.S.-born citizens. Almost half of the tuberculosis cases occurred in young adults between the ages of fifteen and forty-four. In 2008, Philadelphia reported 162 new cases. By 2015, the number of new cases declined to seventy-one. They increased slightly in 2016 to seventy-three when the case rate was 4.7 per 100,000 population. Tuberculosis infected African Americans and foreign-born in proportionally higher numbers than other groups.[21]

Tuberculosis also resurfaced in Argentina in the 1980s. By 1990, the number of new cases began to decline. In 2006, health authorities identified 4,622 cases, of which nearly half were in Buenos Aires. But by 2015, the number of infected people was again increasing and Argentina reported 10,713 new tuberculosis cases. In 2015, Buenos Aires reported 1,154 infected people raising the rate to 37.8 per 100,000 population, eight times the rate of Philadelphia. Buenos Aires faces challenges in continuing to reduce the number of tuberculosis cases and the number of new cases has declined much more gradually than in Philadelphia. Jammed buses probably contribute to the spread of tuberculosis as does the increased number of HIV/AIDS patients, overcrowded living arrangements, and a lower standard of living than in Philadelphia. As in the past, Hospital Muñiz remains the center for treating infectious diseases; it treats all MDR-TB and XDR-TB cases in Buenos Aires.[22]

Tuberculosis remains the biggest infectious killer in the world and the ninth leading cause of death worldwide. In 1994, tuberculosis killed more adults than AIDS, malaria, smallpox and cholera combined. As of 2017, it ranked above HIV/AIDS as a global killer. Philadelphia and, especially, Buenos Aires illustrate that tuberculosis has again become a serious health hazard; the disease is expected to continue to pose a major world health problem in the twenty-first century. The situation in underdeveloped countries is particularly worrisome. In 2016, five countries: India, Indonesia, China, The Philippines and Pakistan accounted for fifty-six percent of the global cases. If untreated, each individual with active tuberculosis infects on average ten to fifteen others.[23] In spite of the availability of effective drug treatments, tuberculosis killed more people in 1995 than in 1900. Some progress has been made since 2000, but many developing nations cannot afford the needed programs. MDR-TB and the combination of tuberculosis and HIV have threatened progress in combating the disease. In 2008, with an increasing number of MDR-TB cases, developing countries could provide treatment to only an estimated ten percent of them. Worldwide, one in every twenty new tuberculosis cases is resistant to two or more drugs. In addition, a cure for (XDR-TB) costs $1,500 to $15,000 in drugs and requires two years of continuous treatment; in comparison, traditional tuberculosis can be cured in six months for $10–$20.[24]

The good news is that the tuberculosis mortality rate has fallen by forty-five percent since 1990. New tuberculosis cases are decreasing in the third world, following the earlier declines in Argentina and the U.S. Many factors explain the decline: in particular, the cresting of the AIDS epidemic in Africa and the increase of foreign aid to treat the ill. However, challenges remain. Tuberculosis killed 1.4 million people worldwide in 2010 and produced 8.8 million new cases (fifty-nine percent of them in Asia, twenty-six percent in Africa and three percent in Latin America). In 2016, 10.4 million people contracted tuberculosis and 1.7 million died. Although eighty-seven percent of the new cases were successfully treated, almost six percent of the new cases were MDR-TB or XDR-TB.[25]

Although globally more men than women died from tuberculosis, in 2009, tuberculosis was the third leading cause of death among women aged fifteen to forty-four. Gender discrimination and poverty affected women's access to health care. China, Russia, India, Pakistan, Thailand and South Africa are among the countries that continue to face serious tuberculosis challenges. Drug-resistant tuberculosis is threatening to reverse India's treatment success through its use of DOT. In South Africa, in 2005, an outbreak of XDR-TB in a rural hospital killed fifty-two out of fifty-three people infected. Tuberculosis is so common in Russia's prisons and detention centers that everyone who has spent time there has latent or active tuberculosis. In countries such as Russia, latent tuberculosis needs to be treated in order to reduce the number of new tuberculosis cases, but treatment is very expensive. Tuberculosis, especially XDR-TB spreads easily in prisons: the disease is generally detected only late, the ill are not isolated and treatment is inadequate. In addition, prisons are overcrowded, serve poor food and compel prisoners to lead stressful lives. The large number and the high turnover of individuals in Russian pre-trial centers and prisons ensure that prisoners' family and friends are also infected. (For example, Gary first developed tuberculosis in Russia.) Tuberculosis kills the majority of Russian HIV/AID patients. (In 2014, WHO estimated that twenty percent of Russian new cases were multi-drug resistant and forty-six percent of previously treated cases.) Social factors, not biological ones, explain the increased tuberculosis in Russian prisons.[26]

Jet travel leads to the rapid spread of the disease; in the U.S., recent arrivals are believed to be responsible for almost half of new tuberculosis cases. XDR-TB is rare in the U.S.; only forty-nine cases were identified between 1998 and 2007, of which at least twelve were fatal. In 1998, a Ukrainian immigrant, who had been treated various times for tuberculosis between 1976 and 1994, walked into a public health clinic in a small town in Erie County, Pennsylvania. When he was diagnosed with tuberculosis, Pennsylvania's health department began a frantic effort to locate the thirty-six passengers seated nearest to the patient on his plane. All but three were located and tested for tuberculosis; of those tested, twenty were negative and thirteen positive, but there was no way to determine when those testing positive had been infected. Similar events will continue to occur. In 2007, Arizona obtained a court order to confine and treat a twenty-seven-year-old with both U.S. and Russian citizenship who had undergone incomplete treatment in Russia and who had developed XDR-TB. When XDR-TB patients are not visibly ill, confirmation often occurs late. Furthermore, the disease is difficult to cure, because it is hard to identify the particular strain and the appropriate drug to treat it.[27]

Patients may fail to heed advice not to travel and thereby increase the number of individuals exposed to the disease. In 1994, a passenger with MDR-TB flew on a commercial airline from Honolulu to Baltimore via Chicago and one month later returned home by the same route. A 1996 *New England Journal of Medicine* study indicated that six percent of those who were on the longest segment of the flight (8.75 hours from Chicago to Honolulu) had a positive tuberculin skin test, whereas less than three percent of the travelers on other segments of the flight (including the Honolulu to Chicago) tested positive. Those seated within two rows of the patient were more likely to have a positive skin test than those seated further away. The result of this study galvanized the U.S. Centers for Disease Control and Prevention in 2007 to quarantine an Atlanta man believed to have XDR-TB (who had traveled in the U.S., Canada and Europe against physician advice), and to locate and test passengers and crew who had been on the same flights. For the first time since 1963, the federal government ordered the quarantining of an infectious individual. Further tests indicated that the Atlanta traveler did not have drug-resistant tuberculosis and had infected no one. As David Barnes has pointed out, in cases like these, there is a tendency to blame the victim and to divert attention away from the underlying causes of the disease: poverty, malnutrition, homelessness, alcoholism, drug abuse and AIDS. He further argues that to control tuberculosis we must not only prevent the transmission of tuberculosis but also improve the lives of the poor. Historically, tuberculosis spreads most rapidly in overcrowded households. For example, in New York City, new cases diminished as the amount of overcrowding housing decreased between 1975 and 1978; but as overcrowding became more common between 1978 and 1990, new cases increased.[28]

Tuberculosis is curable. Currently, low-cost drugs exist that are up to ninety-eight percent effective, but the problem is to get the medication to the infected in time and to make certain that they take the drugs daily for the required six to eight months. Treatment is complex: some medicines must be taken with food and some on an empty stomach. All produce side effects that vary from mild (vomiting and diarrhea) to life-threatening. At the same time, substance abusers, the homeless, the poor and those with HIV/AIDS face major challenges in following the necessary regimen of the antibiotic treatment. Many poor patients stop taking their medications because they cannot afford them, or because their malnutrition leads to illnesses that make the drug regimen difficult. Recognizing that more needs to be done, WHO is promoting a treatment called DOTS (directly observed therapy, short course), which uses a smear test to diagnose tuberculosis and six months of observed therapy with standard drugs. Individuals with drug-resistant tuberculosis increasingly require a much more expensive regimen, treatment lasting for twenty-four months. But because of the cost, WHO has been slow to make the needed medications available in poor countries.[29]

The failure of patients to comply with treatment programs has led some cities to attempt to coerce poor tuberculosis patients to complete their antibiotic regimen. For example, in the 1990s, New York City responded to the tuberculosis epidemic by implementing DOT and detaining those who failed to follow the drug regimen. Between 1993 and 2000, more than 200 noninfectious, noncompliant patients were detained on Roosevelt Island, some for more than two years. The typically detained individuals were poor, Black, HIV-infected and homeless; many were ex-felons and had drug problems. The city's public health efforts led to the decline of MDR-TB and to a lessened incidence of childhood tuberculosis. Unfortunately, in this second tuberculosis epidemic, as in the first one, the poor are too often blamed for contracting and spreading the disease. The detention of noninfectious (primarily poor) individuals raises civil liberties questions. Quarantine is hard to enforce; patients have autonomy, and many of them resist being isolated. The battle against tuberculosis in the U.S. emphasizes new scientific technology, identifies potential tuberculosis carriers and seeks to ensure that treatment regimens are rigorously followed. But the campaign pays less attention to the social issues, that influence who is exposed to the tuberculosis bacteria; it also fails to ensure that poor people receive necessary health care.[30]

Finding new ways to reduce tuberculosis globally requires increased efforts. Specifically, partnerships must be formed between corporations, governments, NGOs and academic institutions; strategies to prevent the rise of drug-resistant bacteria strains must be implemented in underdeveloped countries; and resources must be devoted to research and development. Among the important U.S. public-private partnerships operating as of 2013 were New York's Global Alliance for TB Drug Development, Seattle's Bill & Melinda Gates Foundation's TB Drug Acceleration and the Lilly TB Drug Discovery Initiative. Efforts abroad include the Tres Cantos Open Lab Foundation in the United Kingdom and the Innovative Medicines Initiative in Brussels. Such organizations can encourage trials of new drugs produced by different companies. Universities are being encouraged to forgo profits from their work on antibiotics and to produce not what is most profitable but what is most needed by society.[31]

The WHO and private charities are encouraging underdeveloped countries to adopt a more comprehensive approach to tuberculosis prevention and treatment. Priorities include finding better ways to use existing technologies, promoting more effective new technologies and working to control non-communicable diseases. Often overlooked factors that cause tuberculosis to spread include poor awareness of symptoms, lack of access to diagnosis and treatment, the prohibitive cost of drugs that combat multidrug-resistant strains, medical malpractice, poor quality of health care, broken drug-supply chains and the failure of patients to complete their treatment. These issues need to be considered along with risk factors that are better understood: overcrowded housing, diabetes, tobacco smoking, HIV infection and poor nutrition. The most important factor in stopping the spread of tuberculosis is to detect it early. To promote early detection, public health officials are emphasizing improved medical training, public-health screening and treatment programs. Health officials also seek to identify and treat high-risk individuals such as immigrants from third-world countries who have drug-resistant varieties of the disease. Tuberculosis is a social disease; social factors can prevent a single case from spreading or can lead to an outbreak.[32]

Continued investment in research is necessary to decrease new tuberculosis cases and to lower tuberculosis mortality. Scientists have deciphered the tuberculosis bacterium's genetic code and are currently trying to produce new medications and to develop a more effective tuberculosis vaccine. New drug combinations are needed, in which, medicines that quickly kill tuberculosis interact with slower drugs that reach mycobacteria hiding out in lesions in the lungs. The coming decade looks bright for tuberculosis drug development. In 2010, ten potential vaccines were being tested and two new drugs were slated to be available by 2013. Indeed, Janssen Pharmaceuticals began selling Bedaquiline in the U.S. in June 2013, almost half a century after Rifampicin (1967) was introduced as an addition to the tuberculosis cocktail-drug treatment. Bedaquiline was approved as a treatment for multidrug-resistant tuberculosis under the Federal Drug Administration's guidelines for "accelerated approval" for promising drugs. The drug's success is indicated when there is no detectable mycobacterium in a patient's sputum after six months of treatment. (Formerly, trials would have continued for two and a half years, to ensure that patients were fully recovered from drug-resistant tuberculosis.) Two other developments are also worth noting. First, the European Medicines Agency in London approved in 2013 the use of a new Japanese drug, delamanid which is globally available to treat those with XDR-TB. Pfizer recently sold sutezolid, a drug for treatment of XDR-TB, to a small pharmaceutical company in Rockville for development and testing.[33]

Two other research efforts are also important: finding a cheap test to identify who has tuberculosis; and developing whole-genome sequencing (a laboratory process that determines the DNA sequence of tuberculosis bacteria) to reveal underlying biological and social causes of the disease. By sequencing the entire genome of the tuberculosis bacteria, scientists can differentiate strains and build a reference library to trace where the strain is circulating in the world; with that knowledge, physicians will be better able to prescribe the medications which will destroy the specific strain of bacteria. For public health officials, the most significant issue is to find a cheap and more accurate test for tuberculosis. The standard method for testing for tuberculosis, "smear microscopy," is neither fast nor has it changed much since Robert Koch developed it in the 1880s. It involves staining and examining a sample of sputum under a microscope, counting the bacteria and grading the severity of the infection. Although an easy test to perform, it takes as long as a week to get results which are often inconclusive. It is estimated to accurately detect tuberculosis in less than half of the people with HIV who also have tuberculosis. Two new tests for tuberculosis are being evaluated. Xpert MTB/Rif is an automated machine with a cartridge that detects the DNA sequence specific to *Mycobacterium tuberculosis* in sputum. The machine costs $17,000 and each test requires a cartridge that costs $10. The machine depends on consistent electricity. Thus, it is expensive for developing countries and not always practical, but it can provide an accurate and quick diagnosis. There is also a simple alternative to Xpert MTB/Rif, an improved form of "smear microscopy" that uses light-emitting diode (LED) bulbs and fluorescent dyes, so that bacteria show up more clearly under the microscope; although this method is superior to traditional "smear microscopy," it can still misidentify the bacteria.[34]

In Perspective: Patient Experiences with Tuberculosis

This comparative study has focused on patient experiences, public health responses and tuberculosis developments in Buenos Aires and Philadelphia from 1870 to 1945. It has placed the experience of patients within an urban, national and global context, and has provided evidence of the growing global consensus among physicians and public health officials on how to treat tuberculosis. After physicians accepted Koch's theory that tuberculosis is contagious, patients hoped for a cure—and were disappointed that no cure was at hand. Not surprisingly, patient perspectives on tuberculosis differed from physicians' understanding. The narratives told by the ill and the beliefs held by the families were more diverse than those of orthodox medicine. Whereas physicians accepted Koch's explanation of tuberculosis and science's ability eventually to cure it, patients simultaneously accepted scientific, hereditary and shamanistic causes of the disease and folk, herbal and physician cures for it. The patient view is exemplified in a survey done in 1950, in which fifty-five percent of those questioned wrongly thought that tuberculosis is a hereditary disease.[35]

Patient and physician narratives describe the illness in similar ways, pointing to the disease's symptoms (coughs, fevers, chills, night sweats) and to its consequences (for example, that it made it hard to work). Patient narratives were more emotional; physician narratives were more carefully constructed than those of patients. Patient narratives sometimes ended with a cure, but it was not always the result of a physician's recommendation. Physician narratives in both Buenos Aires and Philadelphia emphasized treatments for tuberculosis that were broadly similar—notwithstanding the differences in care given to people of different classes, genders and ethnicities.

In the 1870 to 1945 era, most patients were treated at clinics or at home. Treatment choices consisted of medication and surgical procedures and fresh air and diet regimens. Men had difficulty coping with raising children and, therefore, expected their tubercular wives to remain at home. The wealthy and middle classes were more likely to travel to improve their health, whereas the working class went to poorly funded public facilities in their neighborhoods. Only a few tuberculosis patients went to sanatoriums and many of those left early. A survey of West Riding Sanatorium (Yorkshire, England) indicated that forty-four percent of the male patients and thirty-two percent of the female patients left early or were discharged for disciplinary reasons. These figures seem high, though, compared with the anecdotal evidence provided by Pennsylvania's and Argentina's sanatoriums.[36] Limited medical technology facilitated the identification of those with tuberculosis. By 1908, the tuberculin skin test determined whether a person had been exposed to the bacterium. By 1909, sputum tests enabled doctors to recognize the active disease in its early stages. The early identification of those with tuberculosis meant that patients could take actions to prevent friends and relatives from contracting tuberculosis and public health officials would develop more intrusive regulations.

After World War I, patients had more options from which to choose for the prevention of tuberculosis. BCG, first used in 1921, became the most widely used vaccine to protect against miliary tuberculosis or tuberculosis meningitis in children. Unfortunately, large-scale clinical trials done in the last forty years call BCG's efficacy into question. BCG is eighty percent effective at protecting healthy children from tuberculous meningitis and miliary tuberculosis, but it does little to protect adolescent, young adults or those with HIV from pulmonary tuberculosis. The result was that unless there was a public health campaign, few individuals chose the vaccine for their children. Since recent studies of populations in different locations have found that the effectiveness of BCG varies, and that protection declines over time, parent choices were reasonable.[37]

From 1870 to 1945, there were few differences in prevention programs between Buenos Aires and Philadelphia. The U.S. had more private charities, public clinics and more wealth than Argentina; Philadelphians had more options for treatment than Porteños. Both Buenos Aires and Philadelphia showed that patients' different classes and ethnicities influenced their experiences more than the differences between the two countries' medical systems. Tuberculosis did economic damage to families, which limited their medical choices. But tuberculosis patients were not always passive participants in efforts of physicians to affect a cure. Patients questioned the need for surgery or specific treatment, but they also welcomed new treatments and at times, willingly endured experimental therapies. Patients who had active tuberculosis often died slow and painful deaths within five years.[38]

Tuberculosis is a social issue as well as a medical problem. In both Buenos Aires and Philadelphia, elite attitude shaped tuberculosis prevention efforts; as a result, the poor, those of African heritage and immigrants were blamed for the disease and thought to need moral reform. Health officials blamed tuberculosis on the living conditions of the poor, who shared beds, used dirty linens, drank too much and lived in crowded slums. Thus, the poor tubercular patients faced not only financial difficulties but also social ostracization. Gradually, research showed that insufficient food, crowded living conditions and inadequate health care—not race or ethnicity—contributed to tuberculosis contagion in both children and adults. However, popular perceptions have been slow to change. With the advent of new medications, tuberculosis rapidly declined among the wealthy and middle classes. However, the failure of the Philadelphia and Buenos Aires governments to recognize the social underpinnings of tuberculosis and to provide needed health services for the poor ensured the disease's reappearance.

Historically, patient treatments have changed. Between 1870 and 1920, physicians told patients to eat healthy food, maintain good hygiene and rest at home or go to rural hotels or sanatoriums. Between 1920 and 1945, physicians sough to identify the tubercular through X-rays and tuberculin, to treat the disease by pneumothorax in sanatoriums and hospitals, and governments expanded public health programs. Between 1945 and 1990, sanatoriums declined in significance and physicians provided chemotherapy in hospitals or through out-patient facilities. Today, we are entering a fourth stage of treatment in which physicians are combining an emphasis on prevention with the development of new, powerful, expensive antibiotics to treat MDR-TB and XDR-TB. The new drugs are often prohibitively costly for poor people especially in underdeveloped nations.

The continuing effort to reduce and eliminate tuberculosis represents the success of both science and medicine and the increasing dependence of physicians and public health officials on technological solutions. Patients have come increasingly to believe that technology and medications by themselves will cure disease. Modern medicine is perceived as always marching forward. Drugs and surgical procedures are expected to become more effective. But the resurgence of tuberculosis shows that this is not always possible. Although the last decade has brought many advances, too often medical science, private organization and public agencies have responded to new medical challenges with only limited success, and have given short shrift especially to the difficulties faced by the poor. Social inequalities often explain who contracts tuberculosis and who recovers from it today, just as in Buenos Aires and Philadelphia between 1870 and 1945.

Although many tuberculosis patients were cured between 1945 and 2018, the emergence of drug-resistance bacteria points to the similarities between patient experiences today and those a century earlier. Pain, isolation and uncertainty characterize the lives of all tuberculosis patients. Tuberculosis patients in 2018 (just like their counterparts in the 1890s) face physical, social, physiological and economic anguish. Anguish and pain are real, and they affect all tuberculosis patients and their families in all time periods. *Beneath the Anguish* is a complicated story of prevention, diagnosis and treatment of tuberculosis in Buenos Aires and Philadelphia. My hope is an historical understanding of tuberculosis practices and treatment between 1870 and 1945 may positively shape current efforts to deal with the disease.

Notes

1 Vance Clark, "TB Sneaks Back: Seven in Family Learn Hard Way," *Spunk* 54, no. 11 (February 1963): 9.
2 Stephanie Aleksanyan, *Washington Post,* 15 February 2016, E1, E6.
3 For Felton's experience, see David Wenner, "Whatever Care We Needed, We Got," *Patriot News*, 25 October 2009, A14–15.

4 From written questionnaire of July 2001 and interview with Marie K. Matteucci in 18 October 2004, Shippensburg, Pennsylvania.

5 Interview with Marie Matteucci, 18 October 2004, Shippensburg, Pennsylvania. For a memoir of another family that suffered tuberculosis in the twentieth century, see Marjorie McVicker Sutcliffe and Judy Sutcliffe, *Grandma Cherry's Spoon: A Story of Tuberculosis* (Santa Barbara, CA: Geronima Press, 1991).

6 Ken Chowder, "How TB Survived Its Own Death to Confront Us again," *Smithsonian* 23, no. 8 (1992): 191; Richard H. Shryock, *National Tuberculosis Association, 1904–1954, A Study of the Voluntary Health Movement in the United States* (New York: National Tuberculosis Association, 1957), 239, 249–50, 300; Barron H. Lerner, *Contagion and Confinement: Controlling Tuberculosis along the Skid Road* (Baltimore: John Hopkins University Press, 1998), 48, 62.

7 "Leading Causes of Death," *World Resources 1998–99* www.wri.org/publication/content/8476 (26 August 2010); also see World Health Organization statistical reports for 1960.

8 David McBride, *From TB to Aids: Epidemics among Urban Blacks since 1900* (Albany, NY: State University of New York Press, 1991), 149; Samuel Kelton Roberts, *Infectious Fear: Politics, Disease and the Health Effects of Segregation* (Chapel Hill, NC: University of North Carolina, 2009), 219–21.

9 Solomon R. Benatar, "Global Poverty and Tuberculosis: Implications for Ethics and Human Rights," in *The Return of the White Plague: Global Poverty and the New Tuberculosis,* eds. Matthew Gandy and Alimuddin Zumla (London: Verso, 2003), 226.

10 Richard Lewontin and Richard Levins, "The Return of the Old Disease and the Appearance of New Ones," in *The Return of the White Plague: Global Poverty and the New Tuberculosis,* eds. Matthew Gandy and Alimuddin Zumla (London: Verso, 2003), 1–6.

11 "South Mountain Restoration Center: And There Was Light," unpublished pamphlet on the center [1968], 1–2; Mary Brady Caverly, "From Cabin to Classic Revival," unpublished paper (17 October 1994), 10; David Wenner," A14–15; "White Haven State School and Hospital," www.asylumprojects.org/index.php?title=White_Haven_State_School_and_Hospital; author's visit to Córdoba in October 1999; Damien Cave, "In Florida, A Lifeline to Patients with TB," *New York Times,* 13 June 2010, 19–21.

12 Author's visits to Hospital "Dr. Enrique Tornú" November 1995 and to the Sanatorio Nacional de Tuberculosis, Santa María, October 1999.

13 Patricia Schaelchin, "'Working for the Good of the Community:' Rest Haven Preventorium for Children," *Journal of San Diego History* 29, no. 2 (1983): 96–113; Cynthia Connolly, *Saving Sickly Children: The Tuberculosis Preventorium in American Life, 1909–1970* (New Brunswick: Rutgers University, 2008), 114–18; "KenCrest," www.kencrest.org/about-us/History.htm (21 March 2007).

14 Sunil Amrith, "In Search of a 'Magic Bullet' for Tuberculosis: South India and Beyond, 1955–1965," *Social History of Medicine* 17, no. 1 (2004): 118–19; Helen Valier, "At Home in the Colonies: The WHO-MRC Trials at the Madras Chemotherapy Centre in the 1950s and 1960," in *Tuberculosis Then and Now*, 222–28.

15 Barron H. Lerner, "New York City's Tuberculosis Control Efforts: The Historical Limitations of the 'War on Consumption,'" *American Journal of Public Health* 83, no. 5 (May 1993): 762; Marilyn Chase, "New, Virulent Forms of Tuberculosis Spur Concerns World-Wide," *Wall Street Journal*

17 (December 1999), sec. B1; Adrian Thomas, "Janssen," *Nature* 502 (10 October 2013): S18–S19; Emily Baumgaertner, "Current TB Treatment May Be Insufficient," *New York Times* (10 April 2018), D 3.

16 Calculations based on Table 2.1: Comparative Demographics, Buenos Aires and Philadelphia suggest a more nuanced view of non-pulmonary tuberculosis deaths. In spite of the increase in pasteurize milk in both cities, non-pulmonary tuberculosis increased in the twentieth century before the AIDS epidemic. In Buenos Aires tuberculosis mortality, as a percent of all tuberculosis deaths, varied between eleven percent in 1900 and twenty-one percent in 1921. Non-pulmonary tuberculosis deaths averaged 14.48 percent of tuberculosis mortality deaths in Buenos Aires between 1900 and 1938. In Philadelphia, 1900–1938, 11 tuberculosis mortality, as a percent of all tuberculosis deaths, varied between 0.44 percent in 1900 and 14.6 percent in 1913. Non-pulmonary tuberculosis deaths averaged 8.98 percent of tuberculosis mortality deaths in Philadelphia between 1900 and 1938.

17 A disease which had once been deadly for women and children was by 1947 mostly fatal for elderly men. In 1907, eleven percent of United States children's deaths resulted from tuberculosis. But by 1947, the figure fell to four percent. From 1907 to 1947, the median age of death due to tuberculosis increased from thirty-three to forty-three. Richard H. Shryock, *National Tuberculosis Association 1904–1954: A Study of the Voluntary Health Movement in the United States* (New York, New York: National Tuberculosis Association, 1957), 62–63, 276–77, 303.

18 Reported Tuberculosis in the United States, 2012, www.cdc.gov/tb/statistics/reports/2012 (August 2014); Shryock, i; Ken Chowder, "How TB Survived Its Own Death to Confront Us again," *Smithsonian* 23, no. 8 (1992): 191.

19 David Brown, "U.S. Tuberculosis Cases Decline as Disease Increases World Wide," *Washington Post* (23 March 1996), sec. A3; Nicholas B. King, "Immigration, Race and Geographies of Differences in the Tuberculosis Pandemic," in *Return of the White Plague,* 50–51.

20 The best source for current information on tuberculosis in the United States is the Centers for Disease Control and Prevention. Their annual reports and updates are posted on the web. See "Table 1. Tuberculosis Cases, Case Rates per 100,000 Population Deaths and Death Rates per 100,000 Population and percentage Change: United States, 1953–2008," www.cdc.gov/tb/statistics/ (26 August 2010); www.tbfacts.org/tb-statistics-united-states/ (12 March 2016); Alan Blinder, "Outbreak Is Fueled by Mistrust in Alabama," *New York Times* (18 January 2016), A 9; "Efforts to eliminate TB in U.S. appear 'stalled'," *Washington Post* (25 March 2016), A3; Aleksanyan, E6.

21 The Philadelphia Department of Public Health issues annual reports on disease since 2004 has included a section on Tuberculosis. For Philadelphia statistics, see *Annual Report: Division of Disease Control, 2007* (Philadelphia, PA: Department of Public Health, 2008), 9. Also see *Annual Summary of Reportable Diseases and Conditions: Division of Disease Control, 2004* (Philadelphia: Division of Disease Control, 2005), 6; for the most recent information, see https://hip.phila.gov/DataReports/Tuberculosis (15 March 2018).

22 The two organizations that provide the most current information on tuberculosis in Argentina are the United Nations and the Pan American Health Organization. www.newswise.com/articles/tuberculosis-spreads-on-crowded-city-buses for a discussion of "Tuberculosis spreads through crowded city buses" (22 December 2014); Viviana Ritacco et al., "Nosocomial Spread of Human Immunodeficiency *Virus-Related Multidrug Resistant Tuberculosis*

in Buenos Aires," *Journal of Infectious Diseases* 176 (September 1997): 637–42; "Tuberculosis: Aumento en la notificación de casos," *El Intransigente Argentina,* www.elintransigente.com/salud/2017/3/17/tuberculosis-aumento-notificacion-casos-427654.html (28 March 2018).

23 The best information on tuberculosis worldwide is provided by the World Health Organization. Their most recent information can be accessed on the Web. See *Global Tuberculosis Report 2017,* 1–6, www.who.int/tb/publications/global_report/en/index.html (15 March 2018).

24 Lisa Belkin, "A Brutal Cure," *New York Times Magazine* (30 May 1999), sec. 6, pp. 36–37; David Brown, "1 in 20 TB Cases Don't React to Some Drugs," *Washington Post* (27 February 2008), sec. A2; Baron H. Lerner, *Contagion and Confinement: Controlling Tuberculosis along the Skid Road* (Baltimore: John Hopkins University Press, 1998), 166–67; World Health Organization, "Tuberculosis," *Fact Sheet* 104, www.who.int/mediacentre/factsheets/fs104/en/ (April 2014).

25 David Brown, "A Breakthrough in the Control of TB," *Washington Post* (12 October 2011), sec.1, p.2; World Health Organization, "Tuberculosis."

26 "Tuberculosis and Gender," (29 March 2018), www.who.int/tb/areas-of-work/population-groups/gender/en/; The global Coalition on Women and AIDS, "Tackling TB and HIV in Women: An Urgent Agenda," www.mchip.net/sites/default/files/Tackling-TB-and-HIV-in-Women.pdf (29 March 2018); Simons Denyer, "Drug-Resistant TB Threatens Health Gains in India," *Washington Post* 6 (September 2012), A 15. Chase, Bl; Belkin, 37; "TB Fights Back," *Washington Post* (17 August 1999), sec. Health, 13; David Brown, "Drug-Resistant Tuberculosis Poses Global Risk, WHO Report Says," *Washington Post* (20 March 2010): A9; Lee B. Reichman with Janice Hopkins Tanne, *Timebomb: The Global Epidemic of Multi-Drug-Resistant Tuberculosis* (New York: McGraw-Hill, 2002), 90, 119–25; Vivien Stern, "The House of the Dead Revisited: Prisons, Tuberculosis and Public Health in the Former Soviet Bloc," in *Return of the White Plague: Global Poverty and the New Tuberculosis,* eds. Matthew Gandy and Alimuddin Zumla (London: Verso, 2003), 185–87; Paul Farmer in *Pathologies of Power,* 123, points out that one million Russians out of a population of 150 million are in prison; Kathy Lally, "HIV/AIDS, TB sapping Russian health, study finds," *Washington Post* (29 March 2013), A6; Aleksanyan, E6.

27 Reichman, 1–10; David Brown, "Man with Rare TB Detained, Isolated," *Washington Post* (30 May 2007), A3.

28 Thomas A. Kenyon, Sarah E. Valway, Walter W. Ihle, Ida M. Onorato, and Kenneth G. Castro, "Transmission of Multi-Resistant Mycobacterium Tuberculosis during a Long Airplane Flight," *New England Journal of Medicine* 334, no. 15 (11 April 1996): 933–38; Brown, "Man with Rare TB," A3; David S. Barnes, "Targeting Patient Zero," 63–68; Deborah Wallace and Roderick Wallace, "The Recent Tuberculosis Epidemic in New York City: Warning from the De-Developing World," in *Return of the White Plague,* 129–35; Gagneux, 853.

29 Susan Ferraro, "Drug-Proof TB New Perils," *New York Daily News* (23 October 1997): 26; Chase, B1; World Health Organization, "Drug-Resistant Tuberculosis Threatens the Western Pacific Region," www.wpro.who.int/mediacentre/releases/2007/20070322/en/ (29 March 2018); "TB Fights Back," 13; Paul Farmer and David Walton, "The Social Impact of Multi-Drug-Resistant Tuberculosis: Haiti and Peru," in *Return of the White Plague,* 164–65.

30 Lerner, *Contagion and Confinement*, 3, 116, 138; Richard Coker, *From Chaos to Coercion: Detention and the Control of Tuberculosis* (New York: St. Martin's Press, 2000), 2, 12, 122–27, 186. Coker also argues that tuberculosis will again be epidemic unless society deals with the underlying issues and improves education, creates jobs and eradicates institutional inequalities, 136–38.

31 Thomas, "Janssen," S18–S20; David G. Russell and Carl F. Nathan, "Graduation Time," *Nature* 502 (10 October 2013): S7.

32 Brown, "A Breakthrough," sec. 1, p. 2; Christopher Dye and Mario Raviglione, "Weigh all TB risks," *Nature* 502 (10 October 2013): S13; Ewen Callaway, "Control Issues," *Nature* 502 (10 October 2013): S16–S17.

33 Amy Maxmen, "A Combined Effort," *Nature* 502 (10 October 2013): S4–S6; Lia D'Ambrosio, et al., "Delamanid and Bedaquiline to Treat Multidrug-Resistant Extensively Drug-Resistant Tuberculosis in Children: A Systematic Review," *Journal of Thoracic Disease* 9 (July 2017): 2093–2101.

34 Catherine De Lange, "Waiting for Results," *Nature* 502 (10 October 2013): S10–S12.

35 Tim Boon, "Lay Disease Narratives, Tuberculosis, and Health Education Films" in *Tuberculosis Then and Now: Perspectives on the History of an Infectious Disease,* eds. Flurin Condrau and Michael Worboys (Montreal: McGill-Queen's University Press, 2010), 24–32.

36 Bryder, *Below the Magic Mountain,* 210; Antonio Cetrángolo, *Treinta años curando tuberculosos* (Buenos Aires: Librería Hachette, 1944), written by a physician who spent his life working in various Argentinean sanatoriums and *Spunk.*

37 Georgina D. Feldberg, *Disease and Class: Tuberculosis and the Shaping of Modern North American Society* (New Brunswick: Rutgers University Press, 1955), 169, 209–10; "Revised BCG Vaccination Guidelines for Infants at Risk for HIV Infection," *Weekly Epidemiological Record* no. 21 (25 May 2007): 193–96; World Health Organization "BCG-the Current Vaccine for Tuberculosis," www.who.int/vaccine_research/diseases/tb/vaccine_development/bcg/en/ (9 December 2011); Sarah Deweerdt, "An Age-Old Problem," *Nature* 502 (10 October 2013): S8–S9.

38 Diego Armus, "Historias de enfermos tuberculosos que protestan Argentina, 1920–1940," in *Avatares de la medicalización en América Latina 1870–1970*, ed. Diego Armus (Buenos Aires: Lugar Editorial, 2005), 84–90; Daniel Priano, "La bacteriología de la tuberculosis vacunación preventiva y curativa," *La Semana Médica* 48, no. 23 (June 5, 1941): 1315–324.

Glossary of Medical Terms

Atropine a medication made from the root and leaf of the belladonna plant; used as a cough remedy for tuberculosis, early twentieth century

Bacille Calmette-Guérin (BCG) a vaccine developed from a weakened form of a live bovine tuberculosis bacillus; in the early 1920s, it proved successful in stimulating the body's immune system to combat tuberculosis

Bedaquiline the first new tuberculosis medication developed in forty years; produced by Janssen Pharmaceuticals to be used with other tuberculosis medications to treat MDR-TB; approved by FDA in December 2012

Cacodylate of soda an ineffective early twentieth-century treatment for tuberculosis

Calcium the most abundant mineral in the body; it was given to tuberculosis patients to increase bone strength

Cholera a bacterial infection of the small intestine that leads to diarrhea and vomiting; it can result in severe dehydration, causing death

Co-infection the simultaneous infection of an individual by two or more viruses or bacteria that causes disease; influences the mortality rates of the disease

Consumption (phthisis) terms used to describe tuberculosis before Robert Koch demonstrated in 1882 that tuberculosis is caused by infectious bacteria

Contagionist one who believes that certain diseases, such as tuberculosis and yellow fever, are transmittable through direct or indirect human contact

Creosote a chemical product distilled from wood and used as an antiseptic and laxative; patients took it orally or inhaled it to reduce coughing during all stages of pulmonary tuberculosis in the 1870–1910 era

Delamanid new drug from the Japanese company, Osteuk, to be used in combination with standard tuberculosis medications to treat XDR-TB patients; approved in Europe in 2014

DOTS (directly observed therapy, short course) tuberculosis treatment presently supported by the World Health Organization which utilizes a smear test for diagnosis and six months of observed therapy (in which an appointed individual watches the patient swallow the dose) with standard tuberculosis drugs

Ergot a type of fungus thought to improve circulation and reduce bleeding in the 1870–1945 era; it may be poisonous

Fluoroquinolones family of broad-spectrum medications which kills bacteria of the respiratory and urinary tracts including tubercle bacilli

Germ theory the scientific explanation that disease is caused by the presence and actions of specific microorganisms which invade the body

Heliotherapy a medical therapy that exposed patients to sunlight for extended periods with the hope of curing tuberculosis

Iodoform a crystalline compound that evaporates easily at room temperature; it was used as a disinfectant and antiseptic and was given orally in the early twentieth century to tuberculosis patients, with the hope of killing tuberculosis bacteria and preventing diarrhea

Isoniazid an organic compound synthesized in the early twentieth century but first used in 1951 in combination with Streptomycin and PAS to cure tuberculosis

Latent tuberculosis an immune response to the tuberculosis bacteria in which individuals test positive to the disease but do not have any symptoms and is not infectious

Maragliano's serum an early twentieth-century ineffective inoculation made from the blood of horses or cattle which contained tuberculosis antibodies; failed to destroy the tuberculosis bacteria in humans

MDR-TB tuberculosis bacteria that is resistant to the two most effective medications against the bacteria: isoniazid and rifampin

Miasma theory the nineteenth-century belief that foul-smelling air, filthy water and decaying animal or vegetable matter caused diseases and epidemics; it was replaced by the germ theory meningeal tuberculosis (tuberculosis meningitis): tuberculosis bacteria travels from the lungs to infect the membrane surrounding the brain and spinal cord

Miliary tuberculosis a form of tuberculosis that is spread from the lungs to other body organs, such as the liver and spleen through the blood and lymph system

***Mycobacterium bovis* (bovine tuberculosis)** bacteria that causes tuberculosis in cattle and may spread to humans who drink unpasteurized milk

***Mycobacterium tuberculosis* (tubercle bacilli)** airborne bacteria that causes tuberculosis; it usually attacks the lungs but can infect any part of the body

Nitroglycerin a nitrate used to improve breathing and decrease the pain of tuberculosis patients

Nutritionist one who believes that an individual's health will improve if the individual eats the right type of food

PAS (para-aminosalicylic acid) antibiotic introduced in 1946 and used in combination with streptomycin to treat tuberculosis

Phosphates chemicals frequently given to nineteenth-century tuberculosis patients that were also used to repair bones and teeth

Pneumothorax (collapse lung therapy) procedure that involved putting air in the pleural cavity to collapse the diseased lung, so it could rest

Potassium iodide a compound used as a nutritional supplement for early twentieth-century tuberculosis patients

Pre-tubercular a term generally used to describe children who appeared malnourished, sickly and physically weak, but did not have any tuberculosis symptoms; it was thought that they might develop tuberculosis

Pueyo vaccine experimental vaccine created by Jesús Pueyo in Buenos Aires in 1936, supported by a euphoric press and public; failed clinical tests

Richet serum a compound separated from animal blood by Charles Richet and utilized unsuccessfully as a tuberculosis cure

Rifampicin (rifampin) antibiotic used to treat tuberculosis; approved for U.S. use in 1971

Scrofula a tuberculosis infection of the neck lymph nodes

Smear microscopy technology developed by Robert Koch in the 1880s; a patient's sputum is fixed to a glass slide and stained with dye and examined under a microscope; if present, the rod-shaped mycobacterium tuberculosis can be identified and counted; the test is often inconclusive

Streptomycin the first effective antibiotic treatment for tuberculosis

Sutezolid antibiotic to treat MDR-TB and XDR-TB that Sequella, a small Rockville, Maryland pharmaceutical company, acquired from Pfizer; it is in clinical trials (2014)

Thoracoplasty the surgical removal of one or more ribs so as to collapse and rest a diseased lung

Tuberculin a sterile liquid that contains the products of substances extracted from the tubercle bacillus; discovered by Robert Koch, it became an effective skin test to diagnose tuberculosis, but proved ineffective as an inoculation to prevent or cure tuberculosis

Typhoid fever a potentially fatal disease transmitted by *Salmonella typhi* bacteria to humans who consume contaminated food or water

XDR-TB tuberculosis bacteria that resist major medications developed to treat it, including isoniazid, rifampin and most fluoroquinolones

Yellow fever a viral infection spread by an infected female mosquito found in tropical and semitropical regions of Africa and South America; it leads to liver and kidney damage and can cause death

Bibliography

Argentina: Manuscript Locations and Primary Materials

Buenos Aires

Academia Nacional de Medicina, Biblioteca
Archivo del Ministerio de Salud Pública de la Nación
Archivo del Protomedicato Facultad de Medicina de Buenos Aires
Archivo General de la Nación Argentina (AGN)
  Archivo Julio Roca
  Fondos de Sociedad de Beneficencia (SB)
  Hospital Vicente López y Planes (HVLP)
  Ministerio del Interior, 1867–1930
  Tribunales Civiles
Archivo Histórico de la Ciudad de Buenos Aires
Archivo y Museo Histórico del Banco de la Provincia de Buenos Aires "Dr. Arturo Jauretche"
Biblioteca del Municipal (Manuel Gálvez)
Biblioteca del Museo Mitre
Biblioteca Facultad de Medicina de Universidad de Buenos Aires
Biblioteca Nacional
Cementerio de la Chacarita
Cementerio de la Recoleta
Hospital Muñiz
Hospital Tornú
Instituto Historia de Ciudad de Buenos Aires
Liga Argentina de Lucha Contra la Tuberculosis
Museo Histórico Nacional
Museo Social Argentino

Province of Córdoba (Argentina)

Archivo Histórico de la Provincia de Córdoba (AHC)
Archivo Municipal de la Provincia de Córdoba
Sanatorio Nacional de Tuberculosos Santa María, Santa María de Punilla (SNSM)

United States: Manuscript Locations and Primary Materials

New York City

New York Academy of Medicine
New York Public Library

Philadelphia, Pennsylvania

American Philosophical Society (APS)
  Eugene Opie Papers (OP)
  Simon Flexner Papers
The Historical Medical Library of the College of Physicians of Philadelphia (CPP)
  Annual Reports of the Henry Phipps Institute
  Hugh M. Kinghorn (HKP)
  Joseph Walsh (JWP)
  Lawrence Francis Flick, collected reprints (FCR)
  Lawrence Francis Flick, Papers (LFP)
  Metropolitan Life Insurance Company. "A War on Consumption"
  Pamphlets and handbills, various 1890–1935
  Spunk, volumes 4–13, 17–18, 20–54
  Transactions of the College of Physicians National Tuberculosis Association (U.S.): Transactions
Historical Society of Pennsylvania (HSP)
  John Seiser Mucklé Papers
  Samuel Gibson Dixon Papers, 1884–1953
Philadelphia City Archives
  Annual Message of the Mayor
  Charities, Bureau of City of Philadelphia
Temple University
  Special Collections Research Center: Annual Message of the Mayor
  Urban Archives (TUUA)
University of Pennsylvania (UP)
  Barbara Bates Center for the Study of the History of Nursing
    Visiting Nurse Society of Philadelphia Records (VNS)
  University Archives and Records Center (GA)
    Alfred Newton Richard Papers (ANRP)
    Phipps Institute (AGPI)

Pennsylvania

Chester County Historical Society (CCHS)
  Joseph Trimble Rothrock Collection (JRC)
South Mountain Restoration Center, Mont Alto, Pennsylvania
State Library of Pennsylvania, Harrisburg
  Annual Report of the Commissioner of Health of the Commonwealth of Pennsylvania
  Bulletin of the National Association for the Study and Prevention of Tuberculosis
  Pennsylvania Health Bulletin

Washington D.C.

Catholic University of America, American Catholic History Research Center and University Archives (CUA)
  Lawrence Francis Flick papers, 1857 to 1938 (FP)

Library of Congress, Hispanic Reading Room
National Library of Medicine
Spunk, volumes 3, 7–17, 19–50, 52–54
International Conference on Tuberculosis, various years

Spain

Archivo General del Ministerio de Asuntos Exteriores
Archivo Histórico Nacional
Biblioteca Nacional de España

United Kingdom

The British Library
The National Archives
The Royal Society of Medicine Library
Wellcome Library: History of Medicine Collection

Argentina: Medical Journals, Newspapers, and Government Documents

Actualidades Médicas Buenos Aires
Anales del Círculo Médico Argentino, 1877–1908
Anuario Estadístico de ciudad de Buenos Aires
Archivos de Medicina Legal
Archivos de Psiquiatría, Criminología y Ciencias Afines
Boletín del Departamento Nacional del Trabajo
Buenos Aires Herald, 1876–1900
Departamento Nacional de Higiene, 1891–1914
El Día Médico
La Lucha Antituberculosa, Revista Argentina del Torax, Revista Argentina de Tuberculosis (Various titles for the Argentine Anti-tuberculosis League journals)
La Nación
La Prensa
La Prensa Médica Argentina
Revista del Círculo Médico Argentino y Centro Estudiantes de Medicina
Revista de Universidad Nacional de Córdoba
Revista Médico-Quirúrgicas (Asociación Médica Bonaerense, Buenos Aires, Argentina)
La Semana Médica (Argentina), 1894–1940
Todo es Historia
La Vanguardia (Argentina)

United States: Medical Journals and Newspapers

American Review of Tuberculosis
Bulletin of the History of Medicine
Journal of the History of Medicine and Allied Sciences
Journal of the Outdoor Life
Journal of Tuberculosis

The Listening Post (Pennsylvania Department of Health)
Proceedings of the Philadelphia County Medical Society
Public Health Reports (1896–1970)
Social History of Medicine
Spunk (Mont Alto), 1909-1963
Transactions of the Medical Society of the State of Pennsylvania

Published Sources

Abel, Emily K. *Hearts of Wisdom: American Women Caring for Kin, 1850-1940*. Cambridge: Harvard University Press, 2002.

———. "Taking the Cure to the Poor: Patients' Responses to New York City's Tuberculosis Program 1894 to 1918."*American Journal of Public Health* 87, no. 11 (November 1997): 1808–15.

———. *Tuberculosis and the Politics of Exclusion: A History of Public Health and Migration to Los Angeles*. Critical Issues in Health and Medicine. New Brunswick: Rutgers University Press, 2007.

Abernethy, Lloyd M. "Progressivism 1905–1919." In *Philadelphia: A 300-Year History*, edited by Russell F. Weigley, 524–65. New York: W.W. Norton & Company, 1982.

Ackerknecht, Erwin H. "Anticontagionism between 1821 and 1867." *Bulletin of the History of Medicine* 22, (1948): 562–93.

Acosta, Leticia. "La Defensa de la infancia contra la tuberculosis." M.D. diss., Facultad de Medicina, Universidad de Buenos Aires, 1918. Buenos Aires: Imp. Vitullo Osurio Hnos., 1918.

Adams, Carolyn, David Bartelt, David Elesh, Ira Goldstein, Nancy Kleiniewski, and William Yancy. *Philadelphia: Neighborhoods, Divisions, and Conflict in a Postindustrial City*. Philadelphia: Temple University Press, 1991.

"After the Sanatorium then What?" *Spunk* 9, no. 11 (February 1918): 34–35.

Aguilar, Oscar P. "La tuberculina como diagnostico pronostico y tratamiento de la tuberculosis pulmonar." M.D. diss., Facultad de Medicina, Universidad de Buenos Aires, 1918.

Aisenberg, Andrew R. *Contagion: Disease, Government and the 'Social Question' in Nineteenth-Century France*. Stanford: Stanford University Press, 1999.

Albarracín, Alejandro. "Consideraciónes sobre la tisis pulmonar." M.D. diss., Facultad de Medicina, Universidad de Buenos Aires, 1875. Buenos Aires: Imprenta de Luis L. Pintos, 1875.

Alderson, Michael. *International Mortality Statistics*. New York: Facts on File, 1981.

Aleksanyan, Stephanie. "When My Brother Got TB, Doctors Said There Was No Hope. How Could That Be?" *Washington Post*, 15 February 2016, E1, E6.

"Algunas formas clínicas especiales de tuberculosis pulmonar en el niño." La Semana Médica 24, no. 17 (26 April 1917): 504–5.

Almeida, Hermione de. R*omantic Medicine and John Keats*. New York: Oxford University Press, 1991.

Alnutt, Brian E. "'The Negro Excursions' Recreational Outings among Philadelphia African Americas, 1876–1926." *The Pennsylvania Magazine of History and Biography* 129, no. 1 (January 2005): 73–104.

Alsina, Juan A. *El Obrero en la República Argentina*. Buenos Aires: Imprenta Calle de Mexico, 1905.

———. "La Santa Cristina en casos avanzados de tuberculosis pulmonar." *La Semana Médica* 4 (November 1926): 1241–42.

Amrith, Sunil. "In Search of a 'Magic Bullet' for Tuberculosis: South India and Beyond, 1955–1965." *Social History of Medicine* 17, no. 1 (2004): 113–30.

Andrews, Bridie J. "Tuberculosis and the Assimilation of Germ Theory in China, 1895–1937." *Journal of the History of Medicine and Allied Sciences* 52, no. 1 (January 1997): 114–57.

Andrews, George Reid. *The Afro-Argentines of Buenos Aires 1800–1900*. Madison: University of Wisconsin Press, 1980.

Anschütz, Germán. "Sobre profilaxis de la tuberculosis: Datos comparativos entre la lucha Argentina y la de otras naciones. *Departamento Nacional de Higiene* 20, no. 2 (March/April 1913): 173–221

Araóz Alfaro, Gregorio. "Bodas de plata." *La Prensa Médica Argentina* 1, no. 1 (10 June 1914): 13.

———. "Tuberculosis difusa de los niños." *Revista de la Sociedad Médica Argentina* 3, no. 14 (March/April 1894): 157–65.

———. "Las tuberculosis ignoradas." *Revisa Médica del Rosario* 3, no. 5/6 (December 1913): 259–60.

———. "Tuberculosis infantil en la República Argentina." *Relación presentada al 2 Congreso Médico Latina América*. Buenos Aires: Imprenta Liberia y Casa Editora de A. Etchepareborda, 1904.

———, and A. Zauchinger. "Consideraciones demográficas sobre la tuberculosis en la República Argentina." *La Prensa Médica Argentina* 14, no. 22 (10 January 1928); 805–21.

Argentina, Comisión directiva del censo nacional. *Segundo censo de la República Argentina, mayo 10 de 1895*. Buenos Aires: J. Peuser, 1896.

——— Comisión directiva del censo nacional. *Tercer censo nacional levantado el 10 junio 1914*. Buenos Aires: Talleres gráficos de L. J. Rosso y cia., 1916.

——— Dirección Nacional de Servicio Estadístico. *Síntesis estadística mensual de la República Argentina*. Buenos Aires: Dirección Nacional de Investigaciones, Estadísticas y Censos, 1947.

Arini, Juan B. *Estudio estadístico del Hospital General de Mujeres*. Buenos Aires: Imprenta de M. Biedma, 1879.

Armus, Diego. *The Ailing City: Health, Tuberculosis, and Culture in Buenos Aires, 1870–1950*. Durham, NC: Duke University Press, 2011.

———. *La ciudad impura: Salud, tuberculosis y cultura en Buenos Aires, 1870-1950*. Buenos Aires: Ensayo Edhasa, 2007.

———. "Historias de enfermos tuberculosos que protestan Argentina, 1920–1940." In *Avatares de la medicalización en América Latina 1870–1970*, edited by Diego Armus, 65–99. Buenos Aires: Lugar Editorial, 2005.

———. "La idea del verde en la ciudad moderna: Buenos Aires, 1870–1940." *Entrepasados: Revista de Historia* 5, no. 10 (1996): 9–22.

———. "'Milonguitas' en Buenos Aires, 1910–1940: tango, ascenso social y tuberculosis." *História Ciêcias, Saúde-Manguinhos* 9, no. 1 (2002): 187–207.

———. "Salud y anarquía: la tuberculosis en el discurso libertario argentino, 1870–1940." In *Salud, Cultura y sociedad en América Latina*, edited by Marcos Cueto, 111–33. Lima: Instituto de Estudios Peruanos, 1996.

———. "Tango, Gender and Tuberculosis in Buenos Aires, 1900–1940." In *Disease in the History of Modern Latin America from Malaria to Aids*, edited by Diego Armus, 101–29. Durham: Duke University Press, 2003.

———. "The Years of Tuberculosis: Buenos Aires, 1870–1950." Ph.D. diss., University of California, Berkeley, 1996.

Arner, Katherine. "Making Yellow Fever American: The Early American Republic, the British and the Geopolitics of Disease in the Atlantic World." *Atlantic Studies* 7, no. 4 (December 2010): 449–63.

Arnold, Marc. *Disease, Class and Social Change: Tuberculosis in Folkestone and Sandgate, 1880–1930*. Newcastle upon Tyre, UK: Cambridge Scholars Publishing, 2012.

Aronowitz, Robert A. *Making Sense of Illness: Science, Society and Disease*. Cambridge: Cambridge University Press, 1998.

Arriaza, Bernardo, et al. "Pre-Columbian Tuberculosis in Northern Chile: Molecular and Skeletal Evidence." *American Journal of Physical Anthropology* 98, no. 1 (September 1995): 37–45.

"La asistencia de los tuberculosos pobres en Buenos Aires." *La Lucha Antituberculosa*, 5, no. 3 (August 1905): 85–87.

"La asistencia de tuberculosos en los hospitales." *La Lucha Antituberculosa* 4, no. 5 (September/October 1903): 98–100.

"La Asistencia de tuberculosos pobres." *Alianza de Higiene Social* 7 (1907–1908): 95–98.

"La asistencia pública de los tuberculosos en Buenos Aires." *Revista de la Tuberculosis* 1, no. 4 (September 1901): 118–19.

"Aspectos social de tuberculosis." *Boletín del Museo Social Argentino* 10, no. 1 (10 July 1921).

Aubel, Harris. "The Mont Alto Business School." *Spunk* 4, no. 12 (July 1920): 10.

Avni, Haim. *Argentina y la historia de la inmigración judía (1810–1950)*. Jerusalén: Editorial Universitaria, AMIA Comunidad de Buenos Aires, 1983.

———. "Argentine Jewry: Its Socio-Political Status and Organizational Patterns." *Dispersion and Unity* 12 (1971): 128–62.

Aznárez, Enrique P. "Historia de la climatoterapia de la tuberculosis en las sierras de Córdoba." *Segundo Congreso Nacional de Historia de la Medicina Argentina* (Córdoba, 21–24 October 1870): 417–22.

———. "La Polémica contagionista de la tuberculosis en el siglo XIX y su repercusión en Córdoba,' La Memoria en contestación del Dr. Francisco Martínez Doblas (1831).'" *Anales de Tisiología y Climatología* 3, (1944): 3–6.

Baer, James A. "Buenos Aires and the Decline of the Liberal State in Argentina". In *Cities of Hope and Despair: People, Protests and Progress in Urbanizing Latin America, 1870–1930*, edited by Ronn Pineo and James A. Baer, 125–52. Boulder: Westview Press, 1998.

Báguena Cervellera, María José. *La Tuberculosis y su historia*. Barcelona: Fundación Uriach, 1992.

Baily, Samuel L. *Immigrants in the Lands of Promise: Italians in Buenos Aires and New York City, 1870–1914*. Ithaca, NY: Cornell University Press, 1999.

Bain, Robert B. "Building an Essential World History Tool: Teaching Comparative History." In *Teaching World History: A Resource Book*, edited by Heidi Roupp, 29–34. Armonk, NY: M.E. Sharpe, 1997.

Balbastro, Arturo. "La Mujer Argentina (Estudio Médico-Social)." M.D. diss., Facultad de Medicina, Universidad de Buenos Aires. Buenos Aires: Imprenta Sud-America, 1892.

Baltzell, E. Digby, Allen Glicksman, and Jacquelyn Litt, "The Jewish Communities of Philadelphia and Boston: A Tale of Two Cities." In Jewish Life in Philadelphia, 1830–1940, edited by Murray Friedman, 290–313. Philadelphia: Institute for the Study of Human Issues, 1983.

Barnes, David S. *The Great Stink of Paris and the Nineteenth-Century Struggle against Filth and Germs*. Baltimore: Johns Hopkins University Press, 2006.

———. *The Making of a Social Disease: Tuberculosis in Nineteenth-Century France*. Berkeley: University of California Press, 1995.

———. "The Rise or Fall of Tuberculosis in Belle-Époque France: A Reply to Allan Mitchell." *Social History of Medicine* 5, no. 2 (August 1992): 279–90.

———. "Targeting Patient Zero." In *Tuberculosis Then and Now: Perspectives on the History of an Infectious Disease*, edited by Flurin Condrau and Michael Worboys, 49–71. Montreal: McGill-Queen's University Press, 2010.

Barry, Carolina. "Cecilia Grierson: Argentina's First Female Doctor." *Irish Migration Studies in Latin America* 6, no. 3 (November 2008): 213–18.

Barton, George. *Little Journeys Around Old Philadelphia*. Philadelphia: Peter Reilly Company, 1925.

Bates, Barbara. *Bargaining for Life; A Social History of Tuberculosis, 1876–1938*. Philadelphia: University of Pennsylvania Press, 1992.

"Battling for Health at Mont Alto." *Pennsylvania Health Bulletin* 39 (October 1912): 1–3.

Baumgaertner, Emily. "Current TB Treatment May Be Insufficient." *New York Times*, 10 April 2018, D3.

Bayne, Ronald. "Ascending the Magic Mountain." *Canadian Medical Association Journal* 159, no. 5 (September 1998): 517–18.

Beaujon, Oscar. "La Ultima enfermedad del Liberador." *Revista de la Sociedad de Bolivariana de Venezuela* 24, no. 82 (1965): 45–50.

Belkin, Lisa. "A Brutal Cure." *New York Times Magazine,* 30 May 1999, sec. 6, 36–37.

Benatar, Solomon R. "Global Poverty and Tuberculosis: Implications for Ethics and Human Rights." In *The Return of the White Plague: Global Poverty and the New Tuberculosis*, edited by Matthew Gandy and Alimuddin Zumla, 222–36. London: Verso, 2003.

Bendix, Reinhard. "The Comparative Analysis of Historical Change." In *Social Theory and Economic Change: Contributions to the Seminar on the Theory of Economic Change held at the University of Edinburgh in March 1965*, edited by Tom Burns and S. B. Saul, 67–86. London: Tavistock Publications, 1967.

Beneficencia 1897–1900. Buenos Aires: Imprenta Litografía y Encuadernación G. Kraft, 1900.

Besio Moreno, Nicolás. *Buenos Aires: Puerto del Río de la Plata, capital de la Argentina: estudio crítico de su población, 1536–1936*. Buenos Aires: Talleres gráficos Tuduri, 1939.

Bermann, Geogorio. *La explotación de los tuberculosos*. Buenos Aries: 1941.

Biggs, Hermann M. "Address of the President," *Transactions of the National Association for the Study and Prevention of Tuberculosis* 3 (1907): 17–18.

———. "The Administrative Control of Tuberculosis in New York City." In *Transactions of the Sixth International Congress on Tuberculosis, Washington, September 28 to October 5, 1908, IV. Philadelphia: William F. Fell Company, 1909, 198–202.*

———. *Brief History of the Campaign against Tuberculosis in New York City.* New York: New York City Department of Health, 1908.

Billings, Jr., John S. *The Registration and Sanitary Supervision of Pulmonary Tuberculosis in New York City.* New York: New York City Department of Health, 1912.

Bjelopera, Jerome P. *City of Clerks: Office and Sales Workers in Philadelphia 1870–1920.* Chicago: University of Illinois Press, 2005.

———. "White Collars and Blackface: Race and leisure among Clerical and Sales Workers in Early Twentieth-Century Philadelphia." *Pennsylvania Magazine of History and Biography* 123, no. 3 (July 2002): 471–90.

Black, C.E. *The Dynamics of Modernization: A Study in Comparative History.* New York: Harper & Row, 1966.

Blanc, Léopold, and Mukund Uplekar. "The Present Global Burden of Tuberculosis." In *The Return of the White Plague; Global Poverty and the "New" Tuberculosis*, edited by Matthew Gandy and Alimuddin Zumla, 95–111. London: Verso, 2003.

Blinder, Alan. "Outbreak Is Fueled by Mistrust in Alabama." *New York Times*, 18 January 2016, A9.

Boffi, Luis L. *Tuberculosis de los viejos.* Buenos Aires: Lotito Hermanos y Cia., 1942.

Bohl, A.J. "Testing for Tuberculosis." *Pennsylvania's Health* 8, no. 5 (September–October, 1930): 20–21.

Bonner, Thomas Neville. *Becoming a Physician: Medical Education in Britain, France, Germany, and the United States, 1750–1945.* New York: Oxford University Press, 1996.

Boon, Tim. "Lay Disease Narratives, Tuberculosis, and Health Education Films." In *Tuberculosis Then and Now: Perspectives on the History of an Infectious Disease*, edited by Flurin Condrau and Michael Worboys, 24–48. Montreal: McGill-Queen's University Press, 2010.

Borges, Jorge Luis. *Evaristo Carriego.* Translated with introduction and notes by Norman Thomas Di Giovanni with the assistance of Susan Ashe. New York: E.P. Dutton, Inc., 1984.

Borkowski, José M. "Tuberculosis en el escolar," M.D. diss., Facultad de Medicina, Universidad de Buenos Aires, 1919.

Brody, Howard. *Stories of Sickness.* New Haven: Yale University Press, 1987.

Brown, David. "A Breakthrough in the Control of TB." *Washington Post,* 12 October 2011, sec. 1: 2.

———. "Drug-Resistant Tuberculosis Poses Global Risk, WHO Report Says," *Washington Post*, 20 March 2010, A9.

———. "Man with Rare TB Detained, Isolated." *Washington Post,* 30 May 2007, A3.

———. "1 in 20 TB Cases Don't React to Some Drugs." *Washington Post*, 27 February 2008, sec. A2.

———. "U.S. Tuberculosis Cases Decline as Disease Increases World Wide." *Washington Post*, 23 March 1996, sec. A3.

Brown, Phil. "Naming and Framing: The Social Construction of Diagnosis and Illness." *Journal of Health and Social Behavior*, 1995 (extra issue): 34–52

Bryce, Benjamin. *To Belong in Buenos Aires: Germans, Argentines, and the Rise of a Pluralist Society*. Sanford: Stanford University Press, 2018.

Bryce, James. *South American Observations and Impressions*. New York: The Macmillan Company, 1923.

Bryder, Linda. *Below the Magic Mountain: A Social History of Tuberculosis in Twentieth-Century Britain*. Oxford Historical Monographs. Oxford: Clarendon Press, 1988.

———. "Papworth Village Settlement—A Unique Experiment in the Treatment and Care of Tuberculosis." *Medical History* 28 (1984): 372–90.

———. "'Wonderlands of Buttercups, Clover and Daisies.' Tuberculosis and the Open-Air School Movement in Britain, 1907–39." In *The Name of the Child: Health and Welfare, 1889–1940,* edited by Roger Cooter. Studies in the social history of medicine, 72–95. London: Routledge, 1992.

Buenos Aires (city). *Anuario estadístico de la ciudad de Buenos Aires*. Buenos Aires: Compañía Sud-Americana de Billetes de Banco, 1885.

———. *Anuario estadístico de la ciudad de Buenos Aires*. Buenos Aires: Compañía Sud-Americana de Billetes de Banco, 1895.

———. *Anuario estadístico de la ciudad de Buenos Aires*. Buenos Aires: Compañía Sud-Americana de Billetes de Banco, 1900.

———. *Anuario estadístico de la ciudad de Buenos Aires*. Buenos Aires: Compañía Sud-Americana de Billetes de Banco, 1910.

———. *Revista de estadística municipal de la ciudad de Buenos Aires* (January–March 1945). Buenos Aires: Dirección General de Estadística Municipal, 1945.

———. *Statistical Year-Book of the City of Buenos Aires*. Buenos Aires: Compañía Sud-Americana de Billetes de Banco, 1910.

———. *Statistical Year-Book of the City of Buenos Aires*. Buenos Aires: Compañía Sud-Americana de Billetes de Banco, 1919.

———. *Year-Book of the City of Buenos Aires, 1910 and 1911*. Buenos Aires: Centenário Alegre, 1912.

Buenos Aires, Dirección General de Estadística Municipal. *Boletín Mensual de Estadística Municipal de la Ciudad de Buenos Aires. Resumen demográfico correspondiente al año 1888*. Buenos Aires: Compañía Sud-Americana de Billetes de Banco, 1889.

Buenos Aires, Dirección General de la Asistencia Pública. *Instrucciones para los inspectores sanitarios*. Buenos Aires: El Correo Español, 1898.

Buenos Aires, Dirección General de Servicio Estadístico Nacional. *Anuario estadístico de la ciudad de Buenos Aires, 1905*. Buenos Aires: Compañía Sud-Americana de Billetes de Banco, 1906.

Bunge, Alejandro Ernesto. "Costo de la vida en la Argentina." *Revista de Economía Argentina* (1918): 39–63.

Bunge, Augusto. "Las Conquistas de la higiene social: los peligros de la industria: II el ambiente del trabajo." *Departamento Nacional de Higiene* 16, no. 6 (June 1909): 243–71.

———. "Las Conquistas de la higiene social: los peligros de la industria: II el ambiente del trabajo." *Departamento Nacional de Higiene* 16, no. 7 (July 1909): 289–381.

———. "Contribución al estudio de la tuberculosis de las serosas." M.D. diss., Facultad de Medicina, Universadad de Buenos Aires, 1900.

———. "El trabajo industrial en Buenos Aires: Informe presentado al Departamento Nacional de Higiene." *Departamento Nacional de Higiene* 11, no. 8 (August 1904): 339–42.

———. "El trabajo industrial en Buenos Aires: Informe presentado al Departamento Nacional de Higiene." *Departamento Nacional de Higiene* 11, no. 9 (September 1904): 399–403.

Burger, T.W. "South Mountain's Sickened City," *Public Opinion* 11 December 2015.

Burke, Gillian, and Peter Richardson. "The Profits of Death: A Comparative Study of Miners' Phthisis in Cornwall and the Transvaal, 1876–1918." *Journal of Southern African Studies* (Great Britain) 4, no. 2 (April 1978): 147–71.

Burke, Peter. *History and Social Theory*. Ithaca: Cornell University Press, 1993.

Burnet, Frank Macfarlane, and David O. White. *Natural History of Infectious Disease*. Cambridge: Cambridge University Press, 1972.

Burt, Nathaniel, and Wallace E. Davies. *"The Iron Age 1876–1905."* In *Philadelphia: A 300-Year History,* edited by Russell Weigley, 471–523. New York: W.W. Norton & Company, 1982.

Bynum, Helen. *Spitting Blood: The History of Tuberculosis*. London: Oxford University Press, 2012.

Cabred, Domingo. *La tuberculosis en la República Argentina. Informe presentado al Ministerio de Relaciones Exteriores y Culto, el 31 de mayo de 1918*. Buenos Aires: Imprenta y Encuadernación del Hospicio de la Mercedes, 1919.

Cafferata, Juan F. "Higiene Social: La vulgarización de la nociones científicas en la lucha contra la tuberculosis." *Revista del Círculo Médico Córdoba* 7, no. 1–2 (January/February 1917).

Callaway, Ewen. "Control Issues." *Nature* 502 (10 October 2013): S16–S17.

Cantón, Eliseo. *Historia de la medicina en el Río de la Plata desde su descubrimiento hasta nuestras días, 1512 á 1925*. Six volumes. Madrid: Imp. G. Hernández y Galo Sáez, 1928.

Cantonnet, Pedro. "La frenicectomía en la tuberculosis pulmonar del niño." *La Semana Médica* 39, no. 15 (14 April 1932): 1191.

Carrillo, Ismael. "La tisis y el clima de nuestras provincias." *Revista Médico-Quirúrgica* 14, nos. 13–14 (8 October 1877): 314–18.

"Carta de un tuberculosos curado en las sierras de Córdoba." *La Lucha Antituberculosa* 5, no. 1 (June 1905): 7–8.

"Cartas de las Sierras: Los nuevos conflictos del sanatorio 'Santa María,' Causa de las causas: la cuestión económica—Mal a comida. Gastos exorbitantes—el empirismo administrativo. Seis meses sin pagar a nadie. . .? La debacle?" *La Vanguardia* 7, February 1922: 2.

"Casas par obreros en el barrio de los Patricios." *Alianza de Higiene Social* 9, no. 3–4 (August/September, 1909): 112–16.

Cassedy, James H. *Charles V. Chapin and the Public Health Movement*. Cambridge: Harvard University Press, 1962.

Casterline, Gail Farr. "St Joseph's and St. Mary's: The Origins of Catholic Hospitals in Philadelphia." *Pennsylvania Magazine of History and Biography* 108, no. 3 (July 1984): 291–314.

Castex, Mariano R. "Nuevos casos de oftalmo-reacción a la tuberculina de Koch." *Departamento Nacional de Higiene* 14, no. 8 (August 1907): 277–78.

Castilla, Caupolicán R. "Hospital de Niños: en el cincuentenario de la fundación de su actual edificio." *La Semana Médica* 50 (9 December 1943): 3331–32.

Cave, Damien. "In Florida, a Lifeline to Patients with TB." *New York Times*, 13 June 2010, 19–21.

Caverly, Mary Brady. "From Cabin to Classic Revival," unpublished paper, 17 October 1994.

Centers for Disease Control and Prevention. "Statistics." http://www.cdc.gov/tb/statistics/ . (26 August 2010).

———. "Tuberculosis Statistics-United States." http://www.tbfacts.org/tb-statistics-united-states/ (12 March 2016).

Ceppi, José. *Guía del emigrante a la República Argentina*. Buenos Aires: Imp. Roma de J. Carbone, 1898.

Cetrángolo, Antonio. "Algunas breves consideraciones sobre la climatoterapia de la tuberculosis en nuestro país." *La Semana Médica* 24, no. 8 (22 February 1917): 242–43.

———. *Treinta años curando tuberculosos*. Buenos Aires: Librería Hachette, 1944.

Charity Organization Society of the City of New York, Committee on the Prevention of Tuberculosis. *Home Treatment of Tuberculosis in New York City; January 8, 1906-October 1, 1907: Being a Report of the Relief Committee of the Committee on the Prevention of Tuberculosis of New York Charity Organization*. New York: Charity Organization Society, 1908.

Chase, Marilyn. "New, virulent forms of tuberculosis spur concerns worldwide." *Wall Street Journal* 17 December 1999, sec. B1.

Chaves, Aaron D. "Motivating Patients to Take Drugs." *Spunk* 54, no. 7 (October 1962): 10–12.

Chaves, G.N. "Consideraciones generales sobre la herencia, el contagio, la profilaxis y el tratamiento de la tuberculosis pulmonar." *La Semana Médica* 6, no. 35 (31 August 1899): 314.

Chemnitz Association. "Protection against Consumption." In *Transactions of the Sixth International Congress on Tuberculosis, Washington, September 28 to October 5, 1908 with an Account of the Catalogue of the Tuberculosis Exhibition*, 5. Philadelphia: W.F. Fell company, 1908.

Chernoviz, Pedro Luis Napoleón. *Diccionario de medicina popular y ciencias accesorias*. Paris: em Casa de autor, 1879.

"Chickens." *Spunk* 14, no. 1 (April 1922): 14.

"Children's Hospital Notes: Wonder of a Child Patient." *Spunk* 18, no. 10 (January 1927): 31–2; 18, no. 11 (February 1927): 44; 19, no. 4 (July 1927): 37; 20, no. 2 (May 1928): 43

Chiocconi, Antonio R. "La tuberculina residual en el tratamiento de la tuberculosis." M.D. diss., Facultad de Medicina, Universidad de Buenos Aires, 1898.

Chowder, Ken. "How TB survived its own death to confront us again." *Smithsonian* 23, no. 8 (1992): 180–94.

"Christmas." *Spunk* 6, no. 9 (December 1914).

"Christmas at Mont Alto." *Spunk* 6, no. 10 (January 1915): 22–23.

"Christmas at the Preventorium." *Spunk* 18, no. 10 (January 1927): 31–33.

Ciafardo, Eduardo O. "Las damas de beneficencia y la participación social de la mujer en la ciudad de Buenos Aires 1880-1920." *Anuario IEHS-Tandil* 5, (1990): 161–70.

———. *Los Niños en la ciudad de Buenos Aires, 1890–1910.* Buenos Aires: Centro Editor de América Latina, 1992.

———. "La práctica benéfica y el control de los sectores populares de la ciudad de Buenos Aries, 1890–1910." *Revista de Indias* 54, no. 201 (May/August, 1994): 383–408.

Cibils Aguirre, Raúl. "El problema de la herencia en tuberculosis." *La Semana Médica* 21, no. 48 (27 November 1924).

Clark, Dennis J. "The Philadelphia Irish: Persistent Presence," In *The Peoples of Philadelphia: A History of Ethnic Groups and Lower Class Life 1790–1940*, edited by Allen F. Davis and Mark H. Haller, 135–54. Philadelphia: Temple University Press, 1973.

Clark, Sydney. *All the Best in South American East Coast.* New York: Dodd Mead, 1956.

Clark, Vance. "TB Sneaks Back: Seven in Family Learn Hard Way." *Spunk* 54, no. 11 (February 1963): 9.

Cleveland, Floyd and Henry Bowditch. "A Clinical Study of the Transmission and Progress of Tuberculosis in Children through Family Associations. In *Transactions of the Sixth International Congress on Tuberculosis, Washington, September 28 to October 5, 1908, 4: 493–502.* Philadelphia: William F. Fell Company, 1909.

Clow, Barbara. "Who's Afraid of Susan Sontag? Or the Myths and Metaphors of Cancer Reconsidered." *Social History of Medicine* 14, no. 2 (August 2001): 293–312.

Coker, Richard. *From Chaos to Coercion: Detention and the Control of Tuberculosis.* New York: St. Martin's Press, 2000.

Colditz, Graham A. and Timothy F. Brewer, Catherine S. Berkey, et al. "Efficacy of BCG Vaccine in the Prevention of Tuberculosis: Meta-analysis of the Published Literature." *Journal of American Medical Association* 271, (1994): 698–702.

Collier, Simon. *The Life, Music and Times of Carlos Gardel.* Pittsburgh: University of Pittsburg Press, 1986.

Commonwealth of Pennsylvania Department of Health, Division of Tuberculosis Sanatoria. *Information and Rules for Patients.* Harrisburg, 1914.

"Comunicación detalles sobre un medicamento contra la tuberculosis, por el profesor R. Koch, de Berlin." *Anales del Círculo Médico Argentino* 14, no. 1 (January 1891): 16–27.

Condrau, Flurin "Beyond the Total Institution: Towards a Reinterpretation of the Tuberculosis Sanatorium." In *Tuberculosis Then and Now: Perspectives on the History of an Infectious Disease*, edited by Flurin Condrau and Michael Worboys, 72–99. Montreal: McGill-Queen's University Press, 2010.

Congrès international de la tuberculose. *Rapports présentés au congrès, Paris 2–7 octobre, 1905.* 3 vols. Paris: Massenet Cie., Éditeur, 1906.

Congreso Internacional de Medicina e Higiene. *Guía Médica de la República Argentina.* Buenos Ares: Gráfica M. Pastor & Cia., 1910.

Coni, Emilio R. "The Antituberculous Campaign in Latin America." *Medical Record* (2 May 1903): 690–91.

———. "Armamento antituberculosos francés y argentina." *Revista de Ciencias Médicas* 8, no. 82 (1925): 260–61.

———. "La asistencia de niños enfermos en Buenos Aires." *Revista de Higiene Infantil* 1 (1892): 597–98.

———. "Asistencia de tuberculosos en la Capital Federal." *Revista de Ciencias Médicas* 8, no. 92 (1925): 214–15.

———. "The Campaign against Tuberculosis in Argentina." *Transactions of the Sixth International Congress on Tuberculosis, Washington, September 28 to October 5, 1908*, 4: 49–61. Philadelphia: William F. Fell Company, 1908.

———. "Campaña contra la tuberculosis en la República Argentina." *La Semana Médica* 16, no. 40 (7 October 1909): 1398–1400; 16, no. 41 (14 October 1909): 1437–52.

———. *Código de higiene y medicina legal de la República Argentina* para uso de los médicos, *abogados, farmacéuticos, etc.*, 2 vols. Buenos Aires: Etchepareborda, 1891.

———. "Colonia de vacaciones de Bella Vista." *Alianza de Higiene Social* 9, no. 7 (December 1909): 195–98.

———. *Higiene Social: Asistencia y previsión social. Buenos Aires caritativo y previsor.* Buenos Aires: Imprenta de Emilio Spinella, Ed., 1918.

———. "Higiene y Salubridad en la República Argentina." In *Primer Congreso Médico Latino-Americano, Santiago de Chile 1 al 9 de enero de 1901*, 76–77. Santiago: Congreso Médico Latino-Americano, 1901.

———. "Hospitalización y aislamiento de los tuberculosos pulmonares en Buenos Aires." *La Semana Médica*, 9, no. 43 (27 October 1904): 1139–40.

———. "La Lucha antituberculosa en la América Latina," *Alianza de Higiene Social* 9, nos. 3–4 (August /September 1909): 75–78, 143–54.

———. "La Lucha antituberculosa en la República Argentina." *La Lucha Antituberculosa* 5, no. 4–8 (1905): 156–78.

———. "Mortalidad infantil en 1891." *Revista de Higiene* 1 (1892): 21–22.

———. "Sanatorio municipal Doctor Tornú." *La Lucha Antituberculosa* 4, no. 12 (12 May 1905): 531.

Coni, Gabriela de L. de. "El Barrio de las ranas." *Alianza de Higiene Social* 7 (1907–1908): 79–80.

Conlogue, Gerald. "More TB in Peruvian Mummies." *Archaeology* 55, no. 2 (March/April 2002): 14.

Connolly, Cynthia A. "Nurses: The Early Twentieth Century Tuberculosis Preventorium's 'Connecting Link.'" *Nursing History Review* 10 (2002): 127–57.

———. "Pale, poor, and 'pretubercular' children: a history of pediatric antituberculosis efforts in France, Germany, and the United States, 1899–1929." *Nursing Inquiry* 11, no. 3 (2004): 138–47.

———. *Saving Sickly Children: The Tuberculosis Preventorium in American Life, 1909-1970.* New Brunswick: Rutgers University, 2008.

———. "The TB Preventorium." *American Journal of Nursing* 100, no. 10 (2000): 62–65.

Contosta, David R. "George Woodward, Philadelphia Progressive." *The Pennsylvania Magazine of History and Biography* 111, no. 3 (July 1987): 341–70.

———. "Suburban Quasi Government in Chestnut Hill, Philadelphia." *The Pennsylvania Magazine of History and Biography* 116, no. 3 (July 1992): 259–94.

Cooper, Clayton Sedgwick. *Understanding South America*. New York: George H. Doran Company, 1918.

Cooper, Frederick. "Race, Ideology, and the Perils of Comparative History." *American Historical Review* 101, no. 4 (1996): 1122–138.

Cooter, Roger. "Anticontagionism and History's Medical Record." In *The Problem of Medical Knowledge: Examining the Social Construction of Medicine*, edited by Peter Wright and Andrew Treacher, 87–108. Edinburgh: Edinburgh University Press, 1982.

Coovadia, H. M., and S. R. Benatar, eds. *A Century of Tuberculosis: South African Perspectives*. Cape Town, South Africa: Oxford University Press, 1991.

Copland, James. The *Forms, Complications, Causes, and Treatment of Bronchitis*. London: Longmans, Green and Co., 1866.

Cortejoso Villanueva, Leopoldo. *Tuberculosis célebres: Grandes personalidades forjadas por la tuberculosis*, 2nd ed. Barcelona: Editorial Mateu, 1958.

Cortés Conde, Roberto. *El progreso argentino, 1880–1914*. Buenos Aires: Editorial Sudamericana, 1979.

Craig, Frank A. *Early Days at Phipps*. Philadelphia: University of Pennsylvania Press, 1952.

———. "The Prognosis in Pulmonary Tuberculosis in Children under Fifteen Years of Age (USA)." In *Transactions of the Sixth International Congress on Tuberculosis*, 2: 652–70. Philadelphia: William F. Fell, Company, 1908.

Crider, Ernest Allen. "Modernization and Human Welfare: The Asistencia Pública and Buenos Aires, 1882–1910." Ph.D. diss., Ohio State University, 1976.

Crnic, Meghan. "Seeking the Salubrious Sea: The Health and Environments of Urban American Families, 1870–1930" (2013). Publicly Accessible Penn Dissertations. 746.

——— and Cynthia Connolly. "'They Can't Help Getting Well Here': Seaside Hospitals for Children in the United States: 1872–1917." *The Journal of the History of Childhood and Youth* 2, no. 2 (Spring, 2009): 220–33.

Croftan, Alfred Careño. *Clinical Therapeutics: A Handbook on the Special Treatment of Internal Disease*. Chicago: Cleveland Press, 1907.

Cummiskey, Julia Ross. "Drugs, Race and Tuberculosis Control in Baltimore, 1950–1978." *Social History of Medicine* 27, no. 4 (November 2014): 728–50.

D'Ambrosio, Lia, Centis, Rosella, Tiberi, Simon, Tadolini, Marina, Dalcolmo, Margareth, Rendon, Adrian, Esposito, Susanna, and Migliori, Battista Giovanni. "Delamanid and Bedaquiline to Treat Multidrug-Resistant and Extensively Drug-Resistant Tuberculosis in Children: A Systematic Review." *Journal of Thoracic Disease* 9, no. 7 (July 2017): 2093–2101.

D'Angelo Anzorena, Antonio. *Tuberculosis de la primera infancia*. M.D. diss., Facultad de Medicina, Universidad de Buenos Aires, 1917. Buenos Aires: Imp. Bossio & Bigliani, 1917.

Daireaux, Emilio. *Industrias y productos*. Vol. 2 of *Vida y Costumbres in el Plata*. Buenos Aires: Félix Lojouane, 1888.

Daniel, Thomas M. *Captain of Death: The Story of Tuberculosis*. Rochester: University of Rochester Press, 1997.

Daughton, J. P. "When Argentina Was "French": Rethinking Cultural Politics and European Imperialism in Belle-Époque Buenos Aires." *The Journal of Modern History* 80, no. 4 (December 2008): 831–64.

Davis, Allen F. and Mark H. Haller, editors. *The Peoples of Philadelphia: A History of Ethnic Groups and Lower class Life, 1790–1940*. Philadelphia: Temple University Press, 1973.

Decoud, Diogène. "El método de Koch en la clínica del Profesor Pirovano." *Anales del Círculo Médico Argentino* 14, no. 2 (February 1891): 43–59.

———. *Les sciences médicales dan la République Argentine*. Buenos Aires: Imprimerie, 1933.

De Lange, Catherine. "Diagnosis: Waiting for Results." *Nature* 502 (10 October 2013): S10–S12.

"Demografía Tuberculosis Pulmonar Mortalidad en el Septenio 1887–93." *Semana Médica 1, no. 28 (26 July 1894): 210.*

"Denuncia de Graves Irregularidades en el Sanatorio 'Santa María,'" *La Vanguardia,* 7 April 1922, p. 2.

"Las denuncias sobre el hospital Tornú." *La Vanguardia*, 16 June 1918, p. 1; 17 June 1918, p. 1; 23 June 1918, p. 1.

Simons Denyer, "Drug-Resistant TB Threatens Health Gains in India," *Washington Post* 6 September 2012, A 15.

"Descriptive Catalogue, the Exhibit of the State Department of Health of Pennsylvania at the International Congress on Tuberculosis, Washington D.C., September 21 to October 12, 1908." In *Third Annual Report of the Commissioner of Health of the Commonwealth of Pennsylvania*, 486–517. Harrisburg, PA: C.E. Aughinbaugh, 1909.

Deutsch, Sandra McGee. "The Catholic Church, Work and Womanhood in Argentina, 1890–1930." *Gender and History* 3:3 (Autumn 1991): 304–25.

Devoto, Fernando J. "Programs and Politics of the First Italian Elite of Buenos Aires, 1852–80." In *Italian Workers of the World: Labor Migration and Formulation of Multiethnic States*, edited by Donna R. Gabaccia, and Fraser M. Otanelli, Translated by Amy Ferlazzo, 41–59. Urbana: University of Illinois Press, 2001.

DeWeerdt, Sarah. "An Age-Old Problem." *Nature* 502 (10 October 2013): S8–S9.

Diamond, Jared and James A Robinson, eds. *Natural Experiments of History.* Cambridge: Belknap Press of Harvard University Press, 2010.

Diccionario Enciclopedia de Medicina y Cirugía Práctico escrito en Alemán bajo la Dirección del Gulenburg. Translated by Isidoro de Miguel y Viguri. Madrid: Saenz de Jubera, Hermanos Editores, 1891.

Dickinson, Joan Younger. "Aspects of Italian Immigration to Philadelphia." *The Pennsylvania Magazine of History and Biography* 90, no. 4 (October 1966): 445–465.

Dietsch, Jorge R. "Sanatorios marítimos: su importancia y necesidad en la asistencia social." *Revista de la Asociación Médica Argentina* 56 (January 1942): 28–36.

Di Liscia, María Silvia. *Saberes, terapias y prácticas médicas en Argentina (1750-1910)*. Biblioteca de historia de América, vol. 24. Madrid: Consejo Superior de Investigaciones Científicas, 2002.

"La Desinfección pública en la tuberculosis." *Revista de la Tuberculosis* 1 (1902): 283–84.

"Dispensario Dr. Enrique Tornú," *La Lucha Antituberculosa* 2, no. 1 (June 1902): 12–14.

Dixon, Samuel Gibson. "The Prevention of Tuberculosis," read before the section of the State Medicine of the British Medical Association at Toronto, Canada, 21 August 1906: 1–12.

Doherty, Peter C. *Pandemics: What Everyone Needs to Know*. Oxford: Oxford University Press 2013.

Doneson, Jules. *Deeds of Love: A History of the Jewish Foster Home and Orphan Asylum of Philadelphia: America's First Jewish Orphanage*. New York: Vantage Press, 1996.

Donze, Pierre-Yves. "Studies Abroad by Japanese Doctors: A Prosopographic Analysis of the Nameless Practitioners, 1862–1912." *Social History of Medicine* 23: 2 (August 2010): 244–60.

Dormandy, Thomas. *The White Death: A History of Tuberculosis*. Washington Square: New York University Press, 2000.

Doyal, Lesley. *What Makes Women Sick: Gender and the Political Economy of Health*. New Brunswick: Rutgers University Press, 1995.

Drake, Anna. L. "Nursing in Tuberculosis." *Listening Post* 5, no. 4 (July–August, 1927): 3–8.

Drolet, Godias J. and Anthony M. Lowell. *A Half Century's Progress against Tuberculosis in New York City, 1900–1950*. New York: New York Tuberculosis and Health Association, 1952.

———. "Tuberculosis Hospitalization." Spunk 18, no. 12 (March 1927): 17–18.

Dubos, René, and Jean Dubos. *The White Plague: Tuberculosis, Man and Society*. New Brunswick: Rutgers University Press, 1987.

Dudden, Arthur P. "The City Embraces 'Normalcy' in 1919–1929." In *Philadelphia: A 300-Year History* edited by Russell F. Weigley, 566–600. New York: W.W. Norton & Company, 1982.

Duffy, John. *A History of Public Health in New York City, 1866–1966*. New York: Russell Sage Foundation, 1974.

Dulles, Charles Winslow. "Consumption Not Contagious," *Transactions of the College of Physicians,* Third series, vol. 19 (1897): 178–90.

Dunn, Mary Maple and Richard S. Dunn. "The Founding, 1681–1701." In *Philadelphia: A 300-Year History,* edited by Russell Weigley, 1–32. New York: W.W. Norton & Company, 1982.

Dunning, Thad. "Improving Causal Inferences: Strengths and Limitations of Natural Experiments." *Political Research Quarterly* 61, no. 2 (2008): 283–93.

Dutton, Gail. "Pre-Columbian Tuberculosis." *Archaeology* 97, no. 4 (July/August 1994): 19.

Dye, Christopher and Mario Raviglione. "Weigh all TB risks." *Nature* 502 (10 October 2013): S13.

Ehrenreich, Barbara, and Deirdre English. *For Her Own Good: 150 Years of Expert Advice to Women*. New York: Doubleday, 1978.

Ellison, David L. *Healing Tuberculosis in the Woods: Medicine and Science at the End of the Nineteenth Century*. Westport: Greenwood Press, 1994.

"En el Hospital Tornú." *La Vanguardia,* 11 August 1918, p. 1.

"En el Hospital Tornú la obra de las enfermeras religiosas." *La Vanguardia*, 9 June 1918, p. 1.

"En el Hospital Tornú: Un Caso Grave." *La Vanguardia*, 28 August 1914, p. 2.

"En el Sanatorio de Tuberculosos de Santa María; Una vista del corresponsal de 'La Vanguardia.'" *La Vanguardia*, 16 January 1920, p. 4; 14 June 1920, p. 5.

"En el Sanatorio 'Santa María,' Ampliando la denuncia de graves irregularidades." *La Vanguardia*, 11 April 1922, p. 6.

"En el Sanatorio Santa María: Extravagancias del doctor Cabred." *La Vanguardia*, 28 December 1919, p. 1.

"En el Sanatorio Santa María; La Inmoralidad de un capellán—inercia de la comisión asesora-La Comida sigue siendo mala-nombramiento excesivo de empleados." *La Vanguardia*, 6 April 1920, p. 8.

"En el Sanatorio 'Santa María.'" *La Vanguardia*, 12 February 1922, p. 2.

"En el Sanatorio Santa María: se renuevan, los hechos bochornos de otras épocas." *La Vanguardia*, 6 October 1922, p. 1.

"Enrique Tornú." *Archivos Argentinos de Tisiología y Neumología* 53, no. 1–4 (1987): 5–8.

Escudé, Carlos Andrés. "Health in Buenos Aires in the Second Half of the Nineteenth Century." In *Social Welfare, 1850–1950: Australia, Argentina and Canada Compared*, edited by D. C. M. Platt, 60–70, 87–106. London: Macmillan Press, 1989.

"Escuelas para niños débiles." *Alianza de Higiene Social* 9, no. 7 (December 1909): 198–99.

Esoin, Sebastián. "Tratamiento de la tuberculosis pulmonar." M.D. diss., Facultad de Medicina, Universidad de Buenos Aires, 1914.

"Estado actual de los tuberculosis pesquisados en el dispensario," *La Semana Médica* 44, no. 41 (14 October 1937): 908.

Etcheverry Boneo, Florencio. "La Sociedad de Beneficencia de la Capital frente a la lucha antituberculosa." *Tercer Congreso Panamericano de Tuberculosis. Montevideo 16–19 Diciembre 1934*, vol. 2: 83–88. Montevideo, 1934–1935.

Farmer, Paul. *Infections and Inequalities: The Modern Plagues*. Berkeley: University of California Press, 1999.

———. *Pathologies of Power: Health, Human Rights, and the New War on the Poor*. Berkeley: University of California Press, 2005.

Farmer, Paul, and David Walton. "The Social Impact of Multi-drug-resistant Tuberculosis: Haiti and Peru." In *The Return of the White Plague: Global Poverty and the 'New' Tuberculosis*, edited by Matthew Gandy and Alimuddin Zumla, 163–77. London: Verso, 2003.

Farrand, Livingston. "Report of the Executive Secretary." *Transactions of the National Association for the Study and Prevention of Tuberculosis* 5 (1909): 17–18.

Fee, Elizabeth, and Evelynn M. Hammonds. "Science, Politics, and the Art of Persuasion: Promoting the New Scientific Medicine in New York City." In *Hives of Sickness: Public Health and Epidemics in New York City*, edited by David Rosner, 155–96. New Brunswick: Rutgers University Press, 1995.

Feldberg, Georgina D. *Disease and Class: Tuberculosis and the Shaping of Modern North American Society*. New Brunswick: Rutgers University Press, 1955.

Feldman, William. "Studies in Chemotherapy of Tuberculosis including Use of Streptomycin." *Transactions and Studies of the College of Physicians of Philadelphia*, Fourth Series 14, no. 3 (December 1946): 81–97.

Fernández, Gladys, Inés Fernández, Susana Jorolinsky, and Norma Míguel. "Los Determinantes sociales de la tuberculosis en la ciudad de Buenos Aires." *Medicina y Sociedad* 7, no. 3 (May/June 1984): 64–70.

Fernández, Ubaldo. "La Mortalidad infantil." *La Semana Médica* 25, no. 24 (13 June 1918): 657–60.
Ferraro, Susan. "*Drug-Proof TB New Perils.*" New York Daily News, 23 October 1997, p. 26.
Ferrer Moratel, C. "Influencia del trabajo en el origen y en el desarrollo de la tuberculosis." *La Prensa Médica Argentina* 36, no. 39 (30 September 1949): 1972–75.
"First Annual Meeting of the National Association for the Study and Prevention of Tuberculosis." *Transactions of the National Association for the Study and Prevention of Tuberculosis,* 1, 1905 (New York: Irving Press, 1906).
First Annual Report of the Henry Phipps Institute for the Study, Treatment, and Prevention of Tuberculosis. Philadelphia: Henry Phipps Institute, 1905.
"First Day Camp in Philadelphia." *Spunk* 3, no. 9 (Dec. 1911): 12–13.
Fishberg, Maurice. *Pulmonary Tuberculosis*, 2nd ed. Philadelphia: Lea & Febiger, 1919.
Flick, Lawrence F. "Address of the Vice-President: The Duties, Responsibilities and Opportunities of the National Association for the Study and Prevention of Tuberculosis," *Transactions of the National Association for the Study and Prevention of Tuberculosis* 2 (1906): 15–20.
———. "Crusade against Tuberculosis." *John Hopkins Hospital Bulletin* 18 (1907): 304–09.
———. "The Crusade against Tuberculosis in Philadelphia." Presented to the Philadelphia County Medical Society on November 23, 1932, privately printed.
———. "Henry Phipps Institute for the Study, Treatment and Prevention of Tuberculosis," *Philadelphia Medical Journal* (31 January 1903): 208–09.
———. "Present Status of the Tuberculosis Campaign and the Essentials for Thorough and Prompt Success." *New York Medical Journal* 91 (1910): 261–64.
———. "Report of the Committee on Tuberculosis." *Annual Report of the American Public Health Association,* (1897): 1–2.
———. "The Work of the First Year." First Annual Report of the Henry Phipps Institute for the Study, Treatment, and Prevention of Tuberculosis. Philadelphia: Henry Phipps Institute, 1905.
———. "The Work of the Year." Second Annual Report of the Henry Phipps Institute for the Study, Treatment, and Prevention of Tuberculosis. Philadelphia: Henry Phipps Institute, 1905.
Floyd, Cleveland, and Henry I. Bowditch. "A Clinical Study of the Transmission and Progress of Tuberculosis in Children through Family Association." In *Transactions of the Sixth International Congress on Tuberculosis*. 2 vols., 493–502. Philadelphia: William F. Fell Company, 1908.
Fones-Wolf, Elizabeth. "Industrial Unionism and the Labor Movement Culture in Depression-Era Philadelphia." *The Pennsylvania Magazine of History and Biography* 109, no. 1 (January 1985): 3–26.
"Formulario." *Anales del Círculo Médico Argentino* 15, no. 8 (August 1892): 575.
Fortuine, Robert. "*Must We All Die?" Alaska's Enduring Struggle with Tuberculosis*. Fairbanks: University of Alaska Press, 2005.
Foster, Enrique. "Dispensario de Lactantes: la Gota de Leche," *Archivos Latinoamericanos de Pediatría*, 1, no. 1 (March 1905): 342–46.

Foucault, Michel. *The Birth of the Clinic: Archaeology of Medical Perception.* Translated by A. M. Sheridan Smith. New York: Vintage Books, 1994.

Fox, Daniel M. "Social Policy and City Politics: Tuberculosis Reporting in New York, 1889–1990." *Bulletin of the History of Medicine* 49, no. 2 (summer 1975): 169–95.

Francine, Albert P. "Results on January 1, 1913 in Philadelphia Patients Discharged from Mont Alto in 1909." In *Transactions of the National Association for the Study and Prevention of Tuberculosis, Ninth Annual Meeting, Washington D.C., May 8-9 1913,* 276–90. Philadelphia: William F. Fell Company, 1913.

———, and H. J. Hartz, "Results with Tuberculin (Dixon's) in Advanced Chronic Ambulatory Tuberculosis." *Journal of the American Medical Association* 60, no. 10 (1913): 717–21.

Frías, Pedro J. "Estudio de algunas cuestiones sobre la herencia de la tisis." M.D. diss., Facultad de Medicina, Universidad de Buenos Aires, 1879. Buenos Aires: Imprenta de M. Biedma, 1879.

Friedman, Murray, ed. *Jewish Life in Philadelphia, 1830–1940.* Philadelphia: Institute for the Study of Human Issues, 1983.

Gabriel, José. *Evaristo Carriego.* Buenos Aires: Agencia Sudamericana de Libros, 1921.

Gache, Samuel. *Climatologie médicale de la République argentine et des principales villes d'Amérique.* Buenos Aires: Imprimerie "Mariano Moreno," 1895.

———. "La lucha antituberculosa en la República Argentina." *La Lucha Antituberculosa* 4, nos. 1–3 (June, July, August 1904): 3–19.

———. *Les logements ouvriers á Buenos Ayres.* Paris: G. Steinhell, 1900.

———. "Profilaxis antituberculosa en Buenos Aires." *La Semana Médica* 10, no. 42 (15 October 1903): 977–84.

———. "Reseña a histórica de la medicina Argentina: 1891–1904." In *Guía médica de la República Argentina*, edited by Congreso Internacional de Medicina e Higiene, 3–38. Buenos Aires: Est. Gráf M. Pastor y Cia., 1910.

———. *La tuberculose dans la République Argentine.* Buenos Aires: Augustín Etchepareborda, 1899.

Gache, Samuel, and J. A. Muñiz, "Sanatorio para mujeres y niños." *La Lucha Antituberculosa* 6, nos. 4/5 (September/October 1906): 149–50.

Gagneux, Sébastien. "Host-pathogen co-evolution in human tuberculosis." *Philosophical Transactions of the Royal Society B. Biological Sciences* 367, no. 1590 (19 March 2012): 850–59.

Gamble, Vanessa Northington. *Making a Place for Ourselves: The Black Hospital Movement, 1920–1945.* New York: Oxford University Press, 1995.

Gandy, Mathew. "Life without Germs: Contested Episodes in the History of Tuberculosis." In *The Return of the White Plague: Global Poverty and the 'New' Tuberculosis*, edited by Matthew Gandy and Alimuddin Zumla, 15–38. London: Verso, 2003.

Gandy, Matthew, and Alimuddin Zumla, eds. *The Return of the White Plague: Global Poverty and the 'New' Tuberculosis.* London: Verso, 2003.

García Esteban, Fernando. *Vida de Florencio Sánchez.* Santiago, Chile: Ediciones Ercilla, 1939.

Garrahan, Juan P. and Octavio M. Pico. "La escuela para niños débiles en la profilaxis antituberculosa, los niños débiles." *La Semana Médica* 27, no. 23 (20 May 1920): 697–701.

Garzón Maceda, Félix. *De los hospitales en Córdoba* desde *1573 hasta 1916*. Vol. 2 *of La Medicina en Córdoba: apuntes para su historia*. Buenos Aires: Talleres Gráficos Rodríguez Giles, 1916.
Gawande, Atul. "Annals of Medicine: Slow Ideas." *New Yorker*, 29 July 2013, 36–45.
Gentry, W. H. "The Laboratory and the Eternal Verities of Tuberculosis." *Spunk* 52, no. 1 (April 1960): 9–13.
Giacobini, Genaro. "La medicina escolar en la lucha contra la tuberculosis." In *Actas y Trabajos*, vol. 5 of *República Argentina, Segundo Congreso Nacional de Medicina, 1 al 8 Octubre de 1922*. Buenos Aires: Las Ciencias, 1927.
———. "La tuberculosis pulmonar en el niño escolar." *Primer Congreso Pan-Americano de la Tuberculosis, Córdoba 10-16 Octubre 1922*, vol. 3. Córdoba: Imprenta de la Universidad, 1922.
Giménez, Angel M. "Consideraciones de higiene sobre el obrero en Buenos Aires" M.D. diss., Facultad de Medicina, Universidad de Buenos Aires, 1901.
Gittings, J. Claxton, Frank Crozer Knowles, and Ashley P.C. Ashhurst. *Tuberculosis in Infancy and Childhood: Lectures Delivered at the Children's Hospital, Philadelphia, under the Auspices of the Philadelphia Pediatric Society*. Philadelphia: J.B. Lippincott Company, 1922.
Giusti, Roberto F. *Florencio Sánchez: su vida y su obra*. Buenos Aires: Sud-Americana de Libros, 1920.
The Global Coalition on Women and AIDS, "Tackling TB and HIV in women: An Urgent Agenda," https://www.mchip.net/sites/default/files/Tackling-TB-and-HIV-in-Women.pdf (29 March 2018).
Global Tuberculosis Report 2017, 1–6, http://www.who.int/tb/publications/global_report/en/index.html. (15 March 2018).
Glynn, Judith R. et.al "Worldwide Occurrence of Beijing/W Strains of Mycobacterium Tuberculosis: A Systematic Review." *Emerging Infectious Diseases* vol. 8, no. 8 (August 2002): 843–49.
Goetz, Thomas. *The Remedy: Robert Koch, Arthur Conan Doyle and the Quest to Cure Tuberculosis*. New York: Gotham Books, 2014.
Golab, Caroline. "The Immigrant and the City: Poles, Italians and Jews in Philadelphia, 1870–1920." In *The Peoples of Philadelphia: A History of Ethnic Groups and Lower-Class Life, 1790–1940*, edited by Allen F. Davis and Mark H. Haller, 203–30. Philadelphia: Temple University Press, 1973.
Gomez, Fernando. "The TB Problem in the Latin American Countries." *Transactions National Tuberculosis Association*, *Fiftieth Annual Meeting, Atlantic City, New Jersey, 1954*: 91–95.
González, José D. "Climatología; a las Sierras Cordobesas: y el Proyectado Sanatorio para tuberculosis." Semana Médica 1, no.30 (9 August 1984): 225–26.
González Carbalho, Loscano. *Fernando Fader*. Buenos Aires: Editorial Poseidon, 1943.
González Leandri, Ricardo. *Curar, persuadir, gobernar: La construcción histórica de la profesión médica en Buenos Aires, 1852–1886*. Madrid: Consejo Superior de Investigaciones Científicas Centro de Estudios Históricos, 1999.
———. "Sujeción y carencia cambio y continuismo en los hospitales de Buenos Aires (1870–1900)." *Asclepio* 42, no. 1 (1990): 291–301.

Goodall, H.S. "Tuberculosis: A Leaflet for Teachers." In *Transactions of the Sixth International Congress on Tuberculosis, Washington, September 28 to October 5, 1908*, 5: 291. Philadelphia W. F. Fell Company, 1908.

Goode, Judith, and Jo Anne Schneider. *Reshaping Ethnic and Racial Relations in Philadelphia: Immigrants in a Divided City*. Philadelphia: Temple University Press, 1994.

Green, Ryland W. *Lippincott's Medical Dictionary: A Complete Vocabulary of the Terms used in Medicine and the Allied Sciences*. Philadelphia: J.B. Lippincott Company, 1897.

Grew, Raymond. "The Case for Comparing Histories." *American Historical Review* 85 (1980): 763–78.

Grygier, Pat Sandiford. *A Long Way from Home: The Tuberculosis Epidemic among the Inuit*.

Montreal: McGill-Queen's University Press, 1994.

Guerrino, Antonio Alberto. "Las primeras legislaciones antituberculosas." *Orientación Médica* 15, no. 713 (15 July 1966): 230.

Guía Médica de la República Argentina, 1890–1891. Buenos Aires: Casa Editora, 1890.

Gutman, Margarita and Jorge Enrique Hardoy. *Buenos Aires: Historia urbana del área metropolitana*. Madrid: Mapfre, 1992.

Gutman, Zacarías. "Diagnóstico de tuberculosis infantil y sus dificultades." M.D. diss., de Ciencia Médicas, Universidad de Buenos Aires, 1904. Buenos Aires: Imprenta Librería y casa editor de A. Etchepareborda, 1904.

Guy, Donna J. "Emilio and Gabriela Coni: Reformers, Public Health, and Working Women." In *The Human Tradition in Latin America: The Nineteenth Century*, edited by Judy Ewell and W. H. Beezley, 233–48. Wilmington, DE: Scholarly Resources, 1989.

———. "Mothers Alive and Dead: Multiple Concepts of Mothering in Buenos Aires." In *Sex and Sexuality in Latin America*, edited by Daniel Balderston and Donna J. Guy, 155–73. New York: New York University Press, 1997.

———. "Niñas en la cárcel; La Casa Correccional de Mujeres como instituto de socorro infantil." In *Historia de las mujeres en la Argentina*, edited by Fernando Gil Lozano, Valeria Silvina Pita, and María Gabriela Ini, vol. 2: 25–45. Buenos Aires: Aguilar Altea Taurus Alfaguara, 2000.

———. "Niños abandonados en Buenos Aires (1880–1914) y el desarrollo del concepto de la madre." In *Mujeres y Cultura en la Argentina del siglo XIX*, edited by Lea Fletcher, 217–26. Buenos Aires: Feminaria Editorial, 1994.

———. "The Politics of Pan-American Cooperation: Maternalist Feminism and the Child Rights Movement, 1913–1960." In *Feminism and Internationalism,* edited by Mrinaline Sinha, Donna J. Guy, and Angela Woollacott, 449-69. Oxford: Blackwell, 1999.

———. *Women Build the Welfare State: Performing Charity and Creating Rights in Argentina. 1880–1955*. Durham: Duke University Press, 2009.

———. "Women, Peonage and Industrialization: Argentina, 1810–1915." *Latin American Research Review* 16, no. 3 (1981): 65–89.

Hacsi, Timothy A. *Second Home: Orphan Asylums and Poor Families in America*. Cambridge: Harvard University Press, 1997.

Haller, Mark H. "Recurring Themes." In *The Peoples of Philadelphia: A History of Ethnic Groups and Lower-Class Life 1790–1940*, edited by Allen F.

Davis and Mark H. Haller, 277–90. Philadelphia: Temple University Press, 1973.

Hanna, Eleanor and Stanley Glaser. "Where to Find...Tuberculosis Mortality and Morbidity Data." *Public Health Reports (1896–1970)* 63, no. 23, Tuberculosis Control Issue No. 28 (4 June 1948): 748–762.

Hansen, Ricardo L., and Leonardo P. Repetti, "La Tuberculosis de la segunda década." *La Prensa Médica Argentina* 29 (23 September 1942): 1517–21.

Hardy, Anne. *The Epidemic Streets: Infectious Disease and the Rise of Preventive Medicine, 1856–1900.* Oxford: Clarendon, 1993.

Harley, David. "Rhetoric and the Social Construction of Sickness and Healing." *Social History of Medicine* 12, no. 3 (December 1999): 407–35.

Harrison, Mark, and Michael Worboys. "A Disease of Civilization: Tuberculosis in Britain, Africa and India, 1900–1939." In *Migrants, Minorities and Health: Historical and Contemporary Studies*, edited by Lara Marks and Michael Worboys, 93–124. London: Routledge, 1997.

Hatfield, Charles. "Report of the Executive Office for the Year Ending May 1, 1920." *Transactions of the National Association for the Study and Prevention of Tuberculosis, Sixteenth Annual Meeting, St. Louis, Mo., April 22, 23 and 24 1920*, 31–41. New York: National Tuberculosis Association, 1920.

Hays, J. N. *The Burden of Disease: Epidemics and Human Response in Western History.* New Brunswick: Rutgers University Press, 1998.

Hepp, John Henry, IV. *The Middle-Class City: Transforming Space and Time in Philadelphia.* Philadelphia: University of Pennsylvania Press, 2003.

Hess, Alfred. "A Tuberculosis Preventorium for Infants." *American Review of Tuberculosis* 1 (January 1918): 669–73.

Hetherington, H. W. "Open-Air Schools for the Treatment of Tuberculosis in Children." In *Tuberculosis in Public School Children*, edited by the Henry Phipps Institute, 512–18. Philadelphia: University of Pennsylvania, 1929.

Hinsdale, Guy. "Tuberculosis in Pennsylvania." *Journal of the American Medical Association* 35, no. 16 (20 October 1900): 996–99.

Historical Society of Pennsylvania. *Day Camp for Tuberculosis* (pamphlet). Philadelphia: William F. Fell Company, 1912.

Historical Society of Pennsylvania. *Pennsylvania Society for the Prevention of Tuberculosis, Annual Report 1913*. Philadelphia: William F. Fell Company, 1913.

Holt, L. Emmett. "A Report on One Thousand Tuberculin Tests in Young Children." In *Transactions of the Sixth International Congress on Tuberculosis*, 2: 551–58. Philadelphia: William F. Fell Company, 1908.

Horowitz, Roger, Jeffrey M. Pilcher, and Sydney Watts. "Meat for the Multitudes: Market Culture in Paris, New York City and Mexico City over the Long Nineteenth Century." *American Historical Review* 109, no. 4 (October 2004): 1055–83.

"Hospital Chat." *Spunk* 9, no. 7 (October 1917): 40–42.

"Hospital Notes: New Arrivals." *Spunk* 52, no. 2 (May 1960): 18; 54, no. 7 (October 1962): 18.

"Hospital para tuberculosos," *La Semana Médica* 11, no. 41 (13 October 1904): 1110.

Howell, Joel D. "Machines and Medicine: Technology Transforms the American Hospital." In *The American General Hospital: Communities and Social*

Context, edited by Diane Elizabeth Long and Janet Golden, 109–34. Ithaca: Cornell University Press, 1989.

"How Must You Live after You Are Apparently Well Again so as to Remain Well." *Spunk* 9, no. 3 (June 1917): 20–22.

Humphries, Courtney. "A Sleeping Giant." *Nature* 502 (10 October 2013): S14–S15.

Hutcheon, Linda, and Michael Hutcheon. *Opera: Desire, Disease, Death*. Lincoln: University of Nebraska Press, 1996.

Hutchinson, Wood. "The Localization of Tuberculosis in Children." In *Transactions of the Sixth International Congress on Tuberculosis*, vol. 2: 417–21. Philadelphia: William F. Fell Company, 1908.

"Information for the Public." *Spunk* 9, no. 1 (April 1917): 1–2.

Iglesia, Rafael E.J. "La vivienda opulenta en Buenos Aires, 1880–1900, hechos y testimonios." In *Primera Jornadas de Historia de Ciudad de Buenos Aires, "La Vivienda en Buenos Aires."* Buenos Aires: Municipalidad de la Ciudad de Buenos Aires, 1985.

"Inspección escolar en la República Argentina, Uruguay, Chile y Brasil." *Alianza de Higiene Social* 9, no. 7 (December 1909): 218–20.

International Congress on Tuberculosis, Washington, September 28 to October 5, 1908. *General Catalogue of the European and American Exhibits*. Philadelphia: William F. Fell Company, 1908.

———. *Official Report of the Executive Committee for Great Britain and Ireland: Report for England and Wales*. London: William Clowes & Sons, 1908.

———. *Transactions of the Sixth International Congress on Tuberculosis, Washington, September 28 to October 5, 1908*, 6 vols. Philadelphia: William F Fell, 1908.

Iribarne, Ramón, and Juan M. Hitache. "La educación antituberculosa." In *Actas y Trabajos: Biología y patología: higiene y medicina pública*, vol. 4 of *República Argentina, Primer Congreso Nacional de Medicina*. Buenos Aires: Imprenta y Casa Editora de Flaiban, 1918.

Jensen, Richard, *<rjensen@uic.edu> "Epidemics in American History,"18 Feb. 1999, H-SCI-MED-TECH@H-NET.MSU.EDU (18 Feb. 1999).*

Johnson, Fred C. "Subdivision of Tuberculosis Sanatoria. Pennsylvania State Sanatorium for Tuberculosis No. 1 Mont Alto." In *Eleventh Annual Report of the Commissioner of Health for the Commonwealth of Pennsylvania* (1916): 895–923. Harrisburg: J. L. L. Kuhn Printer to the Commonwealth, 1920.

Johnston, William. "A Genealogy of Tubercular Diseases in Japan." *Social History of Medicine* 7, no. 2 (1994): 247–67.

———. *The Modern Epidemic: A History of Tuberculosis in Japan*. Cambridge: Harvard University Press, 1995.

———. "Tuberculosis." In *The Cambridge World History of Human Disease*, 1059–67, edited by Kenneth F. Kiple. New York: Cambridge University Press, 1993.

Jones, David S. *Rationalizing Epidemics: Meanings and Uses of American Indian Mortality*

Since 1600. Cambridge: Harvard University Press, 2004.

Jones, Greta. *'Captain of all these Men of Death:' The History of Tuberculosis in Nineteenth and Twentieth Century Ireland*. Welcome Institute Series in the History of Medicine: Clio Medica, 62. Amsterdam, Netherlands: Rodopi, 2001.

Jones, W. Duane. "When Surgery Is Recommended." *Spunk* 54, no. 3 (June 1962): 9–12.

Jordanova, Ludmilla. *Sexual Visions: Images of Gender in Science and Medicine between the Eighteenth and Twentieth Centuries*. Madison: University of Wisconsin Press, 1989.

Jorge, José M. "Estadística del Hospital de Niños correspondiente al año 1878." *Anales del*

Círculo Médico Argentino 2, no. 5 (July 1979): 324–29.

———. "Sanatorio Marítimo y Solarium de Mar del Plata." *La Semana Médica* 28, no. 35 (1 September 1921): 257–96.

Joyce, John St. George. *Story of Philadelphia*. Philadelphia: Rex Printing House, 1919.

Kelynack, T.N. "Tuberculosis in Infancy and Childhood: The Problem Stated." In *Tuberculosis in Infancy and Childhood: Its Pathology, Prevention, and Treatment*, edited by T.N. Kelynack, 2–9. London: Bailliere, Tindall and Cox, 1908.

"KenCrest," http://www.kencrest.org/about-us/History.htm (21 March 2007) Kensington Dispensary for the Treatment of Tuberculosis (Philadelphia). Board of Managers. *Ninth Annual Report of the Kensington Dispensary for the Treatment of Tuberculosis*. Philadelphia: Press of P.C. Stockhausen, 1915.

———. *Seventh Annual Report of the Kensington Dispensary for the Treatment of Tuberculosis*. Philadelphia: Press of P.C. Stockhausen, 1913.

Kenyon, Thomas A., Sarah E. Valway, Walter W. Ihle, Ida M. Onorato, and Kenneth G. Castro. "Transmission of Multi-Resistant Mycobacterium Tuberculosis during a Long Airplane flight." *New England Journal of Medicine* 334, no. 15 (11 April 1996): 933–38.

King, Nicholas B. "Immigration, Race and Geographies of Difference in the Tuberculosis Pandemic." In *The Return of the White Plague: Global Poverty and the New Tuberculosis*, edited by Matthew Gandy and Alimuddin Zumla, 39–54. London: Verso, 2003.

Kingsley, Sherman C., editor. *Open Air Crusaders: A Report of the Elizabeth McCormick Open-Air School together with a General Account of Open-Air School Work in Chicago and a Chapter on School Ventilation*. Chicago: United Charities of Chicago, 1910.

Kirby, Stephanie. "Sputum and the Scent of Wallflowers: Nursing in Tuberculosis Sanatoria, 1920–1970." *Social History of Medicine* 23, no. 3 (December 2010): 602–20.

Klappenbach, E. "Tuberculosis pulmonar: Inyecciones de Gayacol-íodoformado," *Anales del Círculo Médico Argentino* 15, no. 5 (May 1892): 221–38.

Klein, Ira. "Death in India, 1871–1921." *Journal of Asian Studies* 32, no. 4 (August 1973): 639–59.

Kleinberg, S.J. *Widows and Orphans First: Family Economy and Social Welfare Policy, 1880–1930*. Urbana: University of Illinois Press, 2006.

Knopf, S. Adolphus. *Tuberculosis as a Disease of the Masses, and How to Combat It*. New York: M. Firestack, 1901.

———. *Tuberculosis: A Preventable and Curable Disease*. New York: Moffat, Yard and Company, 1909.

Koplik, Henry. "Tuberculosis in Infancy and Childhood." *Johns Hopkins Hospital Bulletin* 23 (April 1912): 113–14.

Krause, Allen K. *Environment and Resistance in Tuberculosis; a presentation of the nature of environment and resistance and their relation to the pathology, diagnosis, symptoms and treatment of tuberculosis*. Baltimore: Williams & Wilkins Company, 1923.

———. *Rest and Other Things: A Little Book of Plain Talks on Tuberculosis Problems*. Baltimore: Williams & Wilkins Company, 1923.

Kress, George H. "Facts a Mother Should Know Concerning Tuberculosis." In *Transactions of the Sixth International Congress on Tuberculosis* 5: 304. Philadelphia: W. F. Fell Company, 1908.

"Laetare Medal Conferred on Lawrence F. Flick M.D. in the Hall of the Society 5 May 1920." *Records of the American Catholic Historical Society of Philadelphia* 31, no. 2 (1920): 117–20.

Lally, Kathy, "HIV/AIDS, TB sapping Russian Health, study finds," Washington Post 29 March 2013, A6.

Landis, Henry R. M. "The Tuberculosis Problem and the Negro," *Virginia Medical Monthly* (January 1923), rpt. in *Sixteenth Report of the Henry Phipps Institute* (Philadelphia, 1924): 1–6.

Lapsansky, Emma Jones. "Feminism Freedom, and Community: Charlotte, Forten and Women Activists in Nineteenth-Century Philadelphia." *The Pennsylvania Magazine of History and Biography* 113, no. 1 (January 1989): 3–20.

"Leading Causes of Death." *World Resources 1998–99*. http://www.wri.org/publication/content/8476 (26 August 2010).

League of Nations, Health Organisation. "Deaths from Specified Causes in Large Towns—Tuberculosis." *Annual Epidemiological Report Corrected Statistics of Notifiable Diseases for the year 1928* (Geneva: Health Section, 1930), 66–67.

———. "Deaths from Specified Causes in Large Towns—Tuberculosis." *Annual Epidemiological Report Corrected Statistics of Notifiable Diseases for the year 1929* (Geneva: Health Section, 1931), 76–77.

———. "Deaths from Specified Causes in Large Towns—Tuberculosis." *Annual Epidemiological Report Corrected Statistics of Notifiable Diseases for the year 1932* (Geneva: Health Section, 1934), 100–104.

———. "Deaths from Specified Causes in Large Towns—Tuberculosis." *Annual Epidemiological Report Corrected Statistics of Notifiable Diseases for the year 1934* (Geneva: Health Section, 1934), 76, 100–104.

———. "Deaths from Specified Causes in Large Towns—Tuberculosis." *Annual Epidemiological Report Corrected Statistics of Notifiable Diseases for the year 1938* (Geneva: Health Section, 1941), 102–5.

———. "Deaths from Specified Causes in Large Town—Tuberculosis." *Epidemiological Report for 1935*, R.E. 177 (Geneva, Health Section, 1935), 36–39.

———. "Deaths from Specified Causes in Large Towns—Tuberculosis." *Epidemiological Report* for 1936, R.E. 182 (Geneva, Health Section, 1936), 95–98.

———. “Deaths from Specified Causes in Large Towns—Tuberculosis.” *Epidemiological Report for 1937,* R.E. 193 (Geneva: Health Section, 1937), 114–16.
———. “Deaths from Specified Causes in Large Town—Tuberculosis.” *Epidemiological Report for 1939,* R.E. 209 (Geneva: Health Section, 1939), 14–16.
———. “List of Notifiable Diseases in each Country, 1925.” *Epidemiological Intelligence, 1925*, No. 10 (Geneva: Health Section, 1926): 189–91.
———. “Mortality from Tuberculosis in Various Cities in 1924 and 1925.” *Epidemiological Intelligence for 1925* (Geneva: Health Section, 1934), 70–71.
———. “Tuberculosis Mortality.” *Weekly Epidemiological Record* for *14 March 1946*, R.H. 1046 (Geneva: Health Section, 1946), 88–92.
———. “Tuberculosis Mortality.” *Weekly Epidemiological Record* for *29 August 1946*, R.H. 1070 (Geneva: Health Section, 1946), 289–93.
———. “Tuberculosis Mortality.” *Weekly Epidemiological Record* for *24 January 1947*, R.H. 1091 (Geneva: Health Section, 1947), 30–34.
———. *Tuberculosis Statistics: Summary of the Report Addressed by Dr. S. Rosenfeld (Vienna) to the Health Committee of the League of Nations, April 1925.* Réunies, Chambéry: Health Section, 1925.
Leake, Eva S. “The Henry Phipps Institute: Recollections of a Foreign Research Fellow.” *Transactions & Studies of the College of Physicians of Philadelphia* 3, no.4 (December 1981): 256–63.
Leavitt, Judith W., And Ronald L. Numbers, editor. *Sickness and Health in America: Readings in the History of Medicine and Public Health.* Madison: University of Wisconsin Press, 1997.
Lehrman, Sally. “The Diabolical Genius of an Ancient Scourge.” *Scientific American 309*, no. 1 (July 2013): 82–85.
Lerner, Barron H. *Contagion and Confinement: Controlling Tuberculosis along the Skid Road.* Baltimore: Johns Hopkins University Press, 1998.
———. “New York City’s Tuberculosis Control Efforts: The Historical Limitations of the ‘War on Consumption.’” *American Journal of Public Health* 83, no. 5 (May 1993): 758–66.
“Let’s Get Acquainted.” *Spunk* 18, no. 8 (November 1926): 20; 21, no. 8 (November 1929): 6–19.
Lewis, Sara A., and Richard V. Kasius. “Tuberculosis Mortality in Major Cities: United States.” *Public Health Reports* (1896–1970) 63, no. 1: 17–18; 38, no. 4: 143–44; 37, no. 46: 28–55.
Lewontin, Richard, and Richard Levins. “The Return of the Old Disease and the Appearance of New Ones.” In *The Return of the White Plague: Global Poverty and the ‘New’ Tuberculosis,* edited by Matthew Gandy and Alimuddin Zumla, 1–6. London: Verso, 2003.
Lezana, Julio. “Elevando los informes parciales sobre investigación de la condición económica de las clases obreras.” *Boletín del Departamento Nacional del Trabajo* 21 (30 November 1912): 297–622.
Lifson, Sol S. “Misunderstanding about TB: To Eradicate TB-These understandings must be eliminated.” *Spunk* 54, no. 10 (January 1963): 9–12.
“Liga Argentina contra la tuberculosis.” *Alianza de Higiene Social* 9, no. 8/9 (January/February 1910): 229–32.
“Liga Argentina contra la tuberculosis: Informe, anual de su presidente correspondiente al año 1907,” *Alianza de Higiene Social* 7 (1907–08): 333.

"La Liga Argentina contra la tuberculosis," *La Lucha Antituberculosa* 2, no. 4 (September 1902): 148–49.

"Liga Argentina contra la tuberculosis." *Revista de la Tuberculosis* 1, no. 6 (November 1901): 217.

Little, Cynthia Jeffress. "The Society of Beneficence in Buenos Aires, 1823–1900." Ph.D. diss., Temple University, 1980.

Liveright, Dorothy. "Tuberculosis among residents of 92 cities of 100,000 or more population: United States, 1939–1941." *Public Health Reports* 59, no 29 (21 July 1944): 942–55.

Lobato, Mirta Zaida. "La Patria degli Italiani and Social Conflict in Early-Twentieth Century Argentina." In *Italian Workers of the World: Labor Migration and Formulation of Multiethnic States*, edited by Donna R. Gabaccia and Fraser M. Otanelli, translated by Amy Ferlazzo, 63–78. Urbana: University of Illinois Press, 2001.

Lomax, Elizabeth. "Hereditary or Acquired Diseases? Early Nineteenth Century Debates on the Cause of Infantile Scrofula and Tuberculosis." *Journal of the History of Medicine and Allied Sciences* 32, no. 4 (June 1997): 356–74.

Lougheed, Kathryn. *Catching Breath: The Making and Unmaking of Tuberculosis*. London: Bloomsbury Sigma, 2017.

Lozano, Nicolás. "Estadística de la mortalidad por tuberculosis en la República Argentina en el decenio de 1911–1920." *La Semana Médica* 29, no 10 (9 March 1922): 370–81.

———. "Estadística de la mortalidad por tuberculosis en la *Revista Argentina* en el decenio de 1911 a 1920," *Actas y trabajos de la tercera conferencia nacional de profilaxis antituberculoso,* 116. La Plata, Argentina: Taller de Impresiones Oficiales, 1922.

Lozano, Nicolás and Carlos Mainini. *El problema de la tuberculosis en la República Argentina: Bases estadísticas de la profilaxis antituberculosa y síntesis de un plan profiláctico*. Buenos Aires: *La Semana Médica*, 1918.

Lupton, Deborah. *Medicine as Culture: Illness, Disease and the Body in Western Society*. London: Sage Publications, 1994.

Madrid Paez, S. "Asistencia preventiva de la infancia en la lucha antituberaculosa." In *Primer Congreso Pan América de la Tuberculosis Córdoba, Octubre 10-16 de 1927*, vol. 3: 166–67. Córdoba: Imprenta de la Universidad, 1927.

Malbrán, Carlos G, and Ezequiel Castilla. "Profilaxia de la tuberculosis en las sierras de Cosquín, Córdoba." *Departamento Nacional de Higiene* 12, no. 8 (August 1905): 391.

Mann, Thomas. *The Magic Mountain*. Translated by H.T. Lowe-Porter. New York: Vintage International, 1992.

Marion, John Francis. *Philadelphia Medica: Being a Guide to the City's Historical Places of Health Interest*. Philadelphia: SmithKline Corporation, 1975.

Marks, Lara, and Michael Worboys, eds. *Migrants, Minorities and Health: Historical and Contemporary Studies*. London: Routledge, 1997.

Martínez, Alberto B. *Censo general de población, edificación, comercio e industrias de la ciudad Buenos Aires, levantado en los días 11 y 18 septiembre de 1904*. Buenos Aires: Cía. Sudamericana de Billetes de Banco, 1906.

———. *Estudio demográfico sobre la tísis en Buenos Aires*. Buenos Aires: Imprenta, litografía y encuadenación de Stiller y Laass, 1886.

Marugo, Federico. "Tratamiento de la Tuberculosis Pulmonar por la recalcificación." M.D. diss., Facultad de Medicina, Universidad de Buenos Aires, 1911. Buenos Aires: Establecimiento Gráfico de Alberto Montes, 1911.

Mastrangelo, Luigi T. "A Patient's View." Spunk 1, no. 3 (June 1909): 10–11.

Matorras, Fenelón. *Tisis tuberculosa y neumónica.* Buenos Aires: Imprenta a Vapor de la Nación, 1878.

Matteucci, Marie. Interview by Vera Blinn Reber. Shippensburg, Pennsylvania, 18 October 2004.

Maxmen, Amy. "A Combined Effort." *Nature* 502 (10 October 2013): S4–S6.

Maxwell, Herbert, and P. H. Pye-Smith. "Report of the Delegates of Her Majesty's Government on the International Congress on Tuberculosis held at Berlin from 24th to 27th May 1899," 3–8.

Great Britain, Parliament, House of Commons, Command Papers. London: Majesty's Stationery Office, 1899.

Mazzeo, Victoria. *Migración internacional en la ciudad de Buenos Aires 1855–1980.* Buenos Aires: Municipalidad de la Ciudad de Buenos Aires, 1988.

———. *Mortalidad infantil en la ciudad de Buenos Aires 1856–1986.* Buenos Aires: Centro Editor de América Latina, 1993.

Mazzini, José. "Profilaxis de la Tuberculosis en las sierras de Córdoba." *Actas y Trabajos.* Vol. 3 of Segunda Conferencia Nacional de Profilaxis Antituberculosa, *Rosario 6-8 de Septiembre 1919.* Rosario de Santa Fe: Talleres de la Biblioteca Argentina, 1920.

McBride, David. *From TB to AIDS: Epidemics among Urban Blacks since 1900.* Albany: State University of New York Press, 1991.

———. "Henry Phipps Institute, 1903-1937: Pioneering Tuberculosis Work with an Urban Minority." *Bulletin of the History of Medicine* 61, no. 1 (Spring 1987): 78–97.

———. *Integrating the City of Medicine: Blacks in Philadelphia Health Care, 1910–1965.* Philadelphia: Temple University Press, 1988.

McCutcheon, R. H. "Mont Alto." *Pennsylvania's Health* 10, no. 1 (January/February 1932): 66–67.

———. "Mont Alto Sanatorium: Past and Present." *The Listening Post* 1, no. 2 (January 1923): 6–9.

Mcivor, Arthur. "Germs at Work: Establishing Tuberculosis as an Occupational Disease in Britain, c. 1900–1951. *Social History of Medicine* 26, no. 4 (Oct. 2012): 812–829.

McKeown, Thomas. *The Modern Rise of Population.* New York: Academic Press, 1976.

———. *The Origin of Human Disease.* London: Basil Blackwell, 1988.

McMillen, Christian W. *Discovery Tuberculosis: A Global History 1900 to the Present.* New Haven: Yale University Press, 2015.

McNeil, Jr., Donald G. "New Tuberculosis Test May Soon Be Possible." *New York Times*, 2 January 2018, D6.

McPhedran, Frederic Maurice. "The Diagnosis and Classification of Pulmonary Tuberculosis in Childhood and Adolescence." *American Review of Tuberculosis* 20, no. 4 (October 1929): 532–36.

Mead, Karen. "Gender, Welfare and the Catholic Church in Argentina: Conferencias de Señoras de San Vicente de Paul, 1890–1916," *The Americas* 58, no. 1 (July 2001): 91–119.

Meckel, Richard A. "Open-Air Schools and the Tuberculous Child in Early 20th-Century America." *Archives of Pediatric and Adolescent Medicine* 150 (January 1996): 91–99.

Metcalf, C. "A History of Tuberculosis." In *A Century of Tuberculosis: South African Perspectives,* edited by H.M. Coovadia and S.R. Benatar, 1–31. Cape Town, South Africa: Oxford University Press, 1991.

Milanesio, Natalia. "Food Politics and Consumption in Perionist Argentina." *Hispanic American Historical Review* 90, no. 1 (2010): 75–108.

Miles, J.A.R. *Infectious Diseases: Colonizing the Pacific.* Dunedin, New Zealand: Otago University Press, 1997.

Miller, Albert G. *History of the German Hospital in Philadelphia and its Ex-Resident Physicians.* Philadelphia: Press of J.B. Lippincott Company.

Mills, Charles K. "The Philadelphia Almshouse and the Philadelphia General Hospital from 1854–1908." *Founders' Week memorial volume: containing an account of the two hundred and twenty-fifth anniversary of the founding of the city of Philadelphia, and histories of its principal scientific institutions, medical colleges, hospitals, etc.*, edited by Frederick P. Henry, 465–516. Philadelphia: City of Philadelphia, 1909.

Mirelman, Victor. *Jewish Buenos Aires 1890-1930:* In *Search of Identity.* Detroit: Wayne State University Press, 1990.

Molero-Mesa, Jorge. "'The right not to suffer consumption:' Health, Welfare, Charity, and the Working Class in Spain during the Restoration Period." In *Tuberculosis Then and Now: Perspectives on the History of an Infectious Disease* edited by Flurin Condrau and Michael Worboys, 171–88. Montreal: McGill-Queen's University, 2010.

Molitor, John. "Educational Hygiene as Applied to School Children." *Spunk* 12, no. 2 (May 1920): 5–10.

"Mont Alto Notes," *Spunk* 8, no. 1 (April 1916): 30–32; 9, no. 6 (September 1917): 32–33; *9, no. 7 (October 1917): 33; 15, no. 2 (May 1923): 25;* 19, *no. 9 (December 1927): 43.*

"Mortalidad por enfermedades infecciosas en la ciudad de Buenos Aries durante los años 1895 y 1896." *Departamento Nacional de Higiene* 6, no. 25 (1 July 1896): 403–9, 424–28; 6, no. 27 (16 July 1896): 494–97; 6, no. 30 (8 August 1896): 522–24; 6, no. 34 (8 September 1896): 610–12, 721–22; 6, no. 42 (8 November 1896): 800-01, 862–66; 7, no. 1, (2 January 1897): 21–23; 7, no. 2 (8 January 1897): 21–23; 7, no. 5 (1 February 1897): 86–89; 7, no. 6 (8 February 1897): 86–89.

"Mortality from Typhoid, Tuberculosis and Pneumonia in 43 Large Cities, 1922. *Public Health Reports (1896–1970)* 38. no. 4 (26 January 1923): 142–44.

Mort, Frank. *Dangerous Sexualities: Medico-Moral Politics in England since 1830.* London: Routledge & Kegan Paul Ltd., 1987.

Mostardini, Gastone. "L'evoluzione della mortalità tubercolare in Europa," *Lotta contro la Tuberculosi* 21, no. 3–4 (March/April 1951): 135–57.

Moya, José C. *Cousins and Strangers: Spanish Immigrants in Buenos Aires, 1850–1930.* Berkeley: University of California Press, 1998.

"Mummy autopsies reveal arthritis, cirrhosis, plaque – but little cancer." *Washington Post*, 29 January 2013, F5.

"Municipalidad y la higiene pública." *El Porteño* (Buenos Aires), 16 February 1877, p. 1.

New, Mitya. "Silent Heroes of Past Not Forgotten in Switzerland's Davos." *North American News Report,* 16 January 1993.

New York (City Department of Health). *Brief History of the Campaign against Tuberculosis in New York City*. New York: Dept. of Health, 1908.

"A Note on the Course of Pulmonary Tuberculosis Mortality since 1914," *Public Health Reports (1896–1970)* 36, no. 21 (27 May 1921): 1178–183.

Noymer, Andrew, and Beth Jarosz. "Second Opinions: Response; Causes of Death in Nineteenth-Century New England: The Dominance of Infectious Disease." *Social History of Medicine* 21, no. 3 (December 2008): 573–78.

"Nuestra asistencia social." *La Vanguardia*, 13 March 1912, p. 1.

"Occupational Therapy." *Spunk* no. 12, no. 6 (September 1920): 51.

O'Hallaron, Alice M. "The Work of the Dispensary Nurse," *Spunk* 6, no. 1 (April 1914): 10–11.

"One Lung Minstrel Company." *Spunk* 6, no. 6 (August 1914): 32–33.

Opie, Eugene L. "Infection with Tuberculosis in Children and in Adults, and the Relations of One to the Other." *Transactions of the College of Physicians* 49, Third Series, vol. 49 (1927): 24–47.

Osler, William. *The Principles and Practice of Medicine*, 2nd ed. New York: D. Appleton and Company, 1895.

Otero, Hernán. *Historia de los franceses en la Argentina*. Buenos Aires: Editorial Biblos, 2012.

Ott, Katherine. *Fevered Lives: Tuberculosis in American Culture since 1870*. Cambridge: Harvard University Press, 1996.

Packard, Randall M. "Tuberculosis and the Development of Industrial Health Policies on the Witwatersrand, 1902–1932." *Journal of Southern African Studies* 13, no. 2 (January 1987): 187–209.

———. *White Plague, Black Labor: Tuberculosis and the Political Economy of Health and Disease in South Africa*. Berkeley: University of California Press, 1989.

Page, Henry F. "The German Hospital of the City of Philadelphia." In *Founders' Week memorial volume: containing an account of the two hundred and twenty-fifth anniversary of the founding of the city of Philadelphia, and histories of its principal scientific institutions, medical colleges, hospitals, etc.*, edited by Frederick P. Henry, 652–59. Philadelphia: City of Philadelphia, 1909.

Panza, Paride T. "Sobre Profilaxis de la tuberculosis." *La Semana Médica*, 28, no. 12 (24 March 1921): 37–47.

Paris, Gloria. *A Child of Sanitariums: A Memoir of Tuberculosis Survival and Lifelong Disability*. Jefferson, NC: McFarland and Company, 2010.

Patroni, Adrián. *Los Trabajadores en la Argentina*. Buenos Aires: Imprenta Litografía Encadernación, 1897.

Paulson, Tom. "A Mortal Foe." *Nature* 502, (10 October 2013): S2–S3.

Penna, José, and Horacio Madero. *La Administración sanitaria y asistencia pública en la ciudad de Buenos Aires*, 2 vols. Buenos Aires: Guillermo Kraft, 1910.

Pennsylvania Society for the Prevention of Tuberculosis, *Annual Report 1896*. Philadelphia, 1897.

———. *Annual Report 1898*. Philadelphia: Society for the Prevention of Tuberculosis, 1898.

———. *Annual Report for the Year Ending April 1, 1908*. Philadelphia: Society for the Prevention of Tuberculosis 1908.

———. *Annual Report for 1911*. Philadelphia: Society for the Prevention of Tuberculosis, 1911.

———. *Annual Report for 1920*. Philadelphia: Society for the Prevention of Tuberculosis. 1920.

———. *Annual Report of the Commissioner of Health of the Commonwealth of Pennsylvania*. Harrisburg: Government Printing Press, 1920.

———. "How Hotel Keepers can Aid in Preventing the Spread of Tuberculosis." Philadelphia: The Historical Society of Pennsylvania, 1910.

———. "Plain Facts about Tuberculosis." In *Transactions of the Sixth International Congress on Tuberculosis, Washington, September 28 to October 5, 1908, 5: 271*. Philadelphia: William F. Fell Company, 1908.

———."Work Among the Negroes of Pennsylvania." *Annual Report 1916*. (Philadelphia, 1916), 10–12.

Pérez, Eugenio. "Opúsculo sobre la tisis pulmonar." M.D. diss., Facultad de Medicina, Universidad de Buenos Aires, 1843.

Pérez, José Antonio. "Gumersindo Sayago y el desarrollo de la tisiología Argentina. In *Segundo Congreso Nacional de Historia de la Medicina Argentina, Córdoba 21 al 24*, edited by Academia Nacional de Medicina, Universidad Nacional de Córdoba, Círculo Médico de Córdoba, 44–53. Córdoba, Argentina: Semana Médica, 1970.

———. "La Tisioneumonología Argentina en los últimos cincuenta años." *Revista Argentina de Tuberculosis, Enfermedades Pulmonares y Salud Pública* 42, nos. 1–4 (1981): 95–105.

Pérez, Norberto. "Asilo de Huérfanos." *Revista de Higiene Infantil* 1 (1892): 601–02.

Perkins, James E. "Isoniazid Effective TB Preventive." *Spunk* 54, no. 3 (June 1962): 13–15.

Persky, Abram H. "The Diagnosis and Treatment of Pulmonary Tuberculosis," *Transactions of the College of Physicians*, Third Series 47 (1925): 567–75.

Philadelphia (Pa.), *Annual Message of the Mayor of the City of Philadelphia with the Annual Reports of Directors of Departments*, various years 1870–1950. Philadelphia: Office of Mayor.

Philadelphia (Pa.), Department of Public Health. *Annual Report: Division of Disease Control, 2007*. Philadelphia: Department of Public Health, 2008.

———. *Annual Summary of Reportable Diseases and Conditions: Division of Disease Control, 2004*. Philadelphia: Department of Public Health, Division of Disease Control, 2005.

———. "Tuberculosis Surveillance." https://hip.phila.gov/DataReports/Tuberculosis (15 March 2018).

"Phipps Institute," *Old Penn (Weekly Magazine of the University of Pennsylvania)* 8 no. 15 (22 January 1910), 2–3.

Piñero, José. "Tisis tuberculosa," M.D. diss., Facultad de Medicina, Universidad de Buenos Aires, 1854.

Plaza, Jorge. *Tratamiento higiénico de la tuberculosis pulmonar*. M.D. diss., Facultad de Medicina, Universidad de Buenos Aires, 1912. Buenos Aires: La Semana Médica, 1912.

Pooley, Siân. "'All We Parents Want Is That Our Children's Health and Lives Should Be Regarded:' Child Health and Parental Concern in England, c. 1860–1910." *Social History of Medicine* 23, no. 3 (December 2010): 528–48.

Prescott, Heather Munro. "The White Plague Goes to College: Tuberculosis Prevention Programs in Colleges and Universities, 1920–1960." *Bulletin of the History of Medicine* 74, no. 4 (Winter 2000): 735–72.

Priano, Daniel. "La bacteriología de la tuberculosis vacunación preventiva y curativa." *La Semana Médica* 48, no. 23 (June 5, 1941): 1315–24.

"Problems of Irregular Discharge: Sanatorium Patients are urged to consider the High Cost of Leaving against Medical Advice." *Spunk* 52, no. 9 (December 1960): 9–10.

Proust, A. J., ed. *History of Tuberculosis in Australia, New Zealand, and Papua New Guinea*. Canberra: Brolga Publishing, 1991.

Puig, Manuel. *Heartbreak Tango*. Translated by Suzanne Jill Levine. New York: E P. Dutton & Co., 1973.

"The Question Box." *Spunk* 13, no. 5 (November 1921): 41; 13, no. 6 (December 1921): 53; 13, no. 7 (January 1922): 50.

Radovanovic, Elisa, and Alicia Busson. "La Vivienda obrera en Buenos Aires en la década de 1880, presupuestos teóricos y realizaciones." In *Primeras Jornadas de Historia de la Ciudad de Buenos Aires: Vivienda en Buenos Aires*, 169–85. Buenos Aires: Municipalidad de la Ciudad de Buenos Aires, Secretaría de Cultura Instituto Histórico de la Ciudad de Buenos Aires, 1985.

Ragno, Francisco. "Manifestaciones anormales de las tuberculosis infantiles." *La Semana Médica* 8, no. 20 (16 May 1901): 285–89.

Raimondi, Alejandro A. "Colocación familiar del recién nacido hijo de padres tuberculosis." *Archivos de Tisiología* 5, no. 2 (January–June 1928): 58–59.

Raimondi, Alejandro A. and Tristán González. "Tuberculosis y embarazo. El nuemotórax en el embarazo y en el parto." *Revista de la Sociedad Argentina de Tisiología* 1 (August 1925): 31–43.

Ramos Mexia, Justino. "Higiene y educación física de la mujer," diss., Facultad de Medicina, Universidad de Buenos Aires, 1898.

Rapoport, Mario, and María Seoane. *Buenos Aires, historia de una ciudad: De la modernidad al siglo XXI: Sociedad, política, economía, y cultura*. 2 vols. Buenos Aires: Planeta-Fundación Banco Ciudad, 2007.

Ravenel, M. F. "Maragliano's method of producing a specific serum for the treatment of tuberculosis and of vaccinating against tuberculosis; with observations upon the treatment carried out with serum in Professor's Maragliano's clinic," in *Second Annual Report of the Henry Phipps Institute for the Study, Treatment, and Prevention of Tuberculosis*, Philadelphia: Henry Phipps Institute, 1905.

Rawson, Guillermo. "Casas de Inquilinato." In *Escritos y Discursos del Doctor Guillermo Rawson*, edited by Alberto B. Martínez. Buenos Aires: Compañía Sud-Americana de Billetes de Banco, 1891, Vol. 1, 113–14.

Reber, Vera Blinn. "Blood, Coughs and Fever: Tuberculosis and the Working Class of Buenos Aires, Argentina, 1884–1915." *Social History of Medicine* 12, no. 1 (April 1999): 73–100.

———. *British Mercantile Houses in Buenos Aires, 1810–1880*. Cambridge: Harvard University Press, 1979.

———. "Misery Pain and Death: Tuberculosis in Nineteenth Century Buenos Aires." *The Americas* 56, no. 4 (April 2000): 497–528.

———. "Poor, Ill and Sometimes Abandoned: Tubercular Children in Buenos Aires, 1880-1920." *Journal of Family History* 27, no. 2 (April 2002): 128–49.

———. "The Sanatorium Age, Pennsylvania and Argentina, 1900–1945." *Pennsylvania History* 73, no. 4 (Autumn 2006): 412–45.

Recalde, Héctor. *Las Condiciones de trabajo.* Vol. 2 of *Mujer condiciones de vida de trabajo y salud.* Buenos Aires: Centro Editión de América Latina, 1988.

———. *La Higiene y el trabajo: 1870–1930.* Vol. 2 of *La Higiene y el trabajo.* Buenos Aires: Centro Editor de América Latina, 1988.

———. *Vida popular y salud en Buenos Aires (1900–1930).* Buenos Aires: Centro Editor de América Latina, 1994.

Reichman, Lee B., with Janice Hopkins Tanne. *Timebomb: The Global Epidemic of Multi-Drug-Resistant Tuberculosis.* New York: McGraw-Hill, 2002.

"Resumen de los trabajos realizados en el primer año de su existencia." *La Lucha Antituberculosa* 2 (May 1901–1902): 29–30.

"Revised BCG Vaccination Guidelines for infants at Risk for HIV infection." *Weekly Epidemiological Record,* no. 21 (25 May 2007): 193–96.

Richardson, Ruth. *Florencio Sánchez and the Argentine Theater.* 1933 Reprint. New York: Gordon Press, 1975.

Riera, Juan P. "Influencia de las costumbres en las enfermedades." M.D. diss., Facultad de Medicina, Universidad de Buenos Aires, 1878.

Riis, Jacob A. "The Story of Sea Breeze." *The Outlook* 197 (May 1914), 85–88.

Rippley, La Vern J. *The German-Americans.* Boston: Twayne Publishers, 1976.

Ritacco, Viviana et al. "Nosocomial Spread of Human Immunodeficiency Virus-Related Multidrug Resistant Tuberculosis in Buenos Aires." *The Journal of Infectious Diseases* 176, no. 3 (September 1997): 637–42.

Roberts, Samuel Kelton. *Infectious Fear: Politics, Disease and the Health Effects of Segregation.* Chapel Hill: University of North Carolina, 2009.

Rock, David. *Argentina, 1516–1987: From Spanish Colonization to Alfonsín.* Berkeley: University of California Press, 1987.

Rodrígues, Laura C., Vinod K. Diwan, and Jeremy G. Wheeler, "Protective Effect of BCG against Tuberculous Meningitis and Miliary Tuberculosis: A Meta-analysis." *International Journal of Epidemiology* 22 (1993): 1154–58.

Rodríguez Castells, Horacio. "Apuntes para la historia de la tuberculosis en la República Argentina." *Revista Argentina de Tuberculosis y Enfermedades Pulmonares* 31, no. 3 (1970): 120–34.

Rodgers, Jimmie. *"TB Blues Lyrics."* http://www.songlyrics.com/jimmie-rodgers/t-b-blues-lyrics/ (20 March 2018).

Rogers, Everett. "Diffusion of preventive innovations." *Addictive Behaviors* 27, no. 6 (November 2002): 989–93.

Rollino, César. "Pronóstico de la tuberculosis pulmonar." M.D. diss., Facultad de Medicina, Universidad de Buenos Aires, 1902. Buenos Aires: Imprenta y Casa Editora de Agustín Etchepareborda, 1902.

Romero, José Luis, and Luis Alberto Romero. *Buenos Aires, Historia de cuatros siglos*, 2 vols. Buenos Aires: Editorial Abril, 1983.

Rosal, Julián, and Manuel Arroyo. *Informe sobre el Congreso Internacional de la Tuberculosis verificado en Paris del 2 al 7 de Octubre de 1905, presentado al Señor Ministro de Relaciones Exteriores*. Guatemala: Tipografía Sánchez y De Guise, 1906.

Rosenberg, Charles E. *The Cholera Years: The United States in 1832, 1849, and 1866*. Chicago: University of Chicago Press, 1962.

———. "Introduction to Framing Disease: Illness, Society and History." In *Framing Disease: Studies in Cultural History* edited by Charles E. Rosenberg and Janet Golden. Health and Medicine in American Society. New Brunswick: Rutgers University Press, 1992.

———. "Inward Vision and Outward Glance: The Shaping of the American Hospital." *Bulletin of the History of Medicine* 53 (1979): 346–91.

———. "What is an epidemic?" In *Living with AIDS* edited by Stephen R. Graubard, 1–17. Cambridge: MIT Press, 1990.

Rosenberg, Clifford. "The International Politics of Vaccine Testing in Interwar Algiers." *American Historical Review* 117 (3 June 2012): 670–97.

Rosenkrantz, Barbara Gutmann, ed. *From consumption to tuberculosis: a documentary history*. New York: Garland Pub., 1994.

Rosner, David. *A Once Charitable Enterprise: Hospitals and Health Care in Brooklyn and New York, 1885–1915*. Cambridge: Cambridge University Press, 1982.

Ross, Paul. "Mexico's Superior Health Council and the American Public Health Association: The Transnational Archive of Porfirian Public Health, 1887–1910." *Hispanic American Historical Review* 89, no. 4 (November 2009): 573–603.

Ross, Stanley R., and Thomas F. McGann, eds. *Buenos Aires 400 Years*. Austin: University of Texas Press, 1982.

Roth, Francis Xavier. *History of St. Vincent's Orphan Asylum, Tacony, Philadelphia: Memoir of its Diamond Jubilee, 1855–1933*. Philadelphia: Nord-Amerika Press, 1934.

Rothman, Sheila M. *Living in the Shadow of Death: Tuberculosis and the Social Experience of Illness in American History*. Baltimore: John Hopkins Press, 1995.

Royer, B. Franklin. "The Work of the State Department of Health in the Tuberculosis Campaign." *Spunk* 5, no. 12 (March 1914): 9–10.

Ruggiero, Kristin. *Modernity in the Flesh: Medicine, Law and Society in Turn-of-the-Century Argentina*. Stanford: Stanford University Press, 2004.

Ruhl, Arthur. *The Other Americans: The Cities, the Countries, and Especially the People of South America*. New York: Charles Scribner's Sons, 1910.

Russell, David G., and Carl F. Nathan. "Graduation time." *Nature* 502 (10 October 2013): S7.

Ryan, Frank. *The Forgotten Plague: How the Battle Against Tuberculosis Was Won – and Lost*. Boston: Back Bay Books, 1994.

Sachs, Theodore B. "Children of the Tuberculosis." In *Transactions of the Sixth International Congress on Tuberculosis*, 2: 479–86. Philadelphia: William F. Fell Company, 1908.

———. "The Official Responsibility of the City in the Tuberculosis Problem." In *Transactions of the Eleventh Annual Meeting, Seattle, Washington, June 14–16*, edited by The National Association for the Study and Prevention of Tuberculosis, 278–87. Baltimore: Williams & Wilkins Company, 1915.

Saggese, Domingo. *Yerbas medicinales Argentinas*, 10th ed. Rosario:Antognazzi y Cia., 1959.

Salo, Wilmar L., Arthur C. Auferheide, Jane Buikstra, and Todd A. Holcomb. "Identification of Mycobacterium tuberculosis DNA in a pre-Columbian Peruvian mummy." *Proceedings of the National Academy of Sciences* 91 (March 1994): 2091–94.

Salvarezza, Domingo. *Tisis Pulmonar. M.D.* diss., Facultad de Medicina, Universidad de Buenos Aires, 1866. Buenos Aires: Imprenta de Buenos Aires, 1866.

Salvatore, Ricardo D. "Stature growth in industrializing Argentina: The Buenos Aires industrial belt 1916–1950." *Explorations in Economic History* 46, no. 1 (January 2009): 70–92.

" Sanatorio de Santa María: Nuevas denuncias." *La Vanguardia,* 29 December 1919, p. 2.

"Sanatorio Marítimo de Mar del Plata." *Revista de la Tuberculosis* 1, no. 8 (January 1902): 284–91.

"Sanatorio Municipal Doctor Tornú," *Lucha Antituberculosa* 4, no. 12 (12 May 1905): 531–35.

"Sanatorio Santa María: La Comida de los enfermos-quejas justificadas." *La Vanguardia*, 4 January 1920, p. 1.

Sánchez Aizcorbe, César. "La cultural fiscal de la mujer en la profilaxis de la tuberculosis." In *Primer Congreso Pan-Americano de la Tuberculosis Córdoba 10-16 Octubre, 1922*, 3: 259–62. Córdoba, Argentina: Imprenta de la Universidad, 1922.

Sánchez, Florencio. *Barranca abajo* (Down in the Gally). In Florencio Sánchez, *Representative plays of Florencio Sánchez*. Translated by Willis Knapp Jones. Washington, D.C.: Pan American Union, 1961.

———. *En Familia*. Buenos Aires: Editorial Moreno, 1965.

Santas, Manuel. "Tratamiento racional de la tuberculosis en la República Argentina." M.D. diss., Facultad de Medicina, Universidad de Buenos Aires, 1898.

Savacool, J. Woodrow. "Philadelphia and the White Plague." *Transactions and Studies of the College of Physicians* ser. 5, vol. 8, no. 3 (1986): 147–81.

Sayago, Gumersindo, Juan B. Rocca and C. Ferrer Moratel. "Influencia del trabajo en el origen y en el desarrollo de la tuberculosis." *La Prensa Médica Argentina* 36, no. 39 (30 September 1949): 1972–75.

Schaelchin, Patricia. "'Working for the Good of the Community': Rest Haven Preventorium for Children." *Journal of San Diego History* 29, no. 2 (1983): 96–113.

Schaffle, Karl. "The State Tuberculosis Dispensary an Asset to the Municipality," *Spunk* 9, no. 7 (October 1917): 8–9.

Schatz, Ricardo. "Higiene pública y policía sanitaria: Profilaxis de la tuberculosis en los tambos de Buenos Aires." *Anales del Círculo Médico Argentino* 18, no. 1 (January 1895): 55–62.

Schenck's almanac. Philadelphia: J. H. Schenck & Son, 1870.
Schiavone, Generoso A. "La Tuberculosis en la primera infancia." *La Semana Médica* 37, no. 14 (3 April 1930): 866–81.
Schneider, Jo Anne. "Patterns for Getting By: Polish women's Employment in Delaware County, 1900–1930." *Pennsylvania Magazine of History and Biography* 114, no. 4 (October 1990): 517–41.
Schneier, Manuel. "Hospital Tornú." *Mundo Hospitalario* 27 (November 1941): 55–56.
Scobie, James R. *Buenos Aires: Plaza to Suburb, 1870–1910*. New York: Oxford University Press, 1974.
Scranton, Philip. "An Immigrant Family & Industrial Enterprise: Seville Schofield and the Philadelphia Textile Manufacture, 1845–1900." *Pennsylvania Magazine of History and Biography* 106, no. 3 (July 1982): 365–92.
———. "Large Firms and Industrial Restructuring: The Philadelphia Region, 1900–1980." *Pennsylvania Magazine of History and Biography* 116, no. 4 (October, 1992): 419–65.
Scrivener, Dr. (John H.). "Argentine Republic, Sanitary Character of the Mountains of Cordova [sic.] and the Andine Heights." *Medical Times and Gazette*, 30 October 1869, 525–26.
Shaw, Ann, and Carole Reeves, eds. *The Children of Craig-y-nos: Life in a Welsh Tuberculosis Sanatorium, 1922–1959*. London: Wellcome Trust Centre for the History of Medicine, 2009.
Sherwood, Frederick Augustus. *Glimpses of South America*. New York: Century Co., 1920.
Shipe, Wilfert, Jr. "First Hand Account: Life in the Children Preventorium Mt. Alto, Pa. 1944–45." Unpublished paper, 23 June 1998, Mt. Alto Archives.
Shryock, Richard H. *National Tuberculosis Association 1904–1954: A Study of the Voluntary Health Movement in the United States*. New York: National Tuberculosis Association, 1957.
Silcox, Harry C. "The Black 'Better Class' Political Dilemma: Philadelphia Prototype Isaiah C. Wears." *Pennsylvania Magazine of History and Biography* 113, no. 1 (January 1989): 45–66.
Silk, Samuel A. "Why do we Give Tuberculin." *Spunk* 6, no. 10 (January 1915): 8–12.
Silvestre, Oliva. *La Mortalidad infantil en Buenos Aires*. Buenos Aires: Imprenta América, 1918.
Simon, Roger D. *Philadelphia: A Brief History*. University Park: Pennsylvania Historical Association, 2003.
Simpson, Eileen. *Orphans: Real and Imaginary*. New York: Weidenfeld & Nicolson, 1987.
Sisto, Genaro. "La escuela preventiva de mar para niños débiles y su importancia en la profilaxis antituberculosa." *La Semana Médica* 26, no. 11 (13 March 1919): 264–69.
"La situación Nacional Santa María: Informe de un telegrama del Centro de estudiantes de medicina." *La Vanguardia*, 23 October 1922, p. 5.
Smallman-Raynor, Matthew R., and Andrew D. Cliff. "War and Disease: Some Perspective on the Spatial and Temporal Occurrence of Tuberculosis in Wartime." In *The Return of the White Plague: Global Poverty and the 'New'*

Tuberculosis, edited by Matthew Gandy and Alimuddin Zumla, 70–92. London: Verso, 2003.

———. *War Epidemics: an Historical Geography of Infectious Diseases in Military Conflict and Civil Strife, 1850–2000*. New York: Oxford University Press, 2004.

Smith, F. B. *The Retreat of Tuberculosis, 1850–1950*. New York: Crom Helm, 1988.

Smith, Gibson. "The Ideal Tuberculosis Clinic." *The Listening Post* 4, no. 35 (Feb. 1926): 16.

Smith, Nicole L. "The Problem of Excess Female Mortality: Tuberculosis in Western Massachusetts, 1850–1910." M.A. thesis, University of Massachusetts-Amherst, 2008.

Sociedad de beneficencia de la capital. *Memoria del año 1905*. Buenos Aires: Imprenta, Litografía y Encuadernación G. Kraft, 1906.

———. *República Argentina: álbum histórico de la Sociedad de Beneficencia de la capital, 1823–1910*. Buenos Aires: Lit. A. Bianche, 1910.

Sofer, Eugene F. *From Pale to Pampa: A Social History of the Jews of Buenos Aires*. New York: Holmes & Meier, 1882.

Sontag, Susan. *Illness as Metaphor and AIDS and Its Metaphors*. New York: New York: Farrar, Straus and Giroux, 1989.

"South Mountain Restoration Center: and There was Light," unpublished pamphlet on the center, [1968].

Spellissy, Joseph M. "The St. Joseph's Hospital" In *Founders' Week memorial volume: containing an account of the two hundred and twenty-fifth anniversary of the founding of the city of Philadelphia, and histories of its principal scientific institutions, medical colleges, hospitals, etc.*, edited by Frederick P. Henry, 613-651. Philadelphia: City of Philadelphia, 1909.

Stahl, Franklin. "St Agnes' Hospital." In *Founders' Week memorial volume: containing an account of the two hundred and twenty-fifth anniversary of the founding of the city of Philadelphia, and histories of its principal scientific institutions, medical colleges, hospitals, etc.*, edited by Frederick P. Henry, 706-09. Philadelphia: City of Philadelphia, 1909.

Stanley, Amy. "Maidservants' Tales: Narrating Domestic and Global History in Eurasia, 1600–1900," *American Historical Review* 121, no.2 (April 2016): 437–60.

Starr, Paul. *The Social Transformation of American Medicine*. New York: Basic Books, 1982.

Stepan, Nancy Leys. "The National and the International in Public Health: Carlos Chagas and the Rockefeller Foundation in Brazil, 1917-1920," *Hispanic American Historical Review* 91, no. 3 (August 2011): 469–502.

Stern, Vivien. "The House of the Dead Revisited: Prisons, Tuberculosis and Public Health in the Former Soviet Bloc." *In The Return of the White Plague: Global Poverty and the New Tuberculosis*, edited by Matthew Gandy and Alimuddin Zumla, 178–91. London: Verso, 2003.

Stockler, Joseph A. "The Contagiousness of Tuberculosis." *Spunk* 6, no. 6 (September 1914): 12–14.

Story, Alistair and Ken Citron. "Private Wealth and Public Squalor: The Resurgence of Tuberculosis in London." *In The Return of the White Plague:*

Global Poverty and the New Tuberculosis, edited by Matthew Gandy and Alimuddin Zumla, 147–62. London: Verso, 2003.
Strauss, Herbert A. "Transplanted and Transformed: German-Jewish Immigrants since 1933." In *America and the Germans: An Assessment of a Three Hundred-Year History*. Volume 2, *The Relationship in the Twentieth Century*, edited by Frank Trommler and Joseph McVeigh, 245–64. Philadelphia: University of Pennsylvania Press, 1985.
"Sucesos del Sanatorio Santa María." *La Vanguardia*, 29 October 1922, p. 6.
"Summary of the Consumptive Department for the Year Ending April 15, 1904." *In 1904: 34th Annual Report: the Philadelphia Protestant Episcopal City Mission.*
Súnico, Antonio. *La tuberculosis en la Sierras de Córdoba*. Buenos Aires: Editorial A. de Martina, 1922.
Sutcliffe, Leroy E. "Mont Alto Jingles." *Spunk* 9, no. 8 (November 1917): 20–22.
Sutcliffe, Marjorie McVicker, and Judy Sutcliffe. *Grandma Cherry's Spoon: A Story of Tuberculosis*. Santa Barbara: Geronima Press, 1991.
Sutherland, John F. "Housing the Poor in the City of Homes: Philadelphia at the Turn of the Century." In *The Peoples of Philadelphia: A History of Ethnic Groups and Lower-Class Life, 1790–1940*, edited by Allen F. Davis and Mark H. Haller, 175-202. Philadelphia: Temple University Press, 1973.
"TB Fights back," Washington Post, 17 August 1999, sec. health, *13*.
Teller, Michael E. *The Tuberculosis Movement: A Public Health Campaign in the Progressive Era*. New York: Greenwood Press, 1988.
Temkin, Owsei. *The Double Face of Janus and other Essays in the History of Medicine*. Baltimore: Johns Hopkins University Press, 1977.
"Teoría y práctica de la historia de Sanatorio Santa María: una vista del corresponsal de 'La Vanguardia.'" *La Vanguardia*, 8 January 1920, p. 4.
Tennant, Margaret. "Children's Health Camps in New Zealand: The Making of a Movement, 1919–1940." *Social History of Medicine* 9, no. 1 (April 1996): 69–87.
Terán, José D. *Pre-Tuberculosis: Contribución a su estudio*. Buenos Aires: Arsenio Guidi Buffarine, 1905.
"Thanksgiving." *Spunk* 6, no. 9 (December 1914): 44–45.
Thomas, Adrian. "Janssen." *Nature* 502 (10 October 2013): S18–S19.
Tinkcom, Margaret B. "Depression and War 1919–1946." In *Philadelphia A 300-Year History*, edited by Russell F. Weigley, 601-48. New York: W.W. Norton & Company, 1981.
Tonina, Teodoro A. "Las escuelas al aire libre." *La Semana Médica* 30, no. 3 (18 January 1923): 104–05.
"Trabajo de la mujer a domicilio." *Boletín del Departamento Nacional del Trabajo* 19 (31 December 1911): 788–91.
Trudeau, Edward L. "Address of the President: National Association for the Study and Prevention of Tuberculosis." *Transactions of the First Annual Meeting, Washington D.C. May 18th and 19th* (1905): 13–19.
"Tuberculosis." Anales del Círculo Médico Argentino 15, no. 9 (September 1892): 667.
"Tuberculosis and Gender," http://www.who.int/tb/areas-of-work/population-groups/gender/en/ (29 March 2018).

"Tuberculosis: Aumento en la notificación de casos." *El Intransigente Argentina*. https://www.elintransigente.com/salud/2017/3/17/tuberculosis-aumento-notificacion-casos-427654.html (28 March 2018).

"Tuberculosis como enfermedad popular: causas; medios de prevenir la y curarla." *La Revista de la Tuberculosis* 1, no. 3 (August 1901): 82–83.

"Tuberculosis en los Hospitales de la Capital." *Revista de Ciencias Médicas* 9, no. 101 (September 1926): 191–92.

"Tuberculosis in the Young." *Spunk* 12, no. 12 (March 1921): 24–25.

"Tuberculosis Mortality in Europe, 1937–44." *Epidemiological Information Bulletin* 1, no. 15 (15 September 1945): 666–72.

"Tuberculosis pulmonar," *La Semana Médica,* 16 July 1894: 210.

Tuberculosis Reference Statistical Yearbook, 1944. New York: Tuberculosis and Health Association, 1945.

Tuberculosis Reference Statistical Yearbook, 1947. New York: Tuberculosis and Health Association 1948

Tuberculosis Reference Statistical Yearbook, Year 1948. New York: Tuberculosis and Health Association, 1949.

Tuberculosis Reference Statistical Yearbook, Year 1949. New York: Tuberculosis and Health Association, 1950.

"Tuberculosis spreads through crowded city buses," (14 December 2014), http://www.newswise.com/articles/tuberculosis-spreads-on-crowded-city-buses.

"Tuberculosis Treatment during Pregnancy, (28 December 2014), http://www.webmd.com/baby/tc/treating-tuberculosis-in-pregnant-women-topic-overview.

"Tuberculosis Trends in Selected Parts of Europe during five-year period 1939–1943," *Tuberculosis Reference Statistical Yearbook*. New York, NY: Sanatorium and Hospital Services, 1944.

"Tuberculosis Work in Philadelphia." *Monthly Bulletin of the Department of Public Health and Charities of the City of Philadelphia* 4, no 6 (June 1919): 85–87.

Túmburus, Juan. *Síntesis histórica de la medicina argentina*. Buenos Aires: El Ateneo, 1926.

Turnbull, William G. "County Tuberculosis Needs." *The Listening Post* 4, no. 37 (April 1926): 4–7.

———. "Heliotherapy," *The Listening Post* 4, no. 41 (November-December 1926): 6–9.

———. "Tuberculosis Sanatoria." *The Listening Post* 3, nos. 24–26 (March-May 1925): 25–27.

"Twenty-first annual Report of the Rush Hospital for Consumption and Allied Diseases from 1 June 1912 to 1 June 1913 and the Women's Board of the Rush Hospital of Philadelphia."

"Últimas incidencias en el sanatorio Santa María: Procedimientos abusivos de la 'Policía interna.'" *La Vanguardia*, 26 July 1924, p. 4.

United Nations Relief and Rehabilitation Administration Health Division. Tuberculosis Mortality in Europe, 1937–44." *Epidemiological Information Bulletin,* 1, no. 15 (September 1945): 666–72.

U.S. Department of Commerce, Bureau of the Census. *Thirteenth Census of the United States*, Vol. 3. Washington, D.C.: Government Printing Office, 1923.

Vaccarezza, Raúl F. *Vida de médicos ilustres*. Buenos Aires: Editoral Troquel, 1980.

Valier, Helen. "At Home in the Colonies: The WHO-MRC Trials at the Madras Chemotherapy Centre in the 1950s and 1960." In *Tuberculosis Then and Now: Perspectives on the History of an Infectious Disease*, edited by Flurin Condrau and Michael Worboys, 213–34. Montreal:

McGill-Queen's University Press, 2010.

Valls, José. "Sanatorios Marítimos." *Revista de la Asociación Médica Argentina* 56, nos. 477–78 (15–30 January 1942): 24–28.

Varbero, Richard A. "Philadelphia's South Italians in the 1920s." *The Peoples of Philadelphia: A History of Ethnic Groups and Lower Class Life 1790–1940*, edited by Allen F. Davis and Mark H. Haller, 255–75. Philadelphia: Temple University Press, 1973.

"Variaciones del salario en la ciudad de Buenos Aires." *Boletín del Departamento Nacional del Trabajo* 19 (31 December 1911): 807–11.

Velásquez, Jacinto. "La mortalidad por enfermedades infecciosas en la capital de la República en 30 años: 1873–1892." *Departamento Nacional de Higiene,* 10 (June 1903): 274–87.

———. "Mortalidad por tuberculosis." *Alianza de Higiene Social*, 9 (1909): 10–11.

Ventura, Ovidio S. *Síntesis demográfica de la Capital Federal*. Buenos Aires: Imprenta Central de Salud Pública de la Nación, 1950.

Vilariño, Idea. *Las letras del tango: la forma, temas y motivos*. Buenos Aires: Editorial Schapire S. R. L., 1965.

Vincent, Frank. *Around and About South America: Twenty Months of Quest and Query*. New York: D. Appleton, 1890.

"A Visit to the Children's Home." *Spunk* 4, no. 7 (October 1912): 27.

Vogliano, Oscar R. C. *Hospital de Niños*. Buenos Aires: Colophon, 1975.

Von Unterberger, Simon Th. "Russian Laws on Tuberculosis." *Transactions of the Sixth International Congress on Tuberculosis, Washington, September 28 to October 5, 1908*, 4: 306–97. Philadelphia: William F. Fell Company, 1908.

Walker, Robin. "The Struggle against Pulmonary Tuberculosis in Australia, 1788–1950." *Historical Studies* (Australia) 20 (April 1983): 439–61.

Wallace, Deborah, and Roderick Wallace. "The Recent Tuberculosis Epidemic in New York City: Warning from the De-Developing World." *In The Return of the White Plague: Global Poverty and the New Tuberculosis*, edited by Matthew Gandy and Alimuddin Zumla, 125–46. London: Verso, 2003.

Walter, Richard J. *Politics and Urban Growth in Buenos Aires, 1910–1942*. New York: Cambridge University Press, 1993.

Walters, F. Rufenacht. *Sanatoria for the Tuberculous: including a description of many existing institutions and sanatorium treatment in pulmonary tuberculosis*. London: George Allen, 1913.

Walsh, John Evangelist. *Darkling I Listen: The Last Days and Death of John Keats*. New York: Palgrave Macmillan, 1999.

Warner, John Harley. *Against the Spirit of System: The French Impulse in Nineteenth Century American Medicine*. Baltimore: John Hopkins University Press, 2003.

Warner, Sam B. *The Private City; Philadelphia in Three Periods of Its Growth.* Philadelphia: University of Pennsylvania Press, 1968.

Weigley, Russell, ed. *Philadelphia: A 300-Year History.* New York: W. W. Norton & Company, 1982.

Weindling, Paul. "International Sanitary Conference," In *International Health Organizations and Movements, 1918–1939*, edited by Paul Weindling, 7–15. New York: Cambridge University Press, 1995.

Wenner, David. "Whatever care we needed, we got." *Patriot News*, 25 October 2009, A14–15.

Werst, Nevin. "Personal Hygiene of Tubercular Patients." *Spunk* 2, no. 5 (August 1910): 21–22.

Wescott, O.D. "Consumption is the Most Common Form of Tuberculosis and is a Germ

Disease," *In International Congress on Tuberculosis, Transactions of the Sixth International Congress on Tuberculosis, Washington, September 28 to October 5, 1908 with an Account and Catalogue of the Tuberculosis Exhibition (Philadelphia, 1908) 5: 277–78.* Philadelphia: W.F. Fell Company, 1908.

Wessel, Henry. N. "The Jewish Hospital Association of Philadelphia." In *Founders' Week memorial volume: containing an account of the two hundred and twenty-fifth anniversary of the founding of the city of Philadelphia, and histories of its principal scientific institutions, medical colleges, hospitals, etc.,* edited by Frederick P. Henry, 663-81. Philadelphia: City of Philadelphia, 1909.

Wheeler, Sandra L. "From Hospital to Sanatorium: Institutional Care of the Tubercular Poor in Hartford, 1900–1910." *Connecticut History* 38, no. 1 (Fall 1997/Spring 1999): 1–11.

Wherrett, G.J. *The Miracle of the Empty Beds: A History of Tuberculosis in Canada.* Toronto: University of Toronto Press, 1978.

White, William C. "The Official Responsibility of the State in the Tuberculosis Problem." In *Transactions of the Eleventh Annual Meeting, Seattle, Washington, June 14–16*, edited by The National Association for the Study and Prevention of Tuberculosis, 209–77. Baltimore: William & Wilkins Company, 1915.

"White Haven State School and Hospital," (28 March 2018), http://www.asylumprojects.org/index.php?title=White_Haven_State_School_and_Hospital;

Whiteman, Maxwell. "Philadelphia's Jewish Neighborhoods." In *The Peoples of Philadelphia: A History of Ethnic Groups and Lower Class Life 1790-1940*, edited by Allen F. Davis and Mark H. Haller, 231–54. Philadelphia: Temple University Press, 1973.

World Health Organization (WHO). "BCG-the current vaccine for tuberculosis. http://www.who.int/tb/vaccinesfaqs/en/ (19 March 2018).

World Health Organization (WHO). "BCG-the current vaccine for tuberculosis," http://www.who.int/vaccine_research/diseases/tb/vaccine_development/bcg/en/. (9 December 2011).

World Health Organization (WHO). "Drug-resistant tuberculosis threatens the Western Pacific Region," http://www.wpro.who.int/mediacentre/releases/2007/20070322/en/ (29 March 2018).

WHO (World Health Organization). Global tuberculosis report, 2013, 2017. http://www.who.int/tb/publications/global_report/en/index.html (19 March 2018).

WHO (World Health Organization), "Tuberculosis," Fact Sheet 104, http://www.who.int/mediacentre/factsheets/fs104/en/ (April 2014).

"Why I am Thankful." *Spunk* 19, no. 10 (January 1928): 43.

Wilcox, J.H. "The Spunk Cure." *Spunk* 1, no. 3 (June 1909): 12.

Wilmot, Frances, and Pauline Saul. *A Breath of Fresh Air: Birmingham's Open-Air Schools, 1911–1970*. Chichester: Phillimore & Co. Ltd, 1998.

Wilson, Leonard G. "The Historical Decline of Tuberculosis in Europe and America: Its Causes and Significance." *Journal of the History of Medicine and Allied Sciences* 45, no. 3 (July 1990): 366–96.

Wingerson, Lois. "Dark History of the White Death." *Archaeology* 97, no. 4, (September/October 2009): 43–47.

Wirth, Thomas. "Urban Neglect: The Environment, Public Health and Influenza in Philadelphia, 1915–1919." *Journal of Pennsylvania History* 73 (2006): 316–42.

Wolfinger, James. *Philadelphia Divided: Race and Politics in the City of Brotherly Love*. Chapel Hill: University of North Carolina Press, 2007.

Worboys, Michael. "Before McKeown: Explaining the Decline of Tuberculosis in Britain, 1880–1930." *In Tuberculosis Then and Now: Perspectives on the History of an Infectious Disease*, edited by Flurin Condrau and Michael Worboys, 148-70. Montreal: McGill Queen's University Press, 2010.

———. "From Heredity to Infection: Tuberculosis, Bacteriology and Medicine, 1870-1900." In *Spreading Germs: Disease Theories and Medical Practice in Britain, 1865–1900,* edited by Michael Worboys, 193-233. Cambridge: Cambridge University Press, 2000.

———. "The Sanatorium Treatment for Consumption in Britain, 1890–1914." In *Medical Innovations in Historical Perspective*, edited by John V. Pickstone, 47–71. New York: St. Martin's Press, 1992.

———. *Spreading Germs: Disease Theories and Medical Practice in Britain, 1865–1900*. Cambridge Studies in the History of Medicine. Cambridge: Cambridge University Press, 2000.

Yujnovsky, Oscar. "Del Conventillo a la villa miseria." In *Buenos Aires historia de cuatro siglos*, edited by José Luis Romero and Luis Alberto Romero, II: 451–64. Buenos Aires: Editorial Abril, 1983.

———. "Políticas de vivienda en la ciudad de Buenos Aires (1880–1914)." *Desarrollo Económico – Revista de Ciencias Sociales* 14, no. 54 (July–September, 1974): 328–71.

Zabatta, Marta M. and Patricia de Forteza. "El Protomedicato y la profilaxis de la tuberculosis en Buenos Aires Virreinal." *La Semana Médica* 152, no. 15 (19 May 1978): 479–83.

Index

For Product Safety Concerns and Information please contact our EU representative GPSR@taylorandfrancis.com
Taylor & Francis Verlag GmbH, Kaufingerstraße 24, 80331 München, Germany

www.ingramcontent.com/pod-product-compliance
Ingram Content Group UK Ltd.
Pitfield, Milton Keynes, MK11 3LW, UK
UKHW022004180926
475701UK00003B/183

9780367585600